Functional Anatomy for Emergency Medical Services

Ann Senisi Scott
Elizabeth Fong
Edited by Richard W.O. Beebe

DELMAR
™
THOMSON LEARNING

Australia Canada Mexico Singapore Spain United Kingdom United States

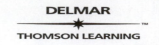

DELMAR
™
THOMSON LEARNING

Functional Anatomy for Emergency Medical Services
Ann Senisi Scott
Elizabeth Fong
Edited by Richard W.O. Beebe

Health Care Publishing Director:
William Brottmiller

Executive Marketing Manager:
Dawn F. Gerrain

Art and Design Coordinator:
Robert Plante

Executive Editor:
Cathy L. Esperti

Developmental Editor:
Darcy M. Scelsi

Project Editor:
Mary Ellen Cox

Editorial Assistant:
Matthew Thouin

Production Editor:
John Mickelbank

For permission to use material from this text or product, contact us by
Tel   (800) 730-2214
Fax   (800) 730-2215
www.thomsonrights.com

Library of Congress Cataloging-in-Publication Data
Scott, Ann Senisi
   Functional anatomy for Emergency Medical Services / Ann Senisi Scott, Elizabeth Fong; edited by Richard W.O. Beebe.
      p. cm.
   Includes index.
   ISBN 0-7668-2757-7 (alk. paper)
      1. Human anatomy. 2. Human physiology. 3. Emergency medical technicians. I. Fong, Elizabeth, 1947-. II. Beebe, Richard W. O. III. Title.

QM23 .2 .S367 2001
612--dc21   2001042520

NOTICE TO THE READER

Contents

① Introduction to the Structural Units / 1

② Chemistry of Living Things / 11

③ Cells / 33

④ Tissues and Membranes / 49

⑤ Integumentary System / 63

Skeletal System / 78

Muscular System / 107

Brain and Central Nervous System / 126

The Peripheral and Autonomic Nervous Systems / 148

Special Senses / 163

11

Endocrine System / 180

12

Blood / 205

13

Heart / 221

14

Circulation and Blood Vessels / 244

15

The Lymphatic System and Immunity / 264

16

Respiratory System / 282

17

Digestive System / 305

18

Nutrition / 335

19

Urinary/Excretory System / 350

Reproductive System / 366

Genetics and Genetically Linked Diseases / 396

Preface

Functional Anatomy for Emergency Medical Services is designed to meet the needs of a growing population of emergency medical services (EMS) students that want more information about anatomy than what they received in their high school biology class. A quick review of the book reveals that it provides a gross but comprehensive overview of anatomy and physiology, such as what might be found in a college survey course in anatomy.

Functional Anatomy for Emergency Medical Services helps prepare students for entry into a paramedic program. Whether it is used as a prerequisite course for the paramedic program or as a supplemental text during a paramedic program, *Functional Anatomy for Emergency Medical Services* provides the paramedic student with a foundational understanding of anatomy and physiology—an understanding that he or she will need to be successful in a paramedic program.

Functional Anatomy for Emergency Medical Services is also useful as an adjunct to existing paramedic textbooks. The textbook can be used to provide background information on anatomy and physiology in preparation for a discussion of pathophysiology. The layout of the text, using a functional approach, lends itself to use in paramedic programs that follow the 1999 National Standard Curriculum for EMT-Paramedics (NSC EMT-P) from the U.S. Department of Transportation.

Functional Anatomy for Emergency Medical Services is an excellent textbook for EMS/Paramedic programs that stand apart from the college setting, for example, hospital-based programs, technical schools and fire academies, and programs that do not enjoy the support of a strong biology department that teaches anatomy.

TO THE STUDENT

EMS students will find that *Functional Anatomy for Emergency Medical Services* is an EMS-friendly book. It reads easily and is organized in a common-sense manner. The challenge in writing a book like this has been to strike a balance between providing too much information and not providing enough. *Functional Anatomy for Emergency Medical Services* is written by a paramedic instructor who knows what is "nice-to-know" and what is "need-to-know." It provides "EMS-specific" information that students need to succeed in a paramedic program.

Functional Anatomy for Emergency Medical Services frequently uses tables and diagrams to help summarize important information and concepts. The artwork is intended to help the student visualize the structures and organs being discussed. The end-of-chapter review questions help the student crystallize important concepts.

TO THE EMS EDUCATOR

The primary purpose of *Functional Anatomy for Emergency Medical Services* is to take subjects like anatomy and physiology and make them more interesting to the EMS student. The editor attempts to do so by integrating some common pathophysiology into the discussion and reintroducing key concepts from an EMS perspective.

Other, more specific, examples of the pedagogical devices used include the following:

Double-Speak Double-speak is the use of both medical and lay terminology. Double-speak helps the EMS student make the transition into the health care professional role and improve his or her understanding of key concepts.

Street-Smart Drawing on more than 25 years of prehospital experience, the editor offers some hard won "pearls of wisdom" in an effort to enlighten the next generation of providers.

EMS Terminology Woven into the text are common EMS terms that have developed as a result of the unique character of EMS.

Changes of Aging These sections bring to the forefront the importance of this population, which is rapidly growing within the health care segment. Integrating the changes of aging into an anatomy book introduces the idea that these changes are natural and not pathological.

● CHAPTER REVIEW

Chapter One—Introduction to the Structural Units The introduction of standard medical/ EMS anatomical terminology.

Chapter Two—Chemistry of Living Things An added discussion of major electrolytes and the signs and symptoms of electrolyte imbalances.

Chapter Three—Cells An expanded discussion of cancer.

Chapter Four—Tissues and Membranes A discussion of tissues and membranes.

Chapter Five—Integumentary System A discussion of common tissue injuries secondary to trauma as well as an expanded discussion of burn trauma.

Chapter Six—Skeletal System An additional discussion of common bone fractures; it is anticipated that EMT-Basics may not have this information.

Chapter Seven—Muscular System An in-depth discussion of compartment syndrome and crush injury.

Chapter Eight—Brain and Central Nervous System A discussion of strokes (brain attacks) and the signs and symptoms including different types of aphasia. Also includes a discussion of intracranial pressure (ICP) and the effects of increased ICP on the brain.

Chapter Nine—The Peripheral and Autonomic Nervous Systems An expanded discussion of the autonomic nervous system and its importance to EMS practice.

Chapter Ten—Special Senses A discussion of the impact of trauma and illness on the special senses, including the changes of aging.

Chapter Eleven—Endocrine System A discussion of diabetes, its types, and complications.

Chapter Twelve—Blood A review of type- and cross-matching, as well as reactions to blood transfusions. Also includes a discussion of the coagulation cascade, including the use of fibrinolytics.

Chapter Thirteen—Heart An in-depth discussion of coronary circulation with specific reference to ventricular walls and infarctions. Utilizes the concept of penumbra and introduces the concept of acute coronary syndrome (ACS).

Chapter Fourteen—Circulation and Blood Vessels A description of the phenomena of shunting and the hypoperfusion/shock syndrome.

Chapter Fifteen—The Lymphatic System and Immunity Cross-references the lymphatic system to infection control. Introduces the concept of bioterrorism.

Chapter Sixteen—Respiratory System An expanded discussion of the airway, including common pathology and treatments.

Chapter Seventeen—Digestive System An introduction to the concepts of medication administration, especially via the enteral route. Also includes a discussion of common digestive disorders.

Chapter Eighteen—Nutrition A discussion of the newest health crisis in the United States, obesity, as well as the importance of good nutrition during periods of high stress to prevent illness.

Chapter Nineteen—Urinary/Excretory System An in-depth discussion of the role of the kidneys in acid-base balance as well as common urinary disorders.

Chapter Twenty—Reproductive System An overview of conception, pregnancy, and the complications of pregnancy.

Chapter Twenty-one—Genetics and Genetically Linked Diseases A discussion of Down's Syndrome and other more common genetic disorders in preparation for lectures on patients with special needs.

How to Study Using Functional Anatomy for Emergency Medical Services

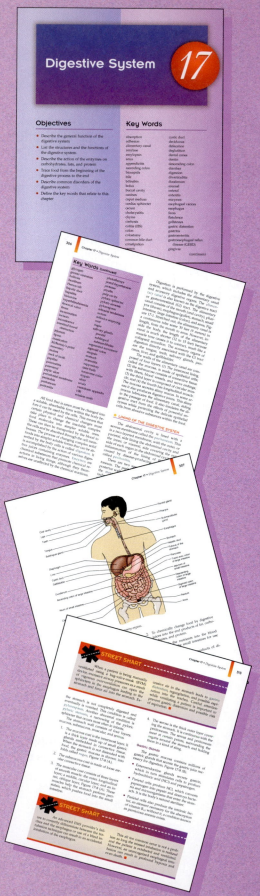

Preview the text before attempting to study the material covered in the individual chapters. By reviewing each section of this textbook, you will better understand its organization and purpose. Reading comprehension and long-term memory levels improve dramatically when you take the time to review the text and learn how it can help you learn.

To get the most from this course, take an active role in your learning by integrating your senses to increase your retention. You may want to:

- *Visually* highlight important material.

- *Read* critically—turn headings, subheadings, and sentences into questions.

- *Recite* important material aloud to stimulate your auditory memory.

- *Draw* your own illustrations of anatomy or function processes and check them for accuracy.

- *Answer* (in writing or verbally) the review questions at the end of the chapter.

Each time you encounter a new chapter, preview it first to understand its overall structure. Review the **Objectives** presented at the beginning of each chapter to easily identify the key facts *before* you read the chapter. These objectives are also useful for review *after* you have completed a chapter. After reading a chapter, test yourself to see whether you can answer each objective. If you can't, you'll know exactly which areas to study again. The **key words** are listed at the beginning of each chapter, are highlighted (at first usage) within the chapter, and are also defined in the glossary.

Read the **main headings, subheadings,** and first sentence of each paragraph—these elements serve as the outline for the whole chapter. Be careful not to overlook the **illustrations, photographs,** and **tables** to help you comprehend the difficult material.

Street Smarts provide information relevant to the care the EMS provider gives while on scene.

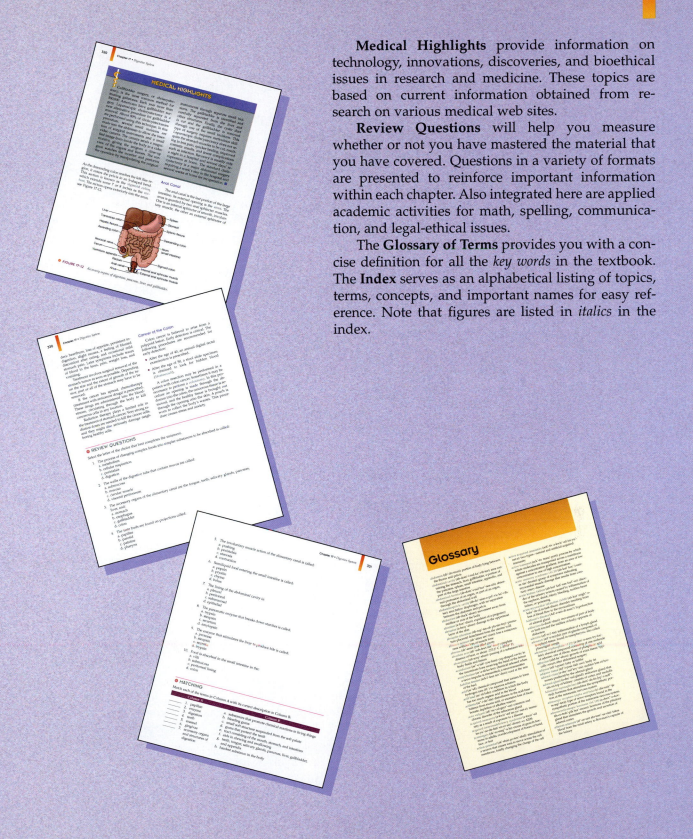

Medical Highlights provide information on technology, innovations, discoveries, and bioethical issues in research and medicine. These topics are based on current information obtained from research on various medical web sites.

Review Questions will help you measure whether or not you have mastered the material that you have covered. Questions in a variety of formats are presented to reinforce important information within each chapter. Also integrated here are applied academic activities for math, spelling, communication, and legal-ethical issues.

The **Glossary of Terms** provides you with a concise definition for all the *key words* in the textbook. The **Index** serves as an alphabetical listing of topics, terms, concepts, and important names for easy reference. Note that figures are listed in *italics* in the index.

How to Use the
Student Activity CD-ROM

The Student Activity CD-ROM was designed as an exciting enhancement to *Functional Anatomy for Emergency Medical Services* to help you learn about the structure and function of the body. As you study each chapter in the text, be sure to explore the corresponding unit on the CD-ROM.

Each chapter is divided into two major sections: exercises and activities. Exercises can be used for additional practice, review, or self-testing. Activities provide an opportunity to play and practice.

Getting started is easy. Follow the simple directions of the CD label to install the program on your computer. Then take advantage of the following features:

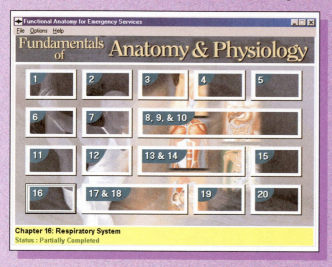

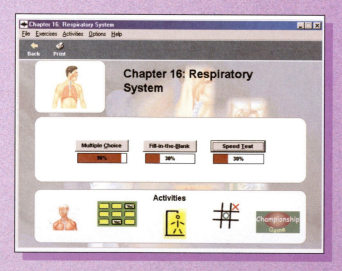

1 **Main Menu** The Main Menu follows the chapter organization of the text—which makes it easy for you to find your way around. Just click on the button for the chapter you want, and you'll come to the chapter opening screen.

Toolbar The Back button at the top left of every screen allows you to retrace your steps, while the Exit button gets you out of the program quickly and easily. As you navigate through the software, check the toolbar for other features that help you use individual exercises or games.

On-Line Help If you get stuck, just press F1 to get help. The on-line help includes instructions for all parts of the Student Activity CD-ROM.

2 **The Chapter Screen** Here you have the opportunity to choose how you want to learn. Select one of the exercises for additional practice, review, or self-testing. Or click on an activity to practice the terms for that chapter in a fun format.

3   Exercises The Student Activity CD-ROM acts as your own private tutor. For each exercise, it chooses from a bank of more than 900 questions. Putting these exercises to work for you is simple:

- Choose a multiple choice, fill-in-the-blank, or matching exercise, whichever one appeals to you.

- You'll encounter a series of 10 questions for each exercise format; each question gives you two chances to answer correctly.

- Instant feedback tells you whether you're right or wrong—and helps you learn more quickly by explaining why an answer was correct or incorrect.

- The Student Activity CD-ROM displays the percentage of correct answers on the chapter screen. An on-screen score sheet (that you can print) lets you track correct and incorrect answers.

- Review your previous questions and answers in an exercise for more in-depth understanding. Or start an exercise over with a new, random set of questions that gives you a realistic study environment.

- When you're ready for an additional challenge, try the timed Speed Test. Once you've finished, it displays your score and the time you took to complete the test, so you can see how much you've learned.

4   Activities To have fun while reinforcing your knowledge, enjoy each of the five simple activities on this disk. You can play alone, with a partner, or on teams.

- **Concentration:** Match terms to their corresponding definitions under the cards as the seconds tick by.

- **Hangman:** Review your spelling and vocabulary by choosing the correct letters to spell anatomy and physiology terms before you're "hanged."

- **Tic-Tac-Toe:** You or your team must correctly answer an anatomy or physiology question before placing an X or an O.

- **Anatomy and Physiology Championship Game:** Challenge your classmates and increase your knowledge by playing this Jeopardy style question-and-answer game.

- **Drag & Drop:** Art labeling exercises are included to help you learn in an interactive environment.

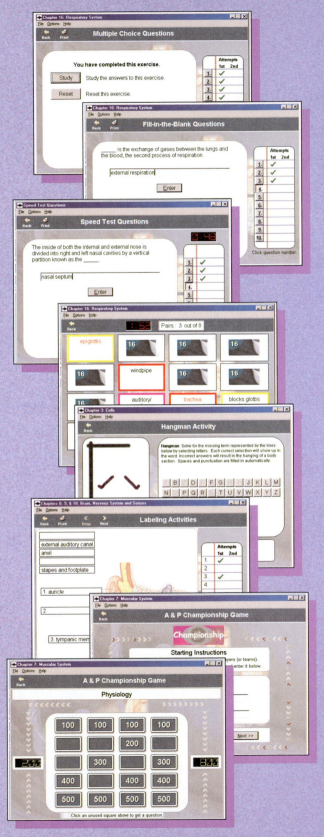

Introduction to the Structural Units

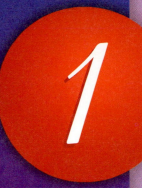

Objectives

- Identify and discuss the different branches of anatomy
- Identify the terms referring to location, direction, planes, and sections of the body
- Identify the body cavities and the organs they contain
- Identify and discuss the life functions and related body systems
- Define the key words that relate to this chapter

Key Words

abdominal cavity
abdominopelvic cavity
anabolism
anatomical position
anatomy
anterior
axilla
biology
buccal cavity
catabolism
caudal
clavicle
coronal (frontal) plane
cranial
cranial cavity
cytology
deep
dermatology
developmental anatomy
distal
dorsal
dorsal cavity
embryology
endocrinology
epigastric

external
gross anatomy
histology
homeostasis
hypogastric
inferior
internal
lateral
life functions
medial
metabolism
microscopic anatomy
midaxillary line (MAL)
midclavicular line (MCL)
midline
midsagittal plane
morphology
nasal cavity
neurology
oral cavity
orbital cavity
organs
organ system
pelvic cavity
physiology

(continues)

Key Words (continued)

planes	superior
posterior	systematic anatomy
proximal	thoracic cavity
retroperitoneal cavity	tissues
sagittal plane	topographic anatomy
section	transverse
spinal cavity	umbilical
superficial	ventral

● ANATOMY AND PHYSIOLOGY

Both anatomy and physiology are branches of a much larger science called **biology**. Biology is the study of all forms of life. Biology studies microscopic one-celled organisms, multicelled organisms, plants, animals, and humans.

Anatomy studies the shape and structure of an organism's body and the relationship of one body part to another. The word anatomy comes from the Greek, *ana*, meaning apart, and *temuein*, to cut; thus the acquisition of knowledge on human anatomy comes primarily from dissection. However, one cannot fully appreciate and understand anatomy without the study of its sister science, **physiology**. Physiology studies the function of each body part and how the functions of the various body parts coordinate to form a complete living organism.

Branches of Anatomy

Anatomy is subdivided into many branches based on the investigative techniques used, the type of knowledge sought after, or the parts of the body under study.

1. **Gross anatomy**. Gross anatomy is the study of large and easily observable structures on an organism. This is done through dissection and visible inspection with the naked eye. In it the different body parts and regions are studied with regard to their general shape, external features, and main divisions. The study of shape is called **morphology**.

2. **Microscopic anatomy**. With the invention and perfection of the microscope, the knowledge of gross anatomy can be extended down to the microscopic level. Microscopic anatomy is subdivided into two branches. One is called **cytology**, which is the study of the structure, function, and development of cells that make up the different body parts. For example, cytology can study the heart cells or the nerve cells composing the brain. The other subdivision is **histology**, which studies the tissues and organs making up the entire body of an organism.

3. **Developmental anatomy**. This part of anatomy studies the growth and development of an organism during its lifetime. More specifically, **embryology** studies the formation of an organism from the fertilized egg to birth.

4. **Topographic anatomy**. The study of the relationship of one body part to another is called **topographic anatomy**. Topographic anatomy utilizes a number of terms that refer to position, direction, and location of planes, sections, and lines of reference.

5. **Systematic anatomy**. Systematic anatomy is the study of the structure and function of various organs or parts making up a particular organ system. Depending on the particular organ system under study, a specific term is applied; for example:

   • **Dermatology**—study of the integumentary system (skin, hair, and nails)

   • **Endocrinology**—study of the endocrine or hormonal system

   • **Neurology**—study of the nervous system

● ANATOMIC TERMINOLOGY

In the study of anatomy and physiology, special words are used to describe the specific location of a structure or organ or the relative position of one body part to another.

The following terms are used to describe the human body as it is standing in the standard **anatomical position**, Figure 1-1. A human being in such a position is standing erect, with face forward, arms at the side, and palms forward.

Terms Referring to Location or Position and Direction

- **Anterior** or **ventral** means "front" or "in front of." For example, the knees are located on the anterior surface of the human body. A ventral hernia may protrude from the front or belly of the abdomen.

- **Posterior** or **dorsal** means "back" or "in back of." For example, human shoulder blades are found on the posterior surface of the body. The dorsal aspect of the foot is the sole of the foot.

- **Cranial** and **caudal** refer to direction; *cranial* refers to the head end of the body; *caudal*

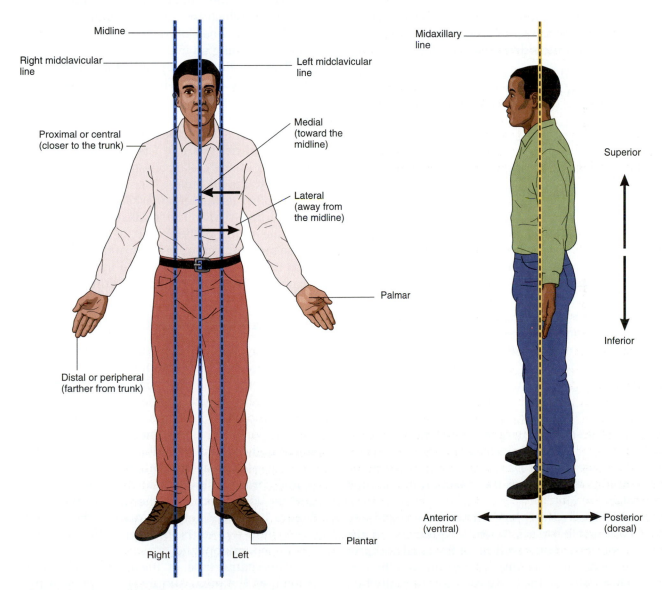

- **FIGURE 1–1** *The standard planes of reference and directional terms.*

refers to the tail end. For example, increased intracranial pressure causes headache. Caudal anesthesia is injected into the lower spine.

- **Superior** and **inferior**—*superior* means "upper" or "above another"; *inferior* means "lower" or "below another." For example, the heart and lungs are situated superior to the diaphragm, whereas the intestines are inferior to it.

- **Medial** and **lateral**—*medial* signifies "toward the midline or median plane of the body," whereas lateral means "away" or "toward the side of the body."

- **Proximal** and **distal**—*proximal* means "toward the point of attachment to the body" or "toward the trunk of the body"; *distal* means "away from the point of attachment or origin" or "farthest from the trunk." For example, the hand is proximal to the wrist; the elbow is distal to the shoulder. NOTE: these two words are used primarily to describe the appendages or extremities.

- **Superficial** or **external** and **deep** or **internal**—*superficial* implies on or near the surface of the body. For instance, a superficial wound just involves an injury to the outer skin. A deep injury involves damage to an internal organ such as the stomach. The terms *external* and *internal* are specifically used to refer to body cavities and hollow organs.

Terms Referring to Body Planes and Sections

Planes are imaginary anatomic dividing lines that are useful in separating body structures, see Figure 1-1. A **section** is a cut made through the body in the direction of a certain plane.

The **sagittal plane** divides the body into right and left parts (refer to Figure 1-1). If the plane starts in the middle of the skull and proceeds down, bisecting the sternum and the vertebral column, the body is divided equally into right and left halves. This is known as the **midsagittal plane**.

A **coronal (frontal) plane** is a vertical cut at right angles to the sagittal plane, dividing the body into anterior and posterior portions. The term *coronal* comes from the coronal suture, which runs perpendicular (at a right angle) to the sagittal suture. A **transverse** or cross section is a horizontal cut that divides the body into upper and lower parts.

Terms Referring to Lines on the Body

EMS providers often use several imaginary lines from which to draw a reference. For example, these lines of reference can be used when describing an injury.

The first line to imagine is the **midline**, as shown in Figure 1-1. The midline runs down the center of the body, equally dividing it into a right and a left half.

To either side of the midline are the **midclavicular lines (MCLs)**. These lines start at the midpoint of the collarbone (**clavicle**) and run parallel to the midline.

Another useful imaginary line is the **midaxillary line (MAL)**. The midaxillary line runs from the middle of the armpit, or **axilla**, parallel to the midline. These are a few of the more common examples of the lines used in topographic anatomy; they are depicted in Figure 1-1.

Terms Referring to Cavities of the Body

The organs that compose most of the body systems are organized into four cavities: cranial, spinal, thoracic, and abdominopelvic, Figure 1-2. The cranial and spinal cavities are within a larger region known as the dorsal (posterior) cavity. The thoracic and abdominopelvic cavities are found in the ventral (anterior) cavity.

The **dorsal cavity** contains the brain and spinal cord. The brain is in the **cranial cavity** and the spinal cord is in the **spinal cavity**, see Figure 1-2. The diaphragm divides the ventral cavity into two parts: the upper thoracic and lower abdominopelvic.

The central area of the thoracic cavity is known as the mediastinum. It is between the lungs and extends from the sternum (breast bone) to the vertebrae of the back. The esopha-

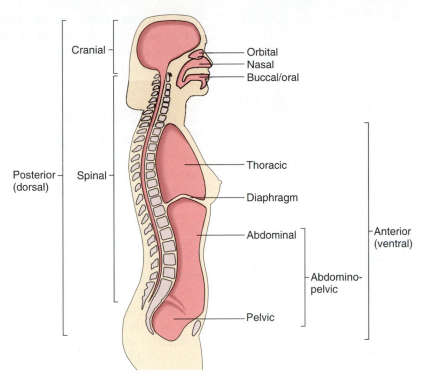

Cranial —
Orbital
Nasal
Buccal/oral

Posterior (dorsal) — Spinal
Thoracic
Diaphragm
Abdominal
Anterior (ventral)
Abdomino-pelvic
Pelvic

● **FIGURE 1–2**   *Cavities of the body.*

gus, bronchi, lungs, trachea, thymus gland, and heart are located in the thoracic cavity. The heart itself is contained within a smaller cavity, called the pericardial cavity.

The **thoracic cavity** is further subdivided into two pleural cavities. The left lung is in the left pleural cavity, the right lung is in the right. Each lung is covered with a thin membrane, which is called the pleura.

The **abdominopelvic cavity** is really one large cavity with no separation between the abdomen and pelvis. To avoid confusion, this cavity is usually referred to separately—as the abdominal cavity and the pelvic cavity. The **abdominal cavity** contains the stomach, liver, gallbladder, pancreas, spleen, small intestine, appendix, and part of the large intestine. The kidneys, aorta, and vena cava are all in a space behind the abdominal cavity called the **retroperitoneal cavity**. Bleeding into the retroperitoneal cavity is often difficult to detect because the abdominal cavity lies over the top of it and the pelvis is behind it. The kidneys are close to but behind the abdominal cavity.

The urinary bladder, the reproductive organs, the rectum, the remainder of the large intestine, and the appendix are in the **pelvic cavity**.

Terms Referring to Regions in the Abdominopelvic Cavity

To locate the abdominal and pelvic organs more easily, anatomists have subdivided the abdominopelvic cavity into nine regions, Figure 1-3.

These regions are located in the upper, middle, and lower parts of the abdomen:

- *Upper*—or **epigastric** region located just below the sternum (breast bone) and the right hypochondriac and the left hypochondriac regions located below the ribs.

- *Middle*—or **umbilical** area located around the navel or umbilicus, the right lumbar region, and the left lumbar region, which extend from anterior to posterior. (A person will complain of back pain or lumbar sprain.)

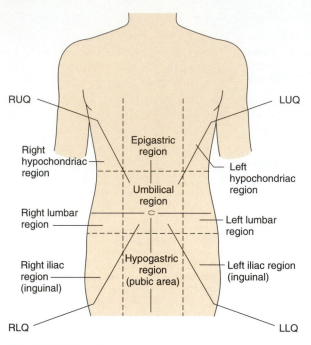

● **FIGURE 1–3**   *The nine regions and four quadrants of the abdominal area.*

- *Lower*—or **hypogastric** region, which may also be referred to as the pubic area, the left iliac, and the right iliac, which may also be called the left inguinal and right inguinal areas.

Smaller Cavities

In addition to the cranial cavity, the skull also contains several smaller cavities. The eyes, eye-ball muscles, optic nerves, and lacrimal (tear) ducts are within the **orbital cavity**. The **nasal cavity** contains the parts that form the nose. The **oral** or **buccal** cavity encloses the teeth and tongue.

● LIFE FUNCTIONS

When we examine humans, plants, one-celled organisms, and multicelled organisms, we recognize that all of them have one thing in common: they are alive.

All living organisms are capable of carrying on life functions. **Life functions** are a series of highly organized and related activities that help living organisms to live, grow, and maintain themselves.

These vital life functions include movement, ingestion, digestion, transport, respiration, synthesis, assimilation, growth, secretion, excretion, regulation (sensitivity), and reproduction, Table 1-1.

● HUMAN DEVELOPMENT

A person is born, grows into maturity, and eventually dies. In the intervening years between birth and death, the body carries on a number of life functions that keep us alive and active. As is true of all living things, each of us inherits a range of size, form, and lifespan. We inherit these many characteristics through the gametes from our parents. Gametes are the sperm and egg cells.

STREET SMART ----------------------------

The only reliable distinguishing landmark on the anterior abdominal wall is the umbilicus. This point is used as a reference when describing areas of injury or pain. Using the umbilicus as the center point, the abdomen has been divided into four quad-rants. Each quadrant is named either left or right and upper or lower. Although other systems of descriptive topographic anatomy exist, this method is the most commonly used in emergency medicine; it is pictured in Figure 1-3. ■

TABLE 1-1 *Review of the Life Functions and Body Systems*

LIFE FUNCTIONS/ BODY SYSTEMS	DEFINITION
Movement/Muscle System	The ability of the whole organism—or a part of it—to move.
Ingestion/Digestive System	The process by which an organism takes in food.
Digestion/ Digestive System	The breakdown of complex food molecules into simpler food molecules.
Transport/Circulatory System	The movement of necessary substances to, into, and around cells, and of cellular products and wastes out of and away from cells.
Respiration/Respiratory System	The burning or oxidation of food molecules in a cell to release energy, water, and carbon dioxide.
Synthesis/Digestive System	The combination of simple molecules into more complex molecules to help an organism build new tissue.
Assimilation/Digestive System	The transformation of digested food molecules into living tissue for growth and self-repair.
Growth/Skeletal System	The enlargement of an organism caused by synthesis and assimilation, resulting in an increase in the number and size of its cells.
Secretion/Endocrine System	The formation and release of hormones from a cell or structure.
Excretion/Urinary System	The removal of metabolic waste products from an organism.
Regulation (sensitivity)/ Nervous System	The ability of an organism to respond to its environment to maintain a balanced state (homeostasis).
Reproduction/ Reproductive System	The ability of an organism to produce offspring with similar characteristics. This is *essential* for species survival, as opposed to individual survival.

Living depends on the constant release of energy in every cell of the body. Powered by the energy that is released from food, the cells are able to maintain their own living condition and thus the life of human beings.

A complex life form like a human being consists of more than fifty thousand billion cells. Early in human development, certain groups of cells become highly specialized for specific functions, like movement or growth.

Special cells, grouped according to function, shape, size, and structure, are called **tissues**. Tissues, in turn, form larger functional and structural units known as **organs**. For example, human skin is an organ made up of epithelial, connective, muscular, and nervous tissue. In much the same way, our kidneys are composed of highly specialized connective and epithelial tissue.

The organs of the human body do not operate independently. They function interdependently with one another to form a live, functioning organism. Some organs are grouped together because they are needed to perform a function. Such a grouping is called an **organ system**. One example is the digestive system, composed of the teeth, esophagus, stomach, small intestine, and large intestine. In this text you will study the various body systems and the organs that make up these systems.

BODY PROCESSES

The functional activities of cells that result in growth, repair, energy release, use of food, and secretions are combined under the heading of **metabolism**. Metabolism consists of two processes that are opposite to each other: anabolism and catabolism. **Anabolism** is the building up of complex materials from simpler ones such as food and oxygen. **Catabolism** is the breaking down and changing of complex substances into simpler ones, with a release of energy and carbon dioxide. The sum of all the chemical reactions within a cell is therefore called metabolism.

The proper function and maintenance of the human body depends on a number of activities. The body must constantly respond to changes in the environment by exchanging substances between its surroundings and its cells. Maintaining the body's cellular environment and function helps to ensure regular body functions. Thus optimum cell functioning requires a stable cellular environment (within very narrow limits of acidity, nutrients, oxygen, temperature, and fluid balance).

The maintenance of such (optimum) internal environmental conditions is known as **homeostasis**. Human survival depends on maintenance or restoration of homeostasis.

● REVIEW QUESTIONS

Select the letter of the choice that best completes the statement.

1. Anatomy is the study of:
   a. the structure of a body part
   b. the structure and function of a body part
   c. the function of a body part
   d. the formation of a body part

2. The study of the function of cells is called:
   a. anatomy
   b. physiology
   c. histology
   d. cytology

3. The anatomical position is described as:
   a. body erect, arms at the side, palms forward
   b. body supine, arms at the side, palms forward
   c. body erect, arms at the side, palms backward
   d. body supine, arms at the side, palms backward

4. A plane that divides the body into right and left parts is the:
   a. transverse plane
   b. coronal plane
   c. sagittal plane
   d. frontal plane

5. If a wound occurs near the surface of the skin, it is:
   a. deep
   b. superficial
   c. medial
   d. lateral

6. The heart is described as superior to the diaphragm because it is:
   a. in back of the diaphragm
   b. in front of the diaphragm
   c. above the diaphragm
   d. below the diaphragm

7. The brain and the spinal cavity are located in the:
   a. ventral cavity
   b. spinal cavity
   c. cranial cavity
   d. dorsal cavity

8. The epigastric region of the abdominal area is located:
   a. just above the sternum
   b. in the umbilical area
   c. just below the sternum
   d. in the pelvic area

9. The sum of the chemical reactions in a cell is known as:
   a. homeostasis
   b. metabolism
   c. anabolism
   d. catabolism

10. The formation and release of hormones from a cell or structure is called:
    a. digestion
    b. excretion
    c. synthesis
    d. secretion

● MATCHING

Match each term in Column A with its correct description in Column B.

Column A	Column B
_____ 1. catabolism	a. balanced cellular environment
_____ 2. pelvic cavity	b. constructive chemical processes that use food to build complex materials of the body
_____ 3. pericardial cavity	c. useful breakdown of food materials, resulting in the release of energy
_____ 4. anabolism	d. contained within the oral cavity
_____ 5. abdominal cavity	e. cavity in which the reproductive organs, urinary bladder, and lower part of the large intestine are located
_____ 6. diaphragm	f. cavity in which the stomach, liver, gallbladder, pancreas, spleen, appendix, cecum, and colon are located
_____ 7. homeostasis	g. cavity containing the heart
_____ 8. tissue	h. group of cells that together perform a particular job
_____ 9. kidneys	i. portion of the dorsal cavity containing the brain
_____ 10. teeth and tongue	j. divides the ventral cavity into two regions
_____ 11. cranial cavity	k. structure located behind the abdominal cavity
_____ 12. organ system	l. organs grouped together because they have a related function
	m. an activity that a living thing performs to help it live and grow

●APPLYING THEORY TO PRACTICE

1. In each of the examples below, choose the bold term that correctly describes the human body according to anatomical position:
    a. In the anatomical position the palms are **forward** or **backward**.
    b. The liver is **superior** or **inferior** to the diaphragm.
    c. The hand is **proximal** or **distal** to the elbow.
    d. The sole of the foot is on the **anterior** or **posterior** part of the body.
    e. *Cranial* refers to the **head** or **tail** end of the body.
    f. The coronal plane divides the body into **front and back** or **right and left** sections.
    g. The arms are located on the **medial** or **lateral** side of the body.
    h. The transverse plane divides the body into **superior and inferior** or **anterior and posterior** parts.

2. Using the correct anatomical term, describe the following to a physician:
    a. the location of an appendectomy scar
    b. a wound that is on the front of the leg
    c. the end of the spine
    d. a pain near the breast bone

3. Think about what your body does within a 24-hour period and name the life functions that take place.

Chemistry of Living Things

2

Objectives

- Relate the importance of chemistry and biochemistry to health care
- Define matter and energy
- Explain the structure of an atom, an element, and a compound
- Describe the four main groups of organic compounds: carbohydrates, fats, proteins, and nucleic acids
- Explain the difference between the DNA molecule and the RNA molecule
- Explain the difference among an acid, a base, and a salt
- Describe why homeostasis is necessary for good health
- Define the key words that relate to this chapter

Key Words

acid
acidosis
alkali
alkalosis
amino acids
atom
base
bicarbonate
biochemistry
buffers
calcium (Ca+)
carbohydrates
carpopedal spasm
chemistry
cholesterol
coagulation
coenzyme
compounds
dehydration
deoxyribonucleic acid (DNA)
disaccharide
diuretics
electrolytes
element

energy
enzymes
extracellular fluid
fasciculations
fats (triglycerides)
gastric tube
glycogen
goit
hydroxide
hypercalcemia
hypermagnesemia
hypernatremia
hypocalcemia
hypokalemia
hypomagnesemia
hyponatremia
hypovolemia
interstitial fluid
intracellular fluid
ions
ionize
isotopes
kidney dialysis
kinetic energy
lipids

(continues)

Key Words (continued)

magnesium (Mg+)	potassium (K+)
malabsorption	potential energy
syndrome	radioactive
malaise	renal compensation
matter	respiratory
milliequivalents (mEq)	compensation
molecule	ribonucleic acid (RNA)
monosaccharides	rickets
multicellular	salt
neutralization	selectively permeable
noncompliance	membranes
nucleic acids	sodium (Na+)
organic catalysts	steroids
organic compounds	tetany
perioral paresthesia	therapeutic level
pH scale	unicellular
phospholipids	ventricular fibrillation
polysaccharides	water intoxication
polyuria	

To be an effective health care professional, an understanding of the normal and abnormal functioning of the human body is essential. A knowledge of basic chemistry and biochemistry is needed.

● CHEMISTRY

Chemistry is the study of the structure of matter, the composition of substances, their properties, and their chemical reactions. There are many chemical reactions that occur in the human body. These reactions range from the digestion of a piece of meat in the stomach and formation of urine in the kidneys to the manufacture of proteins in a microscopic human cell. Ultimately the chemical reactions necessary to sustain life occur in the cells. Thus the study of the chemical reactions of living things is called **biochemistry**.

● MATTER AND ENERGY

Chemistry studies the nature of matter and how its atoms are put together and interact with each other. **Matter** is defined as anything that has weight (mass) and occupies space. Matter exists in the forms of solid, liquid, and gas. An example in our bodies of solid matter is bone; blood is liquid; oxygen is gas.

Matter is neither created nor destroyed, but it can change form through physical or chemical means. A physical change occurs when we chew a piece of food and it breaks up into smaller pieces. A chemical change occurs when the food is acted on by various chemicals in the body to change its composition. For example, imagine a piece of toast that becomes molecules of fat and glucose to be used by the body for energy.

Energy is defined as the ability to do work or to put matter into motion. Energy exists in our body as **potential energy** or **kinetic energy**. Potential energy is energy stored in cells waiting to be released, whereas kinetic energy is work resulting in motion. Lying in bed is an example of potential energy; getting out of bed is an example of kinetic energy.

● ATOMS

An **atom** is the smallest piece of an element. Atoms are invisible to the human eye, yet they are all around us and are part of our human structure. Hydrogen is an example of an atom.

The normal atom is made up of subatomic particles: protons, neutrons, and electrons. The protons have a positive (+) electric charge; the neutrons have no electric charge. The protons and the neutrons make up the nucleus of the atom (which differs from the nucleus of the cell), Figure 2-1. The electrons have a negative (−) electric charge and are arranged around the nucleus in orbital zones or electron shells. Atoms usually have more than one electron shell. The arrangement of the subatomic particles is how the atoms of one element differ from atoms of another element; the structure of the hydrogen atom is different from the structure of the oxygen atom.

The number of protons of an atom is equal to the number of electrons; atoms are electrically neutral, neither negative or positive. An atom can share or combine an electron with

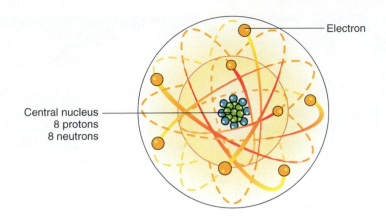

Central nucleus
8 protons
8 neutrons

Electron

🔴 **FIGURE 2–1** *Structure of a typical atom. Eight protons and eight neutrons are tightly bound in the central nucleus, around which the eight electrons revolve.*

another atom to form a chemical bond. If one atom gives up an electron to another atom to form this bond, it will have more protons than electrons and will have a positive charge. The atom that took the extra electron will have more electrons than protons and have a negative charge. These charged atoms are then called **ions**.

Atoms of a specific element that have the same number of protons but different number of neutrons are called **isotopes**. All isotopes of a specific element have the same number of electrons. Certain isotopes are called **radioactive**

isotopes because they are unstable and may decay (come apart). As they decay they give off (emit) energy in the form of radiation, which can be picked up by a detector. The detector not only detects the emission from a radioactive isotope but, with the aid of a computer, can also form the image of its distribution within the body. Radioactive isotopes can be used to study structure and function of particular tissue. In addition, strong radiation from certain isotopes may destroy body tissue. This radiation is useful in the treatment of cancer and other diseases.

MEDICAL HIGHLIGHTS

In 1950, nuclear medicine was introduced that used radionuclides (also known as radioisotopes) to scan the body. This innovative technique was hailed as a diagnostic breakthrough. It can be used to identify abnormal and normal body structures that cannot be seen by x-ray. Since the 1970s we have seen the development of computed tomography (CT scan), positron emission

tomography (PET scan), sonography, and magnetic resonance imaging (MRI).

A CT scan combines x-ray emission with nuclear medicine to look inside the body. The images produced are cross-sectional, patterned much like slices of bread. By taking a series of such images a CT scan can create a multidimensional view of the body. The main feature of the equipment is a large "ring." The patient passes through the ring while the x-ray tube rotates 360 degrees around the patient and takes pictures. After taking many pictures, the computer has enough information to combine segments of the pictures and create views of the internal organs. These views are projected onto a television screen. Still photos are taken to record significant findings. CT scans have all but eliminated exploratory surgery. They are most useful in evaluating brain and abdominal findings.

Positron emission tomography is a procedure in which the patient is given an injection of a short-lived radionuclide and then positioned in the PET scanner. The radionuclides are absorbed by active brain cells and high-energy gamma rays are released as a result. A computer analyzes these rays and produces a color picture of the brain's biochemical activity. The patient must remain alert for this test. Blindfolds and earplugs may be used to reduce external stimuli to the brain. The patient is also asked questions or told to recite to see how the brain activity changes for reasoning and remembering. PET scans are most useful to diagnose the effects of stroke, some aspects of Alzheimer's disease, epilepsy, and mental illness.

Sonography or ultrasound imaging uses high-frequency sound waves for diagnostic purposes. Ultrasound is completely noninvasive and uses no radiation. To date, no harmful effects on living tissue have been noted. Sound waves are sent into the body tissues by a small transducer, which also receives returning sound echoes that are deflected back as they bounce off various internal structures. (A transducer is a device that changes electrical energy into sound waves.) The returning sound waves are converted into electric signals, which are fed into a computer. The computer transforms the signals into scans or graphs that are used to construct visual images of the body. This is the imaging choice for obstetrics to visualize the fetal embryo and placenta. It is useful to examine the pelvic and abdominal areas. The Doppler method is a variation of sonography in which returning sound waves are transformed into audible sounds that can be detected by earphones. Doppler method measures blood flow by moving the transducer along the path of a blood vessel. Data can be obtained concerning the velocity of flow in the area over which the transducer moves.

MRI uses a magnetic field combined with radio frequency waves to produce cross-sectional images of the body. The patient is inserted into a chamber that is built within a huge magnet. The magnetic field causes the atomic ions in the tissue to line up in a parallel fashion. Radio waves are sent into the patient and the aligned ions pick up this energy and change their orientation. When the radio waves are turned off, the ions revert back to the aligned position produced by the magnetic field. These changes in the energy field are sensed and translated by a computer into a visual image. MRI is a good diagnostic tool for degenerative disease such as multiple sclerosis. Caution must be used, however, because strong magnetic fields may damage pacemakers and metal protheses such as hips and knees. Patients must remove all hair clips, jewelry, and watches when receiving an MRI.

EMS providers must be aware of the anxiety people feel when they see the huge CT and MRI machines. Patient education is critical. Explain to patients that they may hear loud noises, which are common during the test. No one can be in the room with them during the test, but a technician will always be in voice contact with the patient. ■

TABLE 2-1 *Some Sample Elements and their Symbols*

ELEMENT	SYMBOL
Calcium	Ca
Carbon	C
Chlorine	Cl
Hydrogen	H
Iodine	I
Iron	Fe
Magnesium	Mg
Nitrogen	N
Oxygen	O
Phosphorus	P
Potassium	K
Sodium	Na
Zinc	Zn

ELEMENTS

Atoms that are alike combine to form the next stage of matter, an **element**. An element is a substance that can neither be created nor destroyed by ordinary means. Elements can exist in more than one phase in our bodies. Our bones are solid and contain the element calcium. The air we take into our lungs contains the element oxygen, which is a gas. Our cells are bathed in fluids that contain the elements hydrogen and oxygen. When these two elements unite they form water.

There are greater than 100 elements found naturally in our world; additional elements have been created by scientists. Each of the elements is represented by a chemical symbol or an abbreviation. Table 2-1 shows a sampling of elements and their chemical symbols.

COMPOUNDS

Various elements can combine together, in a definite proportion by weight, to form **compounds**. A compound has different characteristics or properties from the elements that compose it. For example, the compound water (H_2O) is made of two parts hydrogen and one part oxygen. Separately, hydrogen and oxygen are gaseous elements, but when combined to form water, the resulting compound is a liquid

under normal temperature. Common table salt is a compound made from the two elements sodium (Na) and chlorine (Cl), and it is chemically called sodium chloride (NaCl). Separately, sodium is a metallic element. It is light, silver-white, and shiny when freshly cut, but rapidly becomes dull and gray when exposed to air. Chlorine, on the other hand, is an irritating, greenish-yellow poisonous gas with a suffocating odor. However, the chemical combination of sodium and chlorine results in sodium chloride, table salt, which is a crystalline powder that can be dissolved in water.

Just as elements are represented by symbols, compounds are represented by something called a formula. A formula shows the types of elements present and the proportion of each element present by weight. Some common formulas are H_2O (water), NaCl (common table salt), HCl (hydrogen chloride or hydrochloric acid), $NaHCO_3$ (sodium bicarbonate or baking powder), NaOH (sodium hydroxide or lye), $C_6H_{12}O_6$ (glucose or sugar), $C_{12}H_{22}O_{11}$ (sucrose or common table sugar), CO_2 (carbon dioxide), and CO (carbon monoxide).

A living organism, whether it is a **unicellular** (one-celled) microbe or a **multicellular** animal or plant, can be compared with a chemical factory. Most living organisms will take the 20 essential elements and change them into needed compounds for the maintenance of the organism. In many living organisms, the elements carbon, hydrogen, and oxygen are united to form **organic compounds** (compounds found in living things containing the element carbon). One group of organic compounds manufactured are carbohydrates, such as sugars and starches.

Molecules

The smallest unit of a compound that still has the properties of the compound and has the capability to lead its own stable and independent existence is called a **molecule**. For example, the common compound water can be broken down into smaller and smaller droplets. Finally, when the absolutely smallest unit is reached, one has a molecule of water, H_2O.

IONS AND ELECTROLYTES

In addition to combining to form elements, atoms can share or combine their electrons with other atoms to form chemical bonds. If one atom gives up an electron to another atom to form a bond, it will have more protons than electrons and will have a positive (+) charge (cation). The atom that took the extra electron will now have more electrons than protons and have a negative (−) charge (anion). Such a positively or negatively charged particle is called an ion. The attraction between the opposite charges produces an ionic bond.

When compounds are in solution and they act as if they have broken into individual pieces (ions), the elements of the compound are **electrolytes**. For example, a salt solution consists of sodium (Na^+) ions with a positive charge and chlorine (Cl^-) ions with a negative charge.

In the cells and tissue fluids of the body, ions make it possible for materials to be altered, broken down, and recombined to form new substances or compounds. Electrolytes are responsible for the acidity or alkalinity of solutions and can conduct an electrical charge.

Potassium

The chief electrolyte *inside* the cell is **potassium (K+)**. Potassium controls important cellular functions including osmosis (discussed in the next chapter) and regulation of the acid-base balance (discussed later in this chapter). Potassium also is an important element in several enzyme reactions; enzymes are proteins that act as catalysts that accelerate chemical reactions.

However, the most important function of potassium may be its effect on neuromuscular excitability. *Neuromuscular excitability* refers to the ability of the nervous system to cause the muscles to function. The ability of potassium to help cause muscle contraction is vitally important, especially to cardiac muscle.

The level of potassium in the bloodstream is normally 3.5 to 5.0 mEq/L. A small change in potassium levels outside this narrow range can lead to serious, potentially lifethreatening complications.

Large amounts of potassium in the bloodstream, greater than 6.0 mEq/L, can lead to muscle weakness and **malaise** (French for fatigue). This condition, elevated potassium in the blood, is called **hyperkalemia**.

As the potassium levels continue to increase, the potassium becomes a poison to the heart, irritating the heart muscle and making it beat erratically and ineffectively. Untreated, the potassium-poisoned heart beats more and more weakly until it stops entirely.

Under normal conditions the kidneys dispose of excess potassium in the urine. If the kidneys are unable to perform this task because of kidney failure, excessive amounts of potassium will accumulate, leading to hyperkalemia.

There are many reasons for kidney failure. If the kidneys experience prolonged periods without blood flow because of excessive blood loss secondary to bleeding, for example, then the kidneys may stop functioning and hyperkalemia may occur.

The kidneys also have a limited capacity to rid the body of potassium quickly. A superabundance of potassium caused by massive cell damage can lead to hyperkalemia. Causes of massive cell damage include crushing injury, extensive burns, and myocardial infarction (heart attack).

When the kidneys fail or are overwhelmed, the patient may be placed on a special machine that acts like a kidney. The artificial kidney machine cleanses the blood, eliminating excess potassium in a procedure called **kidney dialysis**.

The body can also rid itself of some potassium via the gastrointestinal tract. Common symptoms of hyperkalemia include nausea and diarrhea, as well as intestinal cramping (colic).

Although hyperkalemia is often seen in emergency medicine, the more common potassium imbalance is low potassium, or **hypokalemia**. When a person's potassium becomes too low, the body's cells, particularly nerve cells and muscles, cannot function properly.

When the blood (serum) potassium falls below 3.5 mEq/L, the muscles become weak. This is similar to the affect that high potassium levels have on muscles. Any potassium imbalance leads to muscle weakness.

Sodium and potassium have a reciprocal relationship. When one is high, the other is low. A large intake of sodium causes normal-functioning kidneys to excrete potassium. Therefore the emergency treatment of hyperkalemia often includes intravenous (IV) administration of sodium bicarbonate. ■

Untreated, hypokalemia can lead to heart irritability and **ventricular fibrillation**, a condition in which the heart just quivers in place, instead of beating normally, and no blood is ejected from the heart. Ventricular fibrillation is a common cause of sudden cardiac death.

Although kidney (renal) disease can cause hypokalemia, the more common cause of hypokalemia is gastrointestinal disturbance. Prolonged vomiting of potassium-rich gastric juices can lead to hypokalemia. A **gastric tube** inserted into the stomach, which mechanically removes gastric contents, has the same effect as prolonged vomiting. These gastric tubes are often inserted to rid the stomach of blood or poison. Prolonged diarrhea of watery, potassium-rich fluid can also lead to hypokalemia.

Medications that increase urine production, called **diuretics**, can also cause a loss of potassium with urine. As a result, potassium supplements, such as K-lor, are often prescribed along with a diuretic. Unfortunately, potassium supplements are often unpleasant tasting, causing the patient to take the diuretic but not the potassium supplement. The patient's failure to take prescribed medications, called **noncompliance**, and specifically the potassium supplement, can lead to hypokalemia.

Potassium is a positively charged electrolyte. When the serum potassium is low, the body starts to excrete hydrogen (H+) to maintain a balance of positive and negative ions in the body. Free hydrogen in the body is an acid. Therefore changes in hydrogen levels affect the acid-base balance. Acid-base balances, and the impact of dramatic shifts in the acid-base balance, are discussed later in this chapter.

Sodium

Whereas potassium is the most abundant intracellular cation, the most abundant *extracellular* cation is **sodium (Na+)**.

Sodium and potassium can be thought of as rivals, each on one side of a wall, the cell membrane; each is trying to get to the other side but cannot. So instead of sodium and potassium crossing the cell membrane, water passes back and forth across the cell membrane trying to maintain a balance of concentrations. This balance occurs because of a process called **osmosis**. Osmosis is discussed in more detail later.

A balance of extracellular sodium, intracellular potassium, and water is essential for good health. When illness causes a loss of sodium in the blood, or **hyponatremia**, then the balance of water within the body is also affected. Therefore whenever there is a loss of sodium, the body cannot maintain a normal level of water and an imbalance occurs. The loss of sodium leads to **dehydration**. The symptoms of dehydration are directly related to the loss of fluid volume in the bloodstream or **hypovolemia**.

Causes of true hyponatremia and dehydration include burns, diarrhea, prolonged vomiting, and renal disorders, especially excessive use of diuretics.

Hyponatremia is, by definition, a deficiency of sodium when compared with the volume of water in the bloodstream. Therefore it is possible to be hyponatremic because there is too much water in the blood, which is called **water intoxication**, as well as being hyponatremic from too little sodium in the bloodstream.

Water intoxication can be caused by a failure of the kidneys to excrete excess water because of renal failure. Water intoxication can also be due to the loss of regulatory mechanisms that control the kidneys.

One of those regulatory mechanisms is a hormone called *antidiuretic hormone (ADH)*. When a malignant tumor or cerebral dysfunction results in excessive levels of ADH, called the *syndrome of inappropriate secretion of antidiuretic hormone (SIADH)*, large quantities of water are retained.

When the serum sodium level falls below 135 mEq/L the patient is technically hyponatremic and will experience muscular weakness and apathy.

Continued loss of excessive amounts of sodium or unabated water intoxication can lead to severe hyponatremia.

The brain is particularly sensitive to hyponatremia. When serum sodium levels drop below 115 mEq/L the patient may start to experience headaches and irritability. Untreated, the patient will become confused and may even convulse or lapse into coma.

When water losses exceed sodium losses, the opposite of what is described above, the patient may become hypernatremic. **Hypernatremia** is a state of excessive sodium in the blood.

Excessive water loss may be due to sweating, diarrhea, or excessive urine production. One cause of excessive urine production (**polyuria**) is diabetes mellitus. In the case of diabetes mellitus, high levels of blood sugar (glucose) pull water out the cells, by osmosis, and into the bloodstream. In turn, the kidneys, sensing this excess fluid volume, excrete it in the form of urine. The result can be that the patient becomes dehydrated and the patient's serum sodium becomes concentrated.

Conversely, hypernatremia can also result from inadequate water intake. Signs of hypernatremia include dehydration symptoms such as a dry tongue and excessive thirst.

Hypernatremia also can be the result of the loss of the regulatory mechanisms that control the kidneys. The hormone *aldosterone* controls the excretion of sodium into the urine. Hyperaldosteronism can cause excessive sodium retention.

As in water intoxication, excessive water loss and the resulting hypernatremia have significant effects on the brain. Confusion, convulsions, and coma may occur as a result of hypernatremia.

Calcium

Although **calcium (Ca+)** is by far the most abundant cation in the human body, it occupies a relatively minor percentage of the blood's electrolytes. That is because 99% of the body's calcium is found within the bones. From this rich store, about 1% of the calcium is released to the bloodstream. Serum calcium is used in blood clotting (**coagulation**), as well as acid-base balance. However, calcium is vital to the function of muscle, especially the heart.

A normal blood calcium level of between 8.8 and 10.4 mg/100 ml is important for proper nervous system function. Calcium levels in the blood are affected by the absorption of calcium from the gastrointestinal tract, the deposit and resorption from the bones, and the excretion in the urine and feces. Any abnormality of calcium levels is often the result of problems with one or more of these three processes.

A low calcium level, or **hypocalcemia**, is relatively rare in the United States, in part because vitamin D is routinely added by commercial diaries to milk. Vitamin D is necessary for the absorption of calcium in the gastrointestinal tract. Before the practice of adding vitamin D to milk, children sometimes developed a bone disorder called **rickets**. Children with rickets grow abnormally shaped bones and have a characteristic bowed leg look.

An even more uncommon cause of hypocalcemia is hypoparathyroidism. The parathyroid glands, located in the neck, are responsible for creating hormones that affect calcium absorption. Without these parathyroid hormones, calcium levels drop, leading to hypocalcemia.

Chronic laxative use can also lead to hypocalcemia. Laxatives interfere with calcium absorption from the gastrointestinal tract.

The symptoms of hypocalcemia include numbness around the mouth (**perioral paresthesia**), cramping of the hands and feet (**carpopedal spasm**), and painful spasms of muscle (**tetany**).

Although elevated calcium levels, or **hypercalcemia**, are more common than hypocalcemia, it is harder to diagnose because the symptoms of hypercalcemia, such as lethargy, nausea, vomiting, and constipation, are common with many other ailments.

Hypercalcemia is most often caused by excessive resorption of calcium from bones. There are many causes of hypercalcemia, including hyperparathyroidism, vitamin D overdose, overuse of certain antacids, and Paget's disease. A common cause of calcium resorption is tumors in bones from cancers elsewhere in the body.

Magnesium

Like calcium, the bulk of the **magnesium (Mg+)** is found in the bones; about 1% is found in the extracellular fluids. Although magnesium is present in relatively small amounts, it still serves important functions in cell metabolism, as well as the activation of enzymes (discussed later in this chapter).

One of the more critical functions of magnesium is its action at the junction of the nerves to skeletal muscles. Without adequate magnesium at the junction the muscles fail to function properly. Interestingly, high levels of magnesium also impair neuromuscular functions.

Most magnesium-related disorders are the result of low magnesium levels, **hypomagnesemia**. Hypomagnesemia is usually the result of either impaired absorption from the gastrointestinal tract or from excessive excretion from the kidneys.

Impaired absorption from the gastrointestinal tract, or **malabsorption syndrome**, leads to insufficient amounts of magnesium in the blood and bones.

Chronic alcoholism can also lead to hypomagnesemia, probably because of both poor absorption and excessive secretion in the urine.

The signs and symptoms of hypomagnesemia are similar to the signs and symptoms of hypocalcemia: carpopedal spasm, tetany, and muscle tremors called **fasciculations**.

Potassium and magnesium are closely related. If the patient has hypokalemia, then the patient may also have hypomagnesemia.

Elevated levels of serum magnesium, or **hypermagnesemia**, are often the result of either kidney failure (an inability to excrete magnesium) or excessive ingestion of magnesium. External sources of magnesium include antacids, cathartics such as Epsom salts, and milk of magnesia.

The symptoms of hypermagnesemia are primarily a function of its action on the nerves. Elevated magnesium interferes with neuromuscular transmission and has a predictable pattern of progression. At first, when serum blood levels are at about 3 to 4 mEq/L, the patient feels flushed and a feeling of warmth comes over the body. As serum levels climb toward 10 mEq/L, hypotension ensues and the patient starts to lose deep tendon reflexes. When the serum magnesium levels approach 15 mEq/L the patient demonstrates a weak, slow pulse; drowsiness; and flaccid extremities (lacking any control). Soon respiratory depression begins and coma sets in. Cardiac arrest is possible when magnesium reaches toxic levels at 25 mEq/L.

Chloride

Chloride is a salt of hydrochloric acid. In other words, chloride is the chemical that remains after the removal of acid (H+) from hydrochloric acid.

Chloride is an important element only because it tends to compete with bicarbonate to combine with acid. Therefore the importance of chloride levels is typically in relation to the acid-base balance of the blood. Acid-base balance is discussed later in this chapter.

Trace Elements

There are more than 50 trace elements in the human body. Examples of trace elements include cobalt, iodine, zinc, manganese, and copper. These trace elements may be relatively negligible compared with the major elements such as sodium, but they are nevertheless important to the physiology of the human body.

For example, iodine is important to the function of the thyroid. Insufficient amounts of the trace element iodine can lead to a medical condition called hypothyroidism, or goit. This condition is rarely seen in the United States because iodine has been added to regular table salt, thereby ensuring that this important trace element is in the diet. Table 2-2 summarizes the normal levels of cations and anions in the body.

Occasionally an EMS provider must administer an electrolyte to a patient. Typically, when a medication is administered to a patient it is measured in weight, usually milligrams (mg), before it is given. That is in part because the medication did not previously exist in the body and a therapeutic level of the medication is desired—that is, so many milligrams per liter of blood.

In the case of electrolytes, the medication is measured in milliequivalents (mEq). That is because electrolytes already exist in the body and the *power* of the electrolyte is being increased. The goal of these efforts is to achieve a balance among the electrolytes. Yet individual electrolytes are not equal in power.

To make the administration of electrolytes easier and more accurate, the unit *milliequivalents* was created. One milliequivalent of *any* electrolyte can combine with 1 milligram of hydrogen. On this basis, all electrolyte amounts to be administered can be standardized.

For example, 1 gram of sodium may not equal 1 gram of chloride in combining power. Yet 1 milliequivalent of sodium does equal 1 milliequivalent of chloride in combining power. The balance of electrolytes, particularly sodium and potassium, is important for homeostatis, and occasionally electrolytes must be furnished to help maintain that balance.

The ability to record electric charges within the tissue are invaluable for diagnostic tools such as an electrocardiogram, which measures the electrical conduction of the heart.

TYPES OF COMPOUNDS

The various elements can combine to form a great number of compounds. All known compounds, whether natural or synthetic, can be classified into two groups: inorganic compounds and organic compounds.

Inorganic Compounds

Inorganic compounds are made of molecules that do not contain the element carbon (C). A few exceptions are carbon dioxide (CO_2) and calcium carbonate ($CaCO_3$). Water is an inorganic compound and makes up 55% to 65% of body weight. Water is the most important inorganic compound to living organisms.

Organic Compounds

Organic compounds are compounds found in living things and the products they make. These compounds always contain the element carbon combined with hydrogen and other elements. Carbon has the ability to combine with other carbons and other elements to form a large number of organic compounds. There are more than a million known organic compounds. Their molecules are comparatively large and very complex. By comparison, inorganic molecules are much smaller. There are four main groups of organic compounds: carbohydrates, lipids, proteins, and nucleic acids.

CARBOHYDRATES

All carbohydrates are compounds composed of the elements carbon (C), hydrogen (H), and oxygen (O). These compounds have twice as many hydrogen as oxygen and carbon atoms. Carbohydrates are divided into three groups. They are the monosaccharides, disaccharides, and polysaccharides.

Monosaccharides

Monosaccharides (from the Greek words *mono*, meaning "one", and *sakcharon*, meaning "sugar") are sugars that cannot be broken down any further. Hence they are also called

TABLE 2-2 *Normal, Elevated, and Depressed Cation and Anion Levels*

ELEMENT	SYMBOL	RANGE	CAUSES	SYMPTOMS
Potassium	K+	Normal 3.5–5.0 mEq/L Elevated	Massive cell damage • Burns • Crush injury Hemorrhagic shock Addison's disease	Malaise Nausea Intestinal colic Diarrhea Flaccid paralysis
		Depressed	Loss of body fluids • Prolonged vomiting • Prolonged diarrhea • Profuse sweating Congestive heart failure Adrenal disorders	Muscle weakness Irregular pulse Hypotension Abdominal distention
Sodium	Na+	Normal 135–145 mEq/L Elevated	Loss of body fluids • Prolonged vomiting • Prolonged diarrhea • Profuse sweating Diabetes Hyperaldosteronism	Thirst Dry tongue Flushed skin Oliguria
		Depressed	Water intoxication • Stroke • Renal failure • Liver cirrhosis Salt loss • Burns • Diarrhea • Prolonged vomiting • Renal disorders SIADH	Confusion Clouded sensorium Convulsions Coma Hypotension
Calcium	Ca+	Normal 8.8–10.5 mg/100ml Elevated	Vitamin D overdose Antacid abuse Hyperparathyroidism Paget's disease	Lethargy Nausea Constipation Coma
		Depressed	Vitamin D deficiency Magnesium deficiency Hypoparathyroidism Chronic laxative use Kidney dialysis	Perioral numbness Carpopedal spasm Tetany Convulsions
Magnesium	Mg+	Normal 1.5–2.5 mEq/L Elevated	Self-medication • Milk of magnesia • Epsom salts • Antacids	Lethargy Flushed Hypotension Paralysis
		Depressed	Impaired absorption • Malabsorption syndrome • Bowel resection Excessive renal loss • Alcoholism -• Diuretics Aldosteronism	Insomnia Muscle weakness Tremors Tetany

single, or simple, sugars. The types of monosaccharide sugars are glucose, fructose, galactose, ribose, and deoxyribose.

Glucose is an important sugar. It is the main source of energy in cells. Glucose, sometimes referred to as blood sugar, is carried by the bloodstream to individual cells, and is stored in the form of **glycogen** in the liver and muscle cells. Glucose combines with oxygen in a chemical reaction called oxidation that produces energy.

Fructose is the sweetest of the monosaccharides and is found in fruit and honey. Deoxyribose sugar is found in deoxyribonucleic acid and ribose sugar is found in ribonucleic acid.

Disaccharides

A **disaccharide** is known as a double sugar because it is formed from two monosaccharide molecules by a chemical reaction called dehydration synthesis. Dehydration synthesis involves the synthesis of a large molecule from small ones by the loss of a molecule of water. Table 2-3 illustrates the process of dehydration synthesis. Examples of disaccharides are sucrose (table sugar), maltose (malt sugar), and lactose (milk sugar).

The opposite reaction to dehydration synthesis is hydrolysis. In this reaction a large molecule is broken down into smaller molecules by the addition of water.

Disaccharides must be broken down by the process of digestion to monosaccharides to be absorbed and used by the body.

Polysaccharides

A large number of carbohydrates found in or made by living organisms and microbes are polysaccharides. **Polysaccharides** are large, complex molecules made up of hundreds to thousands of glucose molecules bonded together in one long chainlike molecule. Examples of polysaccharides are starch, cellulose, and glycogen. Under the proper conditions, polysaccharides can be broken down into disaccharides and then finally into monosaccharides. Starch is a polysaccharide found in grain products and root vegetables such as potatoes. Cellulose is the main structural component of plant tissue.

● LIPIDS

Lipids are molecules containing the elements carbon, hydrogen, and oxygen. Lipids are different from carbohydrates because there is proportionately much less oxygen in relation to hydrogen. Examples of lipids are fats, phospholipids, and steroids.

Characteristics of Lipids

Everywhere you look today you see the words "no fat," and yet lipids or fats are essential to health. Lipids are an important source of stored energy. They make up the essential steroid hormones and help to insulate our bodies. It is when the intake of lipids in the form of fat becomes excessive that a health problem may occur.

Fats (**triglycerides**) are made up of glycerol and fatty acids. This type of lipid is the most abundant in the body.

Phospholipids are lipids that contain carbon, hydrogen, oxygen, and phosphorus. This type of lipid may be found in the cell membranes, the brain, and the nervous tissue.

Steroids are the lipids that contain **cholesterol**. Cholesterol is essential in the structure of

TABLE 2-3 *The Monosaccharide Composition of Sucrose, Maltose, and Lactose*

MONOSACCHARIDE + MONOSACCHARIDE − H_2O (DEHYDRATION SYNTHESIS)	FORMS	DISACCHARIDE
Glucose + Fructose − H_2O	$\longrightarrow$	Sucrose
Glucose + Glucose − H_2O	$\longrightarrow$	Maltose
Glucose + Galactose − H_2O	$\longrightarrow$	Lactose

the semipermeable membrane of the cell. It is necessary in the manufacture of vitamin D and in the production of male and female hormones. Cholesterol is needed to make the adrenal hormone cortisol. However, in certain people, cholesterol can accumulate in the arteries, becoming a problem. The most common food sources of cholesterol are meat, eggs, and cheese. Yet even without these food sources, the liver still manufactures cholesterol.

PROTEINS

Proteins are organic compounds containing the elements carbon, hydrogen, oxygen, nitrogen, and, usually, phosphorus and sulfur. Proteins are among the most diverse and essential organic compounds found in all living organisms. Proteins are found in every part of a living cell, and are also an important part of the outer protein coat of all viruses. Proteins also serve as binding and structural components of all living things. For example, large amounts of protein are found in fingernails, hair, cartilage, ligaments, tendons, and muscle.

The small molecular units that make up the very large protein molecules are called **amino acids**. There are 22 different amino acids that can be combined in any number and sequence to make up the various kinds of proteins.

Table 2-4 gives a list of the nine essential amino acids. Essential amino acids must be ingested because they cannot be made by the body.

Large protein molecules are constructed from any number and sequence of these amino

TABLE 2-4 *The Nine Essential Amino Acids*

ESSENTIAL AMINO ACIDS	SYMBOL
Histidine	His
Isoleucine	Ileu
Leucine	Leu
Lysine	Lys
Methionine	Met
Phenylalanine	Phe
Threonine	Trp
Tryptophan	Try
Valine	Val

acids. The number of amino acids in any given protein molecule can number from 300 to several thousand. Therefore the structure of proteins is quite complicated.

ENZYMES

Enzymes are specialized protein molecules that are found in all living cells. They help to finely control the various chemical reactions occurring in a cell, so each reaction occurs at just the right moment and at the right speed. Enzymes help provide energy for the cell, assist in the making of new cell parts, and control almost every process in a cell. Because enzymes are capable of such activity, they are known as **organic catalysts**. An enzyme or organic catalyst affects the rate or speed of a chemical reaction without itself being changed. Enzymes can also be used over and over again. An enzyme molecule is highly specific in its action. Enzymes are made up of all protein or part protein (**apoenzyme**) attached to a nonprotein part (**coenzyme**). The name of an enzyme usually ends in *-ase*.

NUCLEIC ACIDS

Nucleic acids are important organic compounds containing the elements carbon, oxygen, hydrogen, nitrogen, and phosphorus. There are two major types of nucleic acids: **deoxyribonucleic acid (DNA)** and **ribonucleic acid (RNA)**.

Structure of Nucleic Acids

Nucleic acids are the largest known organic molecules. They are very high molecular weight polymers made from thousands of smaller, repeating subunits called nucleotides. A nucleotide is a complex molecule composed of three different molecular groups. Figure 2-2 shows a typical nucleotide. Group 1 is a phosphate or phosphoric acid group, H_3PO_4, whereas group 2 represents a five-carbon sugar. Depending on the nucleotide, the sugar could be either a ribose or a deoxyribose sugar. Finally, group 3 represents a

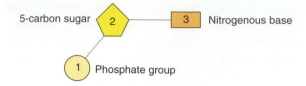

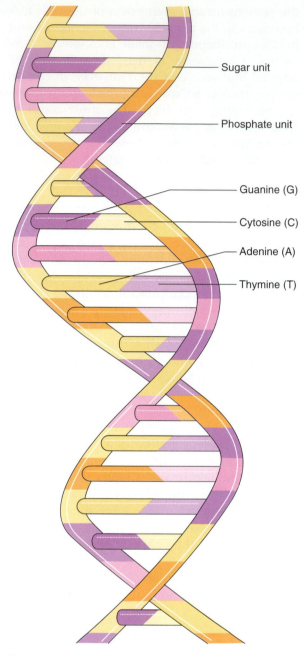

5-carbon sugar — 2

Nitrogenous base — 3

Phosphate group — 1

● **FIGURE 2–2** *Structure of a typical nucleotide.*

nitrogenous base. There are two groups of nitrogenous bases: purines and pyrimidines. The purines are either adenine (A) or guanine (G), whereas the pyrimidines are cytosine (C) and thymine (T).

DNA Structure and Function

DNA is involved in the process of heredity. The nucleus of every human cell contains 46 (23 pairs of) chromosomes, which is a long, coiled molecule of DNA. The chromosomes contain about 100,000 genes. This genetic information tells a cell what structure it will possess and what function it will have. The DNA molecule passes on this genetic information from one generation to the next.

DNA is a double-stranded molecule referred to as a double helix. This structure resembles a twisted ladder. The sides of the ladder are formed by alternating bands of a sugar (deoxyribose) unit and a phosphate unit. The rungs of the ladder are formed by the nitrogenous bases, which always pair in specific ways: thymine pairs with adenine, and cytosine pairs with guanine, Figure 2-3.

RNA Structure and Function

The RNA nucleotide consists of a phosphate group, the ribose sugar, and any one of the following nitrogenous bases: adenine, cytosine, guanine, and uracil instead of thymine. The RNA molecule is a single-stranded molecule, whereas the DNA molecule is a double-stranded molecule.

There are three different types of RNA in a cell: the messenger RNA (m-RNA), the transfer RNA (t-RNA), and the ribosomal

Sugar unit

Phosphate unit

Guanine (G)

Cytosine (C)

Adenine (A)

Thymine (T)

● **FIGURE 2–3** *Schematic of DNA.*

RNA (r-RNA). Messenger RNA carries the instructions for protein synthesis from the DNA molecule located in the nucleus of a cell to the ribosomes in the cytoplasm. The transfer RNA molecule picks up amino acid molecules in the cytoplasm and transfers

TABLE 2-5 *Differences between DNA and RNA Molecules*

TYPE OF NUCLEIC ACID	TYPE OF SUGAR PRESENT	TYPES OF BASES PRESENT	PHOSPHATE GROUP	LOCATION	NUMBER OF STRANDS PRESENT
DNA	Deoxyribose	A, T, G, C	Same as RNA	Cell nucleus, chromosomes	2
RNA	Ribose	A, U, G, C	Same as DNA	Cytoplasm, nucleoli, ribosomes	1

them to the ribosomes, where they are put together to form proteins. The ribosomal RNA helps in the attachment of the m-RNA to the ribosome. Table 2-5 shows the basic differences between the DNA molecule and the RNA molecule.

FLUIDS

Body fluid is made up primarily of water. Sometimes referred to as the "sea within," body fluid accounts for about 60% of an adult's total body weight and up to 80% of an infant's total body weight.

For purposes of discussion, body fluid is divided into two compartments: fluid inside the cell, or **intracellular fluid**, and fluid outside the cell, **extracellular fluid**. Intracellular fluid accounts for about two thirds of the body's fluids, or 25 L in the average 150-pound (70-kg) male.

The remaining one third of body fluid, extracellular fluid, is further divided into two groups. The first fluid group that bathes the cells is called the **interstitial fluid**. Interstitial fluid accounts for about 15% of the total body weight. The remaining fluid is in the intravascular (within the blood) space, which is primarily plasma in the blood.

The average person has 5 to 7 L of blood in his or her system. Loss of as little as 10%, or 4 L, can be devastating despite the presence of another 21 L of fluid in the body. That is in part because the fluids in the body are kept

in their individual compartments by special **selectively permeable membranes**. Movement of fluids between these compartments is closely controlled by several processes described in more detail in the next chapter.

ACIDS, BASES, AND SALTS

Before ending the discussion of basic chemistry and biochemistry, a brief discussion of acids, bases, salts, and pH is essential.

Many inorganic and organic compounds found in living organisms are ones that we use in our daily lives. They can be classified into one of three groups: acids, bases, and salts. We are familiar with the sour taste of citrus fruits (grapefruits, lemons, and limes) and vinegar. The sour taste is due to the presence of compounds called acids. What characteristics do acids have to set them apart from the bases and salts?

Acids

An **acid** is a substance that, when dissolved in water, will **ionize** into positively charged hydronium ions (H_3O^+) or hydrogen ions (H^+) and negatively charged ions of some other element. Basically, an acid is a substance that yields hydronium ions (H_3O^+) in solution. For example, hydrogen chloride (HCl) in pure form is a gas. But when bubbled into water, it becomes hydrochloric acid. How does this happen? Simply. In a water solution, hydrogen chloride ionizes into one hydronium ion and one negatively charged chloride ion.

$$HCl + H_2O \longrightarrow H_3O^+ + Cl^-$$

Hydrogen $\longrightarrow$ Hydronium + Chloride
chloride in   ion   ion
solution

It is the presence of the hydronium ions that gives hydrochloric acid its acidity and sour taste. (However, one should *not* taste any substance to identify it as an acid. There are other more reliable and safer methods for the identification of an acid.) A substance can be tested for its acidity through the use of specially treated paper called litmus paper. In the presence of an acid, blue litmus paper turns red. Table 2-6 gives the name of some common acids, their formulas, and where they are found or how they are used.

Bases

A **base** or **alkali** is a substance that, when dissolved in water, ionizes into negatively charged **hydroxide** (OH^-) ions and positively charged ions of a metal. For example, sodium hydroxide (NaOH) ionizes into one sodium ion (Na^+) and one hydroxide ion (OH^-). The reaction can be shown as follows:

$$NaOH \longrightarrow Na^+ + OH^-$$

Sodium hydroxide $\longrightarrow$ Sodium + Hydroxide
in solution   ion   ion

Bases have a bitter taste and feel slippery between the fingers. They turn red litmus paper blue. Table 2-7 gives the names of some common bases, their formulas, and location or use.

Neutralization and Salts

When an acid and a base are combined, they form a salt and water. This type of reaction is called a **neutralization**, or exchange reaction. In a neutralization reaction, hydrogen ions (H^+) from the acid and hydroxide ions (OH^-) from the base join to form water. At the same time, the negative ions of the acid combine with the positive ions of the base to form a compound called a **salt**. For example, hydrochloric acid and sodium hydroxide combine to form sodium chloride and water. The hydrogen ions from the acid unite with the hydroxide ions from the base to form water. The sodium ions (Na^+) combine with the chloride

TABLE 2-6 *Names, Formulas, Location, and Uses of Some Common Acids*

NAME OF ACID	FORMULA	WHERE FOUND OR USAGE
Acetic acid	CH_3COOH	Found in vinegar
Boric acid	H_3BO_3	Used as weak eyewash
Carbonic acid	H_2CO_3	Found in carbonated beverages
Hydrochloric acid	HCl	Found in stomach
Nitric acid	HNO_3	Used as industrial oxidizing acid
Sulfuric acid	H_2SO_4	Found in batteries and industrial mineral acid

TABLE 2-7 *Names, Formulas, and Locations of Some Common Bases*

NAME OF BASE	FORMULA	WHERE FOUND
Ammonium hydroxide	NH_4OH	Household liquid cleaners
Magnesium hydroxide	$Mg(OH)_2$	Milk of magnesia
Potassium hydroxide	KOH	Caustic potash
Sodium hydroxide	NaOH	Lye

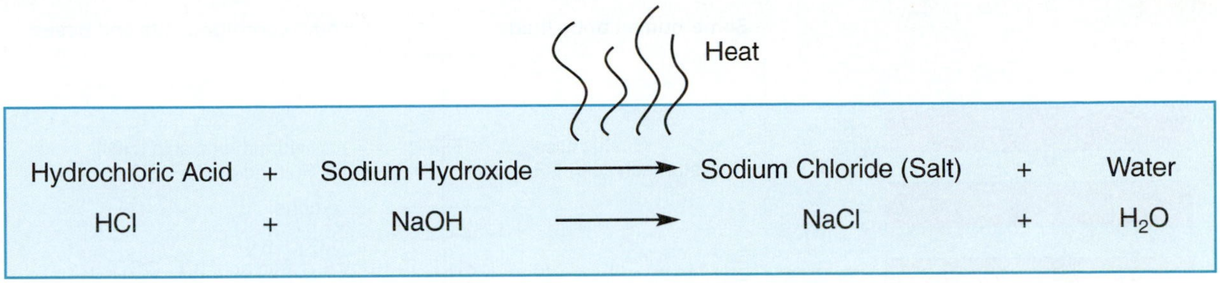

Heat

Hydrochloric Acid	+	Sodium Hydroxide	$\longrightarrow$	Sodium Chloride (Salt)	+	Water
HCl	+	NaOH	$\longrightarrow$	NaCl	+	H_2O

● **FIGURE 2–4** *The neutralization reaction or exchange reaction.*

ions (Cl^-) to form sodium chloride (NaCl). When the water evaporates, solid salt remains. The neutralization reaction is written as shown in Figure 2-4.

● THE pH SCALE

pH is a measure of the acidity or alkalinity (basicity) of a solution. Special pH meters determine the hydrogen or hydroxide ion concentration of a solution on the **pH scale**. The pH scale, which is used to measure the acidity or alkalinity of a solution, ranges from 0 to 14. A pH of 7 indicates that a particular solution has the same number of hydrogen ions as hydroxide ions. This is a neutral pH, and distilled water is neutral with a pH value of 7.0. Any pH value between 0 and 6.9 indicates an acidic solution. The lower the pH number, the stronger the acid or higher hydrogen ion concentration. Any pH value between 7.1 and 14.0 means a solution is basic or alkaline. Thus the greater the number above 7.0, the stronger the base or greater hydroxide ion concentration.

Figure 2-5 shows the pH values of some common acids, bases, and human body fluids. It also shows the color changes that occur on a pH strip.

Acid-Base Balance

For the body's catalysts, especially enzymes, to work, the pH of the body's fluids must be kept nearly neutral, within a pH range of 7.35 to 7.45. Any acids produced by the cells must be neutralized and the acid-base balance restored or serious derangement in bodily functions can occur.

All the body's fluids contain chemicals called **buffers**. Buffers chemically combine with acids and neutralize them. Important buffers in the body include phosphate and blood protein buffers. However, the most important extracellular buffer is **bicarbonate**.

Bicarbonate interacts with the carbon dioxide, created within the cells, to create a weak acid called carbonic acid. This chemical reaction is almost immediate.

STREET SMART

Although an acid can be neutralized with a base, heat is the by-product of that reaction. In cases in which a strong acid or a strong base is spilled on someone, dilution with large amounts of water is in order. Use of the acid or base as an antidote can lead to more serious thermo-chemical burns. ■

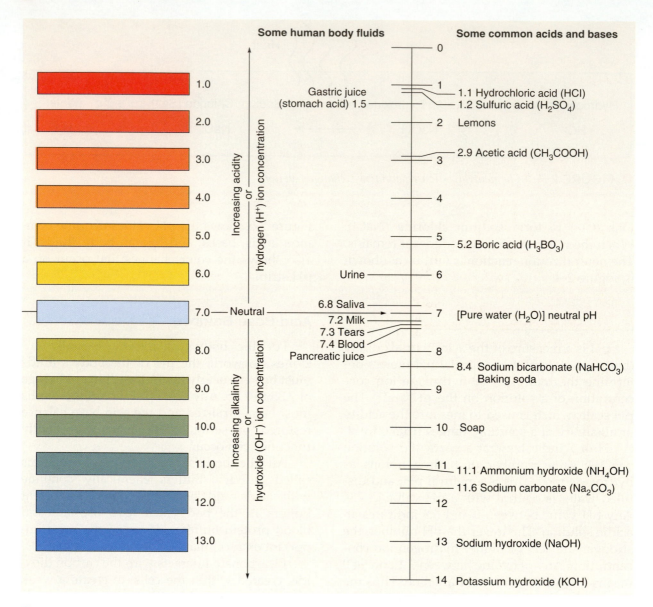

Some human body fluids

Some common acids and bases

Increasing acidity or hydrogen (H^+) ion concentration

Increasing alkalinity or hydroxide (OH^-) ion concentration

- 0
- 1 — 1.1 Hydrochloric acid (HCl)
- Gastric juice (stomach acid) 1.5 — 1.2 Sulfuric acid (H_2SO_4)
- 2 Lemons
- 2.9 Acetic acid (CH_3COOH) — 3
- 4
- 5 — 5.2 Boric acid (H_3BO_3)
- Urine — 6
- 6.8 Saliva — 7 [Pure water (H_2O)] neutral pH
- 7.0 — Neutral
- 7.2 Milk
- 7.3 Tears
- 7.4 Blood
- Pancreatic juice — 8 — 8.4 Sodium bicarbonate ($NaHCO_3$) Baking soda
- 9
- 10 Soap
- 11 — 11.1 Ammonium hydroxide (NH_4OH) — 11.6 Sodium carbonate (Na_2CO_3)
- 12
- 13 Sodium hydroxide (NaOH)
- 14 Potassium hydroxide (KOH)

● FIGURE 2–5 *pH values of some common acids, bases, and human body fluids.*

The carbonic acid is then carried to the lungs, where it is broken down into carbon dioxide to be expelled on expiration, and thus the blood is returned to a normal pH.

Acid-Base Regulation

The acid-base balance is regulated by the respiratory system first and then by the renal system. These two systems interact in an attempt to maintain a nearly neutral pH in the body fluids.

The respiratory system reacts to an increased amount of acid, an increase in acid load, by increasing its rate of ventilation. This in turn causes more carbon dioxide to be exhaled and thus lowers the carbonic acid level. If the increased ventilation rate successfully returns the blood to a normal pH, it is called **respiratory compensation**.

If for some reason the lungs cannot compensate, the kidneys start to withhold more bicarbonate by reabsorbing sodium, which is bound to bicarbonate as sodium bicarbonate.

The kidneys also work by excreting hydrogen ions (acid), primarily from carbonic acid, and other metabolic acids, such as uric acid and keto acids, that form in the body. It takes up to 24 hours for the kidneys to work as a compensatory mechanism, **renal compensation**, in the acid-base balance system.

Acid-Base Imbalance

The amount of acid in the blood largely controls the cells' metabolic functions. An increase (**acidosis**) or decrease (**alkalosis**) of acid in the blood can decrease brain function, alter breathing, cause diarrhea, and even induce a coma.

Acid-base imbalances can usually be traced to problems of either the kidneys or lungs being overwhelmed or failing to function properly. If the problem is not corrected (i.e., compensation does not occur), serious complications will ensue.

Acidosis

The most common acid-base problem is acidosis. Respiratory acidosis can occur because of either problems with the control of ventilation or by failure of the lungs themselves.

Ventilation is controlled in the brain and central nervous system. A severe head injury can cause respiratory depression and hypoventilation, allowing carbon dioxide in the form of carbonic acid to build, leading to respiratory acidosis. A traumatic injury to the cervical spinal cord can sever the phrenic nerve. The phrenic nerve controls the diaphragm, the main muscle of breathing. Without the diaphragm the patient cannot breathe and will become apneic; eventually acidosis will occur.

Certain infections, like polio, affect the nervous system and can also cause paralysis of the diaphragm. Hypoventilation, or apnea, prevents carbon dioxide from being expired and leads to acidosis.

Ingestion of drugs that depress the central nervous system, especially narcotics, can also lead to respiratory depression. The resulting hypoventilation quickly causes respiratory acidosis.

Any blockage or destruction of the lungs prevents exhalation and creates a buildup of carbonic acid. Examples of pulmonary complications that can lead to acidosis include upper airway obstructions, infections such as pneumonia, and swelling of capillary beds surrounding the airways, called pulmonary edema.

One of the most common causes of respiratory failure and acidosis is chronic obstructive pulmonary disease, such as asthma and emphysema. These diseases can plug the airways, preventing exhalation or proper exchange of gases, including carbon dioxide, in the lungs.

Certain diseases can also cause an overproduction of acid, resulting in an acid load that overwhelms the capacity of the acid-base system. Diabetes is one such disease. In diabetes the body's production of insulin, a hormone necessary for carbohydrate metabolism, is either absent or diminished. As a result the body turns to alternative sources for energy such as fat. When fat is metabolized it creates a ketone acid. These acids build up and create a condition called diabetic ketoacidosis.

Some diseases, particularly infections, can cause prolonged diarrhea. Diarrhea, the rapid passage of foodstuffs through the intestinal tract, carries out with it bicarbonate. Unable to absorb bicarbonate from the digestive system, levels of bicarbonate drop in the bloodstream despite the efforts of the kidneys to reabsorb and preserve bicarbonate. The result is an inability of the body to use bicarbonate to balance its normal acid levels.

The intentional or accidental overdose of drugs such as aspirin can also lead to acidosis. Aspirin is an acid, and large amounts of aspirin increase the body's acid load, overwhelming compensatory mechanisms.

The symptoms of acidosis are similar regardless of the mechanism of the acidosis. The brain, being sensitive to acid levels, is often first affected. The patient may complain of headache and may eventually fall into a stupor or coma. The respiratory system, in an attempt to compensate, ventilates faster or deeper. This breathing pattern is called Kussmaul's respiration. Certain acids, like ketones, are aromatic, meaning they will evaporate into the breath.

Diabetic patients in ketoacidosis can have a fruity smell to their breath as a result of keto acids.

Alkalosis

The counterpart to acidosis is alkalosis. Alkalosis is either the result of too much bicarbonate to neutralize acid or loss of large quantities of acids from the body. All causes of alkalosis can be traced to one of these two mechanisms.

Just as there can be respiratory acidosis from inadequate breathing (hypoventilation), there can be respiratory alkalosis from over-breathing (hyperventilation).

There are numerous causes of hyperventilation. The most commonly recognized form of hyperventilation is hysterical hyperventilation. This is when a person becomes excited or experiences a panic attack and starts to breathe rapidly. The resulting constellation of symptoms includes numbness around the lips (peiroral paresthesia) and spasms of the hands (carpopedal spasm); both symptoms are due to transient hypocalcemia, discussed earlier in the chapter.

However, there are a number of medical reasons for hyperventilation. For example, exposure to high elevations, such as in the Rocky Mountains, or flying in a depressurized plane at high altitudes can lead to hyperventilation caused by lower oxygen concentrations. Mild hypoxia occurs, the person hyperventilates to compensate, and the result is respiratory alkalosis.

The complement to respiratory alkalosis is metabolic alkalosis. Metabolic alkalosis can be caused by an excessive loss of acid or a gain of too much buffer like bicarbonate.

Acid can be found in the stomach as hydrochloric acid. Excessive vomiting or excessive gastric suctioning, through a nasogastric tube, causes a loss of hydrochloric acid, leading to metabolic alkalosis.

Conversely, the ingestion of large quantities of bicarbonate can lead to elevated bicarbonate levels. Alka-seltzer is a bicarbonate-based medication used to treat ulcers. Too much Alka-seltzer can lead to metabolic alkalosis.

A clue to a person's acid-base balance lies in the potassium level. When the patient's acid levels drop in the blood, the body attempts to compensate by releasing acid (H+) from the cells to the blood in exchange for potassium (K+). The result is that the patient's blood becomes hypokalemic. Therefore some of the symptoms of alkalosis are directly related to the hypokalemia that occurs. The symptoms of hypokalemia were discussed earlier in the chapter.

The symptoms of metabolic alkalosis include nausea, vomiting, and diarrhea. Unfortunately, these symptoms only worsen the situation. Vomiting causes a loss of more acid from the stomach, and diarrhea prevents the lower intestinal tract from absorbing bicarbonate.

A key physical finding suggesting alkalosis is hypoventilation. Hypoventilation is the body's means of trying to conserve acid in the form of carbonic acid.

A state of homeostasis is required for the body to function at an optimum level of health. If a control system like the acid-base or electrolyte balance is not maintained, cells and tissue will become damaged. A moderate dysfunction causes illness; a severe dysfunction causes death.

● REVIEW QUESTIONS

Select the letter of the choice that best completes the statement.

1. A substance that has weight and occupies space is called:
   a. kinetic energy
   b. catalyst
   c. matter
   d. potential energy

2. Walking is an example of:
    a. a catalyst
    b. kinetic energy
    c. matter
    d. potential energy

3. Water is classified as:
    a. an atom
    b. an element
    c. a mineral
    d. a compound

4. A monosaccharide sugar is:
    a. sucrose
    b. cellulose
    c. maltose
    d. glucose

5. Sugar stored in the liver and muscle cells for energy is called:
    a. glucose
    b. glycogen
    c. fructose
    d. ribose

6. A chemical reaction in the cell is affected by:
    a. enzymes
    b. organic compounds
    c. nucleic acids
    d. energy

7. The strongest acid is found in the stomach. It is:
    a. sulfuric
    b. acetic
    c. hydrochloric
    d. nitric

8. A compound with a pH of 8.4 is alkaline and it is:
    a. milk of magnesia
    b. baking soda
    c. ammonia
    d. lye

9. When proper amounts of an acid and base are combined, the products formed are a salt and:
    a. gas
    b. water
    c. another base
    d. another acid

10. The name given to the atomic particle that is found outside the nucleus of an atom is:
    a. proton
    b. neutron
    c. electron
    d. ion

● MATCHING

Match each term in Column A with its correct description in Column B.

Column A	Column B
_____ 1. glucose	a. fluid within the cell
_____ 2. electrolyte	b. double sugar
_____ 3. intracellular	c. triglycerides
_____ 4. disaccharides	d. chromosomes
_____ 5. HCL	e. conducts an electrical charge in a solution
_____ 6. steroid	f. blood sugar
_____ 7. energy	g. positively or negatively charged particle of an atom
_____ 8. ion	h. ability to do work
_____ 9. DNA	i. cholesterol
_____ 10. fats	j. found in the stomach

● APPLYING THEORY TO PRACTICE

1. Read the label on a loaf of bread and state why the bread can be advertised as "no cholesterol."

2. Compare the fat content in one slice of pizza, a fast food quarter-pound hamburger, a serving of ice cream, and a serving of yogurt.

3. Should DNA identification be required at birth? Have a panel discussion on the "ethics" of DNA testing as part of a pre-employment physical.

Cells

3

Objectives

- Identify the structure of a typical cell
- Define the function of each component of a typical cell
- Relate the function of cells to the function of the body
- Describe the processes that transport materials in and out of a cell
- Describe what a tumor is and define *cancer*
- Define the key words that relate to this chapter

Key Words

0.9% sodium chloride (0.9 NaCl)
3% sodium chloride
5% dextrose in sterile water (D_5W)
action potential
active transport
adenosine triphosphate (ATP)
benign
blood volume expander
cancer
cell
cell membrane
centriole
centrosome
chromatin
chromosome
cytoplasm
cytoskeleton
diffusion
endoplasmic reticulum (smooth and rough)
equilibrium
filtration
Golgi apparatus
hemorrhaging
hyperglycemic
hypertonic solution
hypotonic solution
isotonic solution
keto acid
lactated Ringer's (LR) solution
lysosome
malignant
meiosis
metastases
mitochondria
mitosis
neoplasm
nephrons
normal saline
nuclear membrane
nucleolus
nucleoplasm
nucleus
organelle
osmosis
osmotic pressure

(continues)

Key Words (continued)

perioxisome	sodium-potassium
phagocytosis	pump
pinocytic vesicle	solutes
pinocytosis	somatic cell
protein synthesis	spilling sugar
ribosome	tumor
Ringer's solution	vacuole
selectively permeable	wart (papilloma)
(semipermeable)	
membrane	

TABLE 3-1 *Units of Length in the Metric System*

1 meter = 39.37 inches
1 centimeter (cm) = 1/100 or 0.01 meters
1 millimeter (mm) = 1/1000 or 0.001 meters
1 micrometer (μm) or micron (μ) = 1/1,000,000 or 0.000001 meters
1 nanometer (nm) = 1/1,000,000,000 or 0.000000001 meters
1 angstrom (Å) = 1/10,000,000,000 or 0.0000000001 meters

When a field of grass is seen from a distance it looks just like a solid green carpet. Closer observation, however, shows that it is not a solid mass but is made up of countless separate blades of grass. So it is with the body of a plant or animal; it seems to be a single entity, but when any portion is examined under a microscope it is found to be made up of many small, discrete parts. These tiny parts, or units, are called cells. (NOTE: These units were first discovered in the 1600s by Robert Hook. When examining a piece of cork under a crude microscope, the units reminded him of a monk's room, which was called a cell). All living things, whether plant or animal, unicellular or multicellular, large or small, are composed of cells. A cell is microscopic in size. *The cell is the basic unit of structure and function of all living things.*

Because cells are microscopic, a special unit of measurement is employed to determine their size. This is the micrometer (μm) or micron (μ). It is used to describe both the size of cells and their cellular components, Table 3-1.

To better understand the structure of a cell, let us compare a living entity—such as a human being—with a house. The many individual cells of this living organism are comparable with the many rooms of a house. Just as each room is bounded by four walls, floor, and ceiling, a cell is bounded by a specialized cell membrane with many openings. Cells, like rooms, come in a variety of shapes and sizes. Every kind of room or cell has its own unique function. A house can be made up of a single room or many. In much the same fashion, a living thing can be made up of only one cell (unicellular) or many cells (multicellular).

Basic and *typical* are terms used to identify structures common to most living cells.

CELL MEMBRANE

Every cell is surrounded by a cell membrane. It is sometimes called a plasma membrane. The cell membrane separates the cell's cytoplasm from its external environment and from the neighboring cells. It also regulates the passage or transport of certain molecules into and out of the cell, while preventing the passage of others. This is why the cell membrane is often called a *selectively semipermeable membrane.* The cell membrane is made of protein and lipid (fatty substance) molecules arranged in a double layer. This arrangement is rather like a sandwich: the lipid molecules are the filling, and the two layers of protein molecules are the slices of bread.

NUCLEUS

The nucleus is the most important organelle within the cell. It has two vital functions: to control the activities of the cell and to facilitate cell division. This spherical organelle is usually located in or near the center of the cell. Various dyes or stains, like iodine, can be used to make the nucleus stand out. The nucleus stains vividly because it contains deoxyribonucleic acid (DNA) and protein. Both readily absorb stains. Surrounding the nucleus is the nuclear membrane.

The DNA and protein are arranged in a loose and diffuse state called chromatin. When the cell is ready to divide, the chromatin condenses to form short, rodlike structures called chromosomes. There is a specific number of chromosomes in the nucleus for each species. The number of chromosomes for the human being is 46, or 23 pairs.

When a cell reaches a certain size, it may divide to form two new cells. When this occurs, the nucleus divides first by a process called mitosis. During this process, the nuclear material is distributed to each of the two new nuclei. This is followed by division of the cytoplasm into two approximately equal parts through the formation of a new membrane between the two nuclei. It is only during the process of nuclear division that the chromosomes can be seen.

Chromosomes are important because they store the hereditary material—DNA—that is passed on from one generation of cells to the next.

Nuclear Membrane

The nuclear membrane, or nuclear envelope, is a double-layered membrane that has openings at regular intervals. Through these pores materials can pass from either the nucleus to the cytoplasm or from the cytoplasm to the nucleus. The outer layer of the nuclear membrane is continuous with the endoplasmic reticulum of the cytoplasm and may have small round projections on it called ribosomes. (A discussion of the ribosomes and endoplasmic reticulum follows.)

Nucleoplasm

The nucleoplasm is a clear, semifluid medium that fills the spaces around the chromatin and the nucleoli.

Nucleolus and the Ribosomes

Within the nucleus are one or more nucleoli. Each nucleolus is a small, round body, Figure 3-1. It contains ribosomes made up of ribonucleic acid and protein. The ribosomes can pass from the nucleus through the nuclear pores into the cytoplasm. There the ribosomes aid in protein synthesis. They may exist freely in the cytoplasm, be in clusters called polyribosomes, or be attached to the walls of the endoplasmic reticulum.

CYTOPLASM

The cytoplasm is a sticky semifluid material found between the nucleus and the cell membrane. Chemical analysis of the cytoplasm shows that it consists of proteins, lipids, carbohydrates, minerals, salts, and water (70% to 90%). Each of these substances, other than water, varies greatly from one cell to the next and from one organism to the next. The cytoplasm is the background for all the chemical reactions that take place in a cell, such as protein synthesis and cellular respiration. Molecules are transported around the cell by the circular motion of the cytoplasm. Embedded in the cytoplasm are organelles, structures that help a cell to function. Table 3-2 summarizes the organelles and their functions.

Centrosome and Centrioles

The centrioles are two cylindrical organelles found near the nucleus in a tiny round body called the centrosome. The centrioles are perpendicular to each other. Figure 3-1 shows two centrioles near the nucleus. During mitosis, or cell division, the two centrioles separate from each other. In the process of separation, thin cytoplasmic spindle fibers form between the two centrioles. This structure is called a spindle-fiber apparatus. The spindle fibers attach themselves to individual chromosomes to help in the even and equal distribution of these chromosomes to two daughter cells.

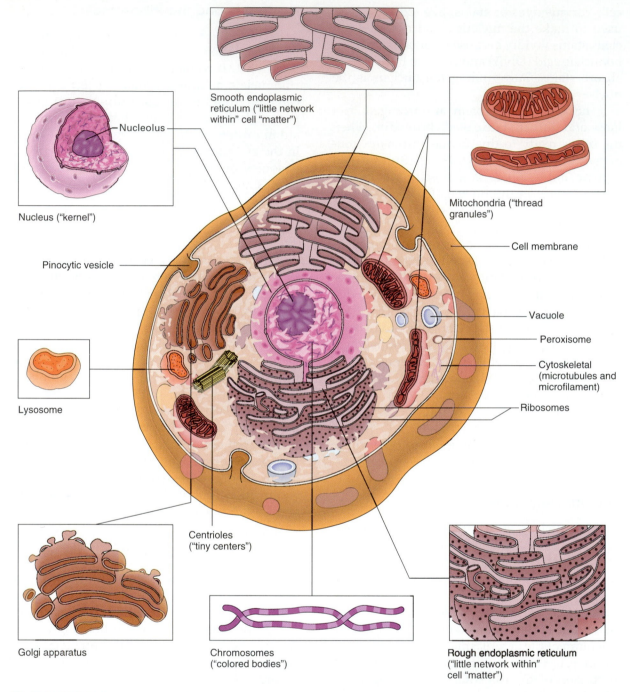

● **FIGURE 3–1**   *Structure of a typical animal cell.*

Endoplasmic Reticulum

Crisscrossing the cellular cytoplasm is a fine network of tubular structures called the **endoplasmic reticulum** (*reticulum* means "network"). Some of this endoplasmic reticulum connects the nuclear membrane to the cell membrane. Thus it serves as a channel for the transport of materials in and out of the nucleus. Sometimes the endoplasmic reticulum accumulates large masses of proteins and acts as a storage area.

TABLE 3-2 *Cell Organelles and their Functions*

ORGANELLE	FUNCTION
Cell membrane	Regulates transport of substances into and out of the cell.
Cytoplasm	Provides an organized watery environment in which life functions take place by the activities of the organelles contained in the cytoplasm.
Nucleus	Serves as the "brain" for the control of the cell's metabolic activities and cell division.
Nuclear membrane	Regulates transport of substances into and out of the nucleus.
Nucleoplasm	A clear, semifluid medium that fills the spaces around the chromatin and the nucleoli.
Nucleolus	Functions as a reservoir for ribonucleic acid (RNA).
Ribosomes	Serve as sites for protein synthesis.
Endoplasmic reticulum	Provides passages through which transport of substances occurs in cytoplasm.
Mitochondria	Serve as sites of cellular respiration and energy production; store ATP.
Golgi apparatus	Manufactures carbohydrates and packages secretions for discharge from the cell.
Lysosomes	Serve as centers for cellular digestion.
Peroxisomes	Contain enzymes that oxidize cell substances.
Centrosome	Contains two centrioles that are functional during animal cell division.
Cytoskeleton	Forms internal framework.

There are two types of endoplasmic reticulum: **rough** and **smooth**. Rough endoplasmic reticulum has ribosomes studding the outer membrane. The ribosomes are the sites for protein synthesis in the cell. The smooth endoplasmic reticulum has a role in cholesterol synthesis, fat metabolism, and detoxification of drugs.

Mitochondria

Most of the cell's energy comes from spherical or rod-shaped organelles called **mitochondria** (singular, mitochondrion; *mito* means "thread", *chondrion* means "granule"). These mitochondria vary in shape and number. There can be as few as a single one in each cell or as many as a thousand or more. Cells that need the most energy have the greatest number of mitochondria. Because they supply the cell's energy, mitochondria are also known as the "powerhouses" of the cell.

The mitochondria have a double-membraned structure that contains enzymes. These enzymes help to break down carbohydrates, fats, and protein molecules into energy to be stored in the cell as **adenosine triphosphate**, otherwise known as **ATP**. All living cells need ATP for their activities.

Golgi Apparatus

The **Golgi apparatus** is also called Golgi bodies or the Golgi complex. It is an arrangement of layers of membranes resembling a stack of pancakes. Scientists believe that this organelle synthesizes carbohydrates and combines them with protein molecules as they pass through the Golgi apparatus. In this way the Golgi apparatus stores and packages secretions for discharge from the cell. These organelles are abundant in the cells of gastric glands, salivary glands, and pancreatic glands.

Lysosomes

Lysosomes are oval or spherical bodies found in the cellular cytoplasm. They contain powerful enzymes that digest protein molecules. The lysosome thus helps to digest old, wornout cells; bacteria; and foreign matter. If a lysosome should rupture, as sometimes happens, it starts digesting the cell's proteins, causing it to die. For this reason lysosomes are also known as "suicide bags."

Perioxisomes

Membranous sacs that contain oxidase enzymes are called **perioxisomes**. These enzymes help to digest fats and detoxify harmful substances.

Cytoskeleton

The **cytoskeleton** is the internal framework of the cell; it is made up of microtubules, intermediate filaments, and microfilaments. The filaments provide support for the cells, and the microtubules are thought to aid in movement of substances through cytoplasm.

Pinocytic Vesicles

Large molecules such as protein and lipids, which cannot pass through the cell membrane, enter a cell by way of the pinocytic vesicles. The **pinocytic vesicles** form by the cell membranes folding inward to form a pocket. The edges of the pocket then close and pinch away from the cell membrane, forming a bubble or **vacuole** in the cytoplasm. This process by which a cell forms pinocytic vesicles to take in large molecules is called pinocytosis, or "cell drinking."

● CELL DIVISION

Both the growth and the maintenance of all the cells in the human body are achieved through cell division. Some human body cells (**somatic cells**) live only a short time, whereas others are subjected to continual "wear and tear" and are destroyed. The process of cell division or mitosis produces new cells. All cells do not reproduce at the same rate. Blood-forming cells of the bone marrow, the cells of the skin, and the cells of the intestinal tract reproduce continuously. Muscle cells only reproduce every few years; however, muscle tissue may be enlarged with exercise. Neurons, or nerve cells, essentially do not reproduce.

Mitosis

Cell division, or mitosis, is divided into two distinct processes: the first stage is the division of the nucleus, and the second stage is the division of the cytoplasm.

Mitosis essentially is an orderly series of steps by which the DNA in the nucleus of a cell is precisely and equally distributed to two daughter nuclei. The process of cell division of the sex cell, or gamete, is called **meiosis**. During meiosis, the ovum from the female and the spermatozoa from the male *reduce* their respective chromosomes to 23, or half the normal amount. When fertilization (the union of the ovum and sperm) occurs, the two cells combine to form a simple cell called the zygote, which then has the full set of 46 chromosomes, 23 from each parent, Figure 3-2.

● PROTEIN SYNTHESIS

Cells produce proteins that are essential to life, such as albumin or globulin, through a process called **protein synthesis**. Within each cell is the DNA that determines the kinds of proteins that are produced. The blueprint for each individual kind of protein is contained within a specific gene that resides in the DNA chain.

● MOVEMENT OF MATERIALS ACROSS CELL MEMBRANES

The cell membrane controls passage of substances into and out of the cell. This is important because a cell must be able to acquire materials from its surrounding medium, after which it either secretes synthesized substances or excretes wastes. The physical processes that control the passage of materials through the cell membrane are diffusion, osmosis, filtration, active transport, phagocytosis, and pinocytosis. Diffusion, osmosis, and filtration are passive processes, which means they do not need energy to function. Active transport, phagocytosis, and pinocytosis are active processes that do require energy.

Diffusion

Diffusion is a physical process in which molecules of gases, liquids, or solid particles spread or scatter themselves evenly through a

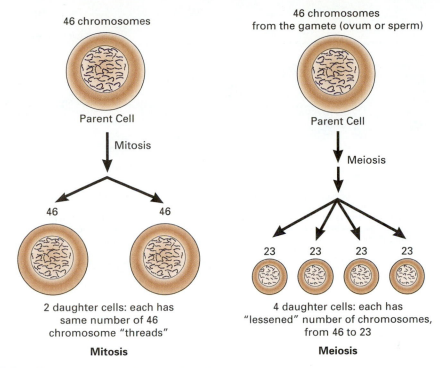

46 chromosomes

Parent Cell

Mitosis

46   46

2 daughter cells: each has
same number of 46
chromosome "threads"

Mitosis

46 chromosomes
from the gamete (ovum or sperm)

Parent Cell

Meiosis

23   23   23   23

4 daughter cells: each has
"lessened" number of chromosomes,
from 46 to 23

Meiosis

● **FIGURE 3–2**   *The processes of mitosis and meiosis.*

medium. When solid particles are dissolved within a fluid, they are known as solutes. Diffusion also applies to a slightly different process in which solutes and water pass across a membrane to distribute themselves evenly throughout the two fluids, which remain separated by the membrane. Generally, *molecules move from an area where they are greatly concentrated to an area where they are less concentrated.* The molecules eventually will distribute themselves evenly within the space available; when this happens, the molecules are said to be in a state of equilibrium, Figure 3-3.

The three common states of matter are gases, liquids, and solids. Molecules diffuse more quickly in gases and more slowly in solids. Diffusion occurs because of the heat energy of molecules. As a result, molecules are always in constant motion, except at absolute zero ($-273°$ C). In all cases, the movement of molecules increases with an increase in temperature.

A few familiar examples of the rates of diffusion may be helpful. For instance, if one thoroughly saturates a wad of cotton with ammonia and places it in a far corner of a room, the entire room will soon smell of ammonia. Air currents quickly carry the ammonia fumes throughout the room. Another test for diffusion is to place a pair of dye crystals on the bottom of a water-filled beaker. Eventually they will uniformly permeate and color the water. This diffusion process takes quite a while, especially if no one stirs, shakes, or heats the beaker. In still another test, a dye crystal placed on an ice cube moves even more slowly through the ice. Diffusion of the dye can be accelerated by melting the ice.

The diffusion rate of molecules in the various media (gas, liquid, and solid) depends on the distances between each molecule and how freely they can move. In a gas, molecules can move more freely and quickly; within a liquid, molecules are more tightly held together. In a solid substance, molecular movement is highly restricted and thus very slow.

Diffusion plays a vital role in permitting molecules to enter and leave a cell. Oxygen diffuses from the bloodstream, where it dwells in greater concentration. From the bloodstream,

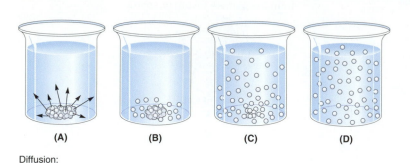

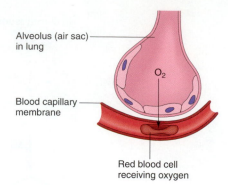

Diffusion:

(A) A small lump of sugar is placed into a beaker of water; its molecules dissolve and begin to diffuse outward. **(B & C)** The sugar molecules continue to diffuse through the water from an area of greater concentration to an area of lesser concentration. **(D)** Over a long period; the sugar molecules are evenly distributed throughout the water, reaching a state of equilibrium.

Example of diffusion in the human body: Oxygen diffuses from an alveolus in a lung where it is in greater concentration, across the blood capillary membrane, into a red blood cell where it is in lesser concentration.

⬤ **FIGURE 3–3** *The process of diffusion. The sugar molecules eventually reach a state of equilibrium.*

the oxygen enters the fluid surrounding a cell, then into the cell itself, where it is far less concentrated. In this manner the flow of blood through the lungs and bloodstream provides a continuous supply of oxygen to the cells. Once oxygen has entered a cell, it is used in metabolic activities.

Osmosis

Osmosis is the diffusion of water or any other *solvent* molecule through a selectively permeable membrane (like the cell membrane). A **selectively permeable (semipermeable) membrane** is any membrane through which some solutes can diffuse, but others cannot.

Sausage casing is a selectively permeable membrane that can be used as a substitute for a cell membrane. A solution of salt, sucrose (table sugar), and gelatin is placed into the sausage casing. This mixture is then suspended in a beaker filled with distilled water, Figure 3-4. The sausage casing is permeable to water and salt, but not to gelatin and sucrose. Thus only the water and salt molecules can pass through the casing. Eventually more salt molecules move out because the experiment began with a greater concentration of these molecules inside. At the same time, more water molecules move into the casing because there were more outside when the experiment began.

Initial stage

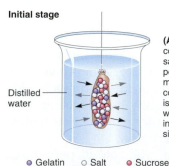

(A) Initially the sausage casing contains a solution of gelatin, salt, and sucrose. The casing is permeable to water and salt molecules only. Because the concentration of water molecules is greater outside the casing, water molecules diffuse into the casing. The opposite situation exists for the salt.

Distilled water

⬤ Gelatin ○ Salt ⬤ Sucrose

10-12 hours later

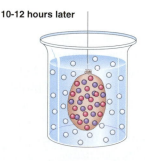

(B) The sausage casing swells because of the net movement of water molecules inward. However, the volume of distilled water in the beaker remains constant.

⬤ **FIGURE 3–4** *Osmosis: the diffusion of water through a selectively permeable membrane. (A sausage casing is an example of a selectively permeable membrane.)*

The volume of water increases inside the casing, causing it to expand because of the entry of water molecules. When the number of water molecules entering the casing is equal to the number exiting, equilibrium has been achieved: the casing will expand no further.

The pressure exerted by the water molecules within the casing at equilibrium is called the **osmotic pressure**.

Osmosis is the movement of water molecules across a semipermeable membrane from an area of higher concentration of a solution to an area of lower concentration of a solution. The key word is *solute*, the amount of concentration of a dissolved substance.

In the human body this is well illustrated by a red blood cell in blood plasma, Figure 3-5. If a red blood cell is put into blood plasma, which has the same number of sodium particles as a red blood cell, the osmotic pressure of the red blood cell and that of the plasma are the same, representing an **isotonic solution**.

If a red blood cell is put into fresh water, which has fewer sodium particles than the red blood cell, water rushes into the red blood cell. The fresh water represents a **hypotonic solution**.

If a red blood cell is put into sea water, which has more sodium particles than the red blood cell, water leaves the red blood cell to dilute the sea water. The sea water represents a **hypertonic solution**.

Filtration

Filtration is the movement of solutes and water across a semipermeable membrane. This results from some mechanical force, such as blood pressure or gravity. The solutes and water move from an area of higher pressure to an area of lower pressure. The size of the membrane pores determines which molecules are to be filtered. Thus filtration allows for the separation of large and small molecules. Such filtration takes place in the kidneys. The process allows larger protein molecules to remain within the body and smaller molecules to be excreted as waste, Figure 3-6.

Active Transport

Active transport is a process in which molecules move across the cell membrane from an area of lower concentration against a concentration gradient to an area of higher concentration. This process requires the high energy chemical compound ATP (adenosine triphosphate). The ATP is supplied by cell metabolism.

How does active transport work? One theory suggests that a molecule is picked up from outside the cell membrane and is brought inside by a carrier molecule. Both molecule and carrier are bound together, forming a temporary carrier-molecule complex. This carrier-molecule complex shuttles across the cell membrane; the molecule is released at the inner surface of the membrane, from which it enters

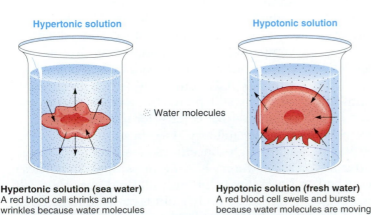
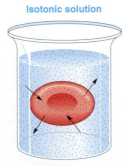

Hypertonic solution

Hypotonic solution

Isotonic solution

Water molecules

Hypertonic solution (sea water)
A red blood cell shrinks and wrinkles because water molecules are moving out of the cell.

Hypotonic solution (fresh water)
A red blood cell swells and bursts because water molecules are moving into the cell.

Isotonic solution (human blood serum)
A red blood cell remains unchanged, because the movement of water molecules into and out of the cell are the same.

● **FIGURE 3–5** *Movement of water molecules in solutions of different osmotic pressure.*

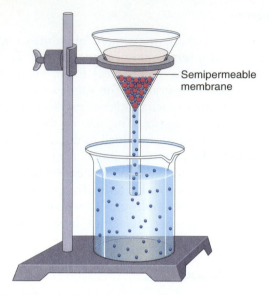

Filtration: Small molecules are filtered through the semipermeable membrane, while the large molecules remain in the funnel.

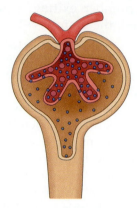

Example of filtration in the human body: Glomerulus of kidney, large particles such as red blood cells and proteins remain in the blood, and small molecules such as urea and water are excreted as a metabolic excretory product—urine.

● **FIGURE 3-6**   *Example of filtration: a passive transport process.*

STREET SMART

Advanced Emergency Medical Technicians (AEMTs) are occasionally called on to administer intravenous (within the vein) fluids for a variety of medical conditions.

For example, if the patient is dehydrated, the AEMT administers a hypotonic solution like 5% dextrose in sterile water (D_5W). Because the solution is hypotonic, it quickly leaves the bloodstream by osmosis, and rehydrates the cells within the tissues.

If the patient is hemorrhaging (bleeding), the AEMT should replace the blood loss with another readily available solution until the blood can be replaced.

The most common solution used for this purpose is 0.9% sodium chloride (0.9 NaCl) in sterile water. The other name for this solution is normal saline because blood and 0.9% NaCl have the same tonicity (isotonic). Normal saline has a tendency to stay in the

bloodstream for a longer period and is therefore considered a blood volume expander.

Early attempts were made to duplicate the chemical makeup of blood. The first solution was created by Sydney Ringer, a British physiologist (1835–1910), and was called Ringer's solution. It contained potassium chloride, sodium chloride, and calcium chloride.

Later physicians added the chemical compound lactate, in an attempt to counteract the lactic acid in the blood, and lactated Ringer's (LR) solution was invented. Many surgeons still prefer the *balanced* electrolyte solution—that is, LR—for trauma patients.

The military has been experimenting with high-concentration sodium solutions, 3% sodium chloride in sterile water. These *supersaline* solutions pull fluid out of the cell (60% of the body's fluids are within the cells) and into the bloodstream temporarily. The intent is to keep the soldier alive until the blood loss can be replaced.

There are many different intravenous solutions available. Some are hypotonic so-lutions, some are hypertonic solutions, and most are isotonic solutions. The choice of fluids depends on the patient's physical condition. ■

the cytoplasm. At this point the carrier acquires energy at the inner surface of the cell membrane. Then it returns to the outer surface of the cell membrane to pick up another molecule for transport. Accordingly, the carrier can also convey molecules in the opposite direction, from the inside to the outside, Figure 3-7.

These carrier-molecule complexes, in essence, create a *biological pump* that moves chemicals against the concentration gradient in violation of the natural law of diffusion.

The most important of these pumps is the sodium-potassium pump. After a nerve cell or muscle cell acts, the sodium-potassium pump reacts and pushes sodium back into the cell and potassium out of the cell. The result is that two chemicals are lined up across the cell membrane from each other, ready to move fluid across the membrane. This chemical urge to cross the cell membrane is called an action potential.

Facilitated Transport

In some instances hormones, such as insulin, help carry large molecules, such as glucose, across the cell membrane. Similar to active transport, these hormones form carrier-molecule complexes, using the hormone as a carrier to cross the cell membrane.

Phagocytosis

Phagocytosis, or "cell eating," is quite similar to pinocytosis, with an important differ-

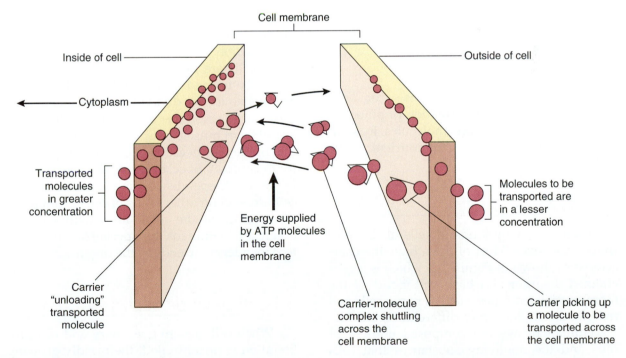

Cell membrane

Inside of cell

Outside of cell

Cytoplasm

Transported molecules in greater concentration

Molecules to be transported are in a lesser concentration

Energy supplied by ATP molecules in the cell membrane

Carrier "unloading" transported molecule

Carrier-molecule complex shuttling across the cell membrane

Carrier picking up a molecule to be transported across the cell membrane

● **FIGURE 3–7**   *The active transport of molecules from an area of lesser concentration to an area of greater concentration, according to one theoretical model.*

STREET SMART

When the pancreas stops secreting insulin, a hormone needed to actively transport sugar across the cell membrane, the cells change their metabolism from aerobic (oxygen using) to the much less efficient anaerobic (without oyxgen). Anaerobic metabolism creates as a byproduct a large amount of acid, called **keto acid**. At the same time the sugar in the blood continues to build, and the pa-

tient becomes **hyperglycemic** (exhibiting an increase in blood sugar) as well.

The acids in the blood then cause the membrane pores in the kidney's functional units, the **nephrons**, to dilate, and sugar starts to be excreted with the urine. This passage of sugar with urine is called **spilling sugar** and is a cardinal sign of diabetes mellitus. ■

ence: In pinocytosis the substances engulfed by the cell membrane are in solution; however, in phagocytosis the substances engulfed are within particles. Human white blood cells undergo phagocytosis. The particulate substance is engulfed by an enfolding of the cell membrane to form a vacuole enclosing the material. When the material is completely enclosed within the vacuole, digestive enzymes pour into the vacuole from the cytoplasm to destroy the trapped substance.

Pinocytosis

As stated earlier, **pinocytosis**, or "cell drinking," involves the formation of pinocytic vesicles that engulf large molecules in solution. The cell then ingests the nutrient for its own use.

● SPECIALIZATION

There are many kinds of cells of different shapes and sizes. Most of them have the characteristics shown in Figure 3-1, which is a generalized diagram of a basic cell. Some of the more specialized types, such as nerve cells and red blood cells, look very different, Figure 3-8.

Human beings are composed entirely of cells and the nonliving substances that cells build up around themselves. The interaction of

the various parts of the cell within the cellular structure constitutes the life of the cell. These interactions result in the life activities, life processes, or life functions that were discussed in Chapter 1. However, in complex organisms, groups of cells become specialists in a particular function. Nerve cells, for example, have become specialized in response; red blood cells, in oxygen transport.

Specialized cells may lose the ability to perform some of the other functions, such as reproduction (cell division). Normally, when nerve cells are destroyed or damaged, others cannot be formed to replace them. Heart muscle cells no longer divide when they reach maturity. If a person has a heart attack, there is a loss of heart muscle cells, which are replaced by scar tissue. The heart then loses some of its ability to contract. Specialization also has resulted in an interdependence among cells—certain cells depend on other kinds of cells to aid them in carrying on the total life activities of the organism. In humans this specialization and interdependence extends to the organs.

● DISORDERS OF CELL STRUCTURE

When cell growth goes awry and cell proliferation is uncontrolled, the rapidly growing mass of cells is called a cancer. Cancer is the pri-

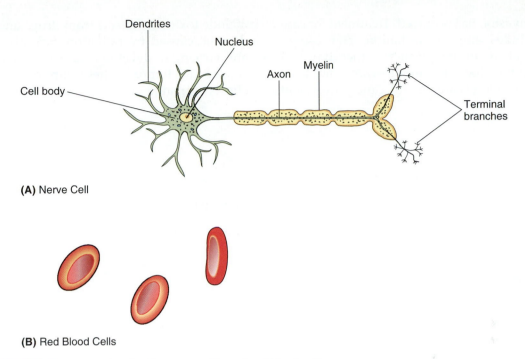

(A) Nerve Cell

(B) Red Blood Cells

● **FIGURE 3–8**   *Specialized cells: nerve cells and red blood cells.*

mary cause of death for approximately one quarter of all U.S. residents. In fact, cancer is the second leading cause of death in the United States overall.

Causes of cancer are varied, depending on the site of the cancer. For example, lung cancer, the most common type, is thought to be caused by cigarette smoking. On the other hand, the specific cause of breast cancer, a common cancer among women, is unknown, but the incidence increases dramatically after a woman goes through menopause.

Tumor

A **tumor** results when cell division does not occur in the usual pattern. If the pattern is interrupted by an abnormal and uncontrolled growth of cells, the result is a tumor. Tumors are also known as **neoplasms**, and they can be divided into two groups: benign or malignant.

In a **benign** tumor, cells are confined to the local area. Benign tumors are given other names, depending on their type or location (e.g., a **wart**, or **papilloma**, is a type of tumor of the epithelial tissue). Most benign tumors can be surgically removed.

A **malignant** tumor, or **cancer**, is when cells move rapidly from one place to another. This process is called **metastases**. These tumors cause death. In some cases, if the cancer is detected early, it may be treated and the person may recover. It is important for EMS providers to know the early signs of cancer. Some of these signs are weight loss, general feeling of poor health, abnormal bleeding, wounds that are slow to heal, and some type of abnormal function.

Diagnostic tests can detect the early stages of cancer. Some of these tests are x-ray, mammogram, sonogram, and biopsy. These tests can be conducted on an outpatient basis. If you are working in a medical office, get the procedures from your local testing center. Give the patient this information before any testing begins.

Treatment of cancer depends on the type of tumor and where it is located. Cancers may also be classified according to stages. Each stage reflects the size of the cancer and how much invasion has occurred. Treatment for cancer includes surgery, radiation, and use of drugs called antineoplastics. Other types of treatment include immunotherapy and laser treatment. Disadvantages of cancer treatment include toxic side effects from drugs and tissue damage caused by radiation. Scientists today are working to develop cancer treatments specific to the tumor to help eliminate the side effects of treatment.

● REVIEW QUESTIONS

Select the letter of the choice that best completes the statement.

1. Structures found in cytoplasm to help cells function are called:
   a. nucleolus
   b. organelles
   c. ribosomes
   d. vacuoles

2. Regulating transport of substances in and out of the cell is the:
   a. cell membrane
   b. nuclear membrane
   c. cytoplasm
   d. nucleus

3. A structure that digests worn out cells and bacteria is called:
   a. perioxisome
   b. ribosome
   c. lysosome
   d. mitochondria

4. The function of Golgi apparatus of the cell is:
   a. protein synthesis
   b. destroying bacteria
   c. digesting fats
   d. storing and packaging secretions

5. The internal framework of the cell is called:
   a. mitochondria
   b. cytoskeleton
   c. endoplasmic reticulum
   d. ribosomes

● COMPLETION

Fill in the blank with the correct word.

1. The powerhouse of the cell stores _____ and is called _____.

2. The rough endoplasmic reticulum is studded with _____ , which serve as a site for _____ synthesis.

3. The perioxisomes contain _____ enzymes, which help digest
   _____.

4. The _____ for each individual's kind of protein is contained within a specific
   _____ in the _____ chain.

● MATCHING

Match each term in Column A with its correct description in Column B.

Column A	Column B
_____ 1. solute	a. cells confined to local area
_____ 2. isotonic solution	b. has a higher concentration of Na than red blood cells
_____ 3. diffusion	c. needs ATP for energy
_____ 4. phagocytosis	d. malignant tumor
_____ 5. osmosis	e. solid particles dissolved within a fluid
_____ 6. benign	f. cell reproduction
_____ 7. hypertonic solution	g. molecules move from higher concentration to lower
_____ 8. cancer	h. has same concentration of Na as red blood cells
_____ 9. mitosis	i. engulfs bacteria
_____ 10. active transport	j. diffusion of water molecules

●APPLYING THEORY TO PRACTICE

1. The cell is a miniature of how the body works. Name the cellular structure responsible
   for each: digestion, respiration, energy, circulation, and the reproductive process.

2. Describe how the cell takes in nutrients and name at least three products that the cell
   manufactures.

3. Explain to the patient presenting with a heart attack what happens to the cells of the heart
   muscle when someone has a heart attack and what the difference is between scar tissue and
   heart tissue.

4. You are working in an emergency care center. A person comes in dehydrated and the doctor
   orders a hypotonic solution. Explain why this solution is used instead of an isotonic
   solution.

● LABELING

Study the following diagram of a typical cell. Enter the names of the structures after the properly numbered callouts, as listed below.

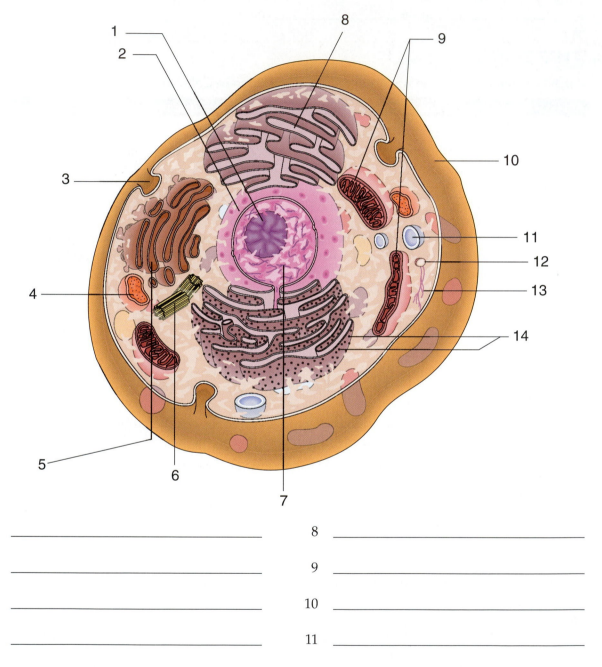

1 _____   8 _____

2 _____   9 _____

3 _____   10 _____

4 _____   11 _____

5 _____   12 _____

6 _____   13 _____

7 _____   14 _____

Tissues and Membranes

Objectives

- List the four main types of tissues
- Define the function and location of tissues
- Define the function and location of membranes
- Define the terms *organ* and *organ system*
- Relate various organs to their respective systems
- Describe the processes involved in the two types of tissue repair
- Describe the process of granulation
- Define the key words that relate to this chapter

Key Words

aponeuroses
bactericidal
cicatrix
clean wound
collagen
connective tissue
elastin
epithelial
fasciae
gastric mucosa
graft
granulation
intestinal mucosa
ligament
membrane
mucosa
mucous membrane
muscle tissue
nervous tissue
organ system
parietal membrane
pericardial membrane
peritoneal membrane
pleural membrane
primary repair
respiratory mucosa
scab
secondary repair
serosa
serous fluid
serous membrane
sutures
synovial membrane
tendon
tissue
visceral membrane

TISSUES

Multicellular organisms are composed of many different types of cells. Although they are not randomly arranged, each of these cells performs a special function. These millions of cells are grouped according to their similarity in shape, size, structure, intercellular materials, and function. Cells so grouped are called tissues. There are four main types of tissue. (1) Epithelial tissue protect the body by covering internal and external surfaces. The cells of the epithelial tissue also produce secretions such as digestive juices. The epithelial tissue is named according to its structure. (2) Connective tissue supports and connects organs and tissue. (3) Muscle tissue contains cells that have the ability to contract and move the body. (4) Nervous tissue contains cells that react to stimuli and conduct an impulse.

Specialization of cells can be seen in a study of the epithelial cells, which make up epithelial tissue. Epithelial cells that cover the body's external and internal surfaces have a typical shape, either columnar, cubical, or platelike. This variation is necessary so the epithelial cells can fit together smoothly to line and protect the bodily surface. Muscle cells making up muscle tissue are long and spindle-like so they can contract.

Some tissues are composed of both living cells and various nonliving substances that the cells build up around themselves. The variations, functions, and locations of each type are described in Table 4-1.

MEMBRANES

A membrane is formed by putting two thin layers of tissue together. The cells in the membrane may secrete a fluid. Membranes are classified as epithelial or connective.

Epithelial Membranes

Epithelial membranes are classified as mucous or serous, depending on the type of secretions produced, Figure 4-1.

Mucous membranes. These structures line surfaces and spaces that lead to the outside of the body, as well as the respiratory, digestive, reproductive, and urinary systems. The mucous membrane produces a substance called mucous, which lubricates and protects the lining. For example, the mucous in the digestive tract protects the lining of the stomach and small intestines from the digestive juices. The term mucosa is used for a specific mucous membrane, namely:

- respiratory mucosa, which lines the respiratory passages

- gastric mucosa, which lines the stomach

- intestinal mucosa, which lines the small and large intestines

Serous membrane. This is a double-walled membrane that produces a watery substance, called serous fluid, and lines closed body cavities. The outer part of the membrane that lines the cavity is known as the parietal serous membrane; the part that covers the organs within is known as the visceral serous membrane. The fluid produced allows the organs within to move freely and prevents friction. The name serosa is given to the specific serous membranes, all beginning with the letter *p*. Following are the serous membranes:

- pleural membrane, which lines the thoracic or chest cavity and protects the lungs; the fluid is called pleural fluid

- pericardial membrane, which lines the heart cavity and protects the heart; the fluid is called pericardial fluid

- peritoneal membrane, which lines the abdominal cavity and protects the abdominal organs; the fluid is called peritoneal fluid

Cutaneous membrane (skin). This is a specialized type of epithelial membrane; it will be discussed in Chapter 5.

TABLE 4-1 *Different Kinds of Human Tissue*

TYPE OF TISSUE	FUNCTION	CHARACTERISTICS AND LOCATION	MORPHOLOGY
I. EPITHELIAL	Cells form a continuous layer covering internal and external body surfaces, provide protection, produce secretions (digestive juices, hormones, perspiration), and regulate the passage of materials across themselves. **A. Covering and lining tissue** These cells can be stratified (layered), ciliated, or keratinized.	**1. Squamous epithelial cells** These are flat, irregularly shaped cells. They line the heart, blood and lymphatic vessels, body cavities, and alveoli (air sacs) of lungs. The outer layer of the skin is composed of stratified and keratinized squamous epithelial cells. The stratified squamous epithelial cells on the outer skin layer protect the body against microbial invasion. **2. Cuboidal epithelial cells** These are the cube-shaped cells that line the kidney tubules and cover the ovaries and secretory parts of certain glands. **3. Columnar epithelial cells** Elongated, with the nucleus generally near the bottom and often ciliated on the outer surface. They line the ducts, digestive tract (especially the intestinal and stomach lining), parts of the respiratory tract, and glands.	

(continues)

TABLE 4-1 (*continued*)

TYPE OF TISSUE	FUNCTION	CHARACTERISTICS AND LOCATION	MORPHOLOGY
I. EPITHELIAL (*continued*)	**B. Glandular or secretory tissue** These cells are specialized to secrete materials like digestive hormones, milk, perspiration, and wax. They are columnar or cuboidal shaped.	**Endocrine gland cells** These cells form ductless glands that secrete their substances (hormones) directly into the blood-stream. For instance, the thyroid gland secretes thyroxin, whereas adrenal glands secrete adrenaline. **Exocrine gland cells** These cells secrete their substances into ducts. The mammary glands, sweat glands, and salivary glands are examples.	
II. CONNECTIVE	Cells whose intercellular secretions (matrix) support and connect the organs and tissues of the body. **A. Adipose tissue** This tissue stores lipid (fat); acts as filler tissue; and cushions, supports, and insulates the body.	Connective tissue is found almost everywhere within the body: bones, cartilage, mucous membranes, muscles, nerves, skin, and all internal organs. A type of loose, connective tissue composed of saclike adipose cells; they are specialized for the storage of fat. Adipose cells are found throughout the body: in the subcutaneous skin layer, around the kidneys, within padding around joints, and in the marrow of long bones.	
	B. Areolar (loose) connective This tissue surrounds various organs and supports both nerve cells and blood vessels, which transport nutrient materials (to cells) and wastes (away from cells). Areolar tissue also (temporarily) stores glucose, salts, and water.	Areolar tissue is composed of a large, semifluid matrix, with many different types of cells and fibers embedded in it. These include fibroblasts (fibrocytes), plasma cells, macrophages, mast cells, and various white blood cells. The fibers are bundles of strong, flexible white fibrous protein called **collagen** and elastic single fibers of **elastin**. It is found in the epidermis of the skin and in the subcutaneous layer with adipose cells.	

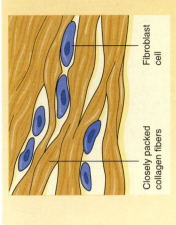

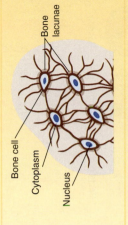

Fibroblast cell

Closely packed collagen fibers

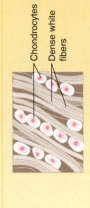

Bone lacunae

Bone cell

Cytoplasm

Nucleus

Cells (chondrocytes)

Matrix

Lacunae (space enclosing cells)

Chondrocytes

Dense white fibers

C. Dense fibrous

This tissue forms ligaments, tendons, and aponeuroses. **Ligaments** are strong, flexible bands (or cords) that hold bones firmly together at the joints. **Tendons** are white, glistening bands attaching skeletal muscles to the bones. **Aponeuroses** are flat, wide bands of tissue holding one muscle to another or to the periosteum (bone covering). **Fasciae** are fibrous connective tissue sheets that wrap around muscle bundles to hold them in place.

Dense fibrous tissue is also called white fibrous tissue, because it is made from closely packed white collagen fibers. Fibrous tissue is flexible but not elastic. This tissue has a poor blood supply and heals slowly.

D. Supportive

1. Bone (osseous) tissue—

Comprises the skeleton of the body, which supports and protects underlying soft tissue parts and organs and also serves as attachments for skeletal muscles.

Connective tissue whose intercellular matrix is calcified by the deposition of mineral salts (like calcium carbonate and calcium phosphate). Calcification of bone imparts great strength. The entire skeleton is composed of bone tissue.

2. Cartilage—

Provides firm but flexible support for the embryonic skeleton and part of the adult skeleton.

a. Hyaline—

Forms the skeleton of the embryo.

Hyaline cartilage is found on articular bone surfaces and also at the nose tip, bronchi, and bronchial tubes. Ribs are joined to the sternum (breastbone) by the costal cartilage. It is also found in the larynx and the rings in the trachea.

b. Fibrocartilage—

A strong, flexible, supportive substance, found between bones and wherever great strength (and a degree of rigidity) is needed.

Fibrocartilage is located within intervertebral discs and in the pubic symphysis between the pubic bones.

(continues)

TABLE 4-1 *(continued)*

TYPE OF TISSUE	FUNCTION	CHARACTERISTICS AND LOCATION	MORPHOLOGY
II. CONNECTIVE *(continued)*	**D. Supportive** *(continued)* **c. Elastic cartilage—** The intercellular matrix is embedded with a network of elastic fibers and is firm but flexible.	Elastic cartilage is located inside the auditory ear tube, external ear, epiglottis, and larynx.	Elastic fibers / Chondrocyte / Nucleus
	E. Vascular (liquid blood tissue) **1. Blood—** Transports nutrient and oxygen molecules to cells and metabolic wastes away from cells (can be considered a liquid tissue). Contains cells that function in the body's defense and in blood clotting.	Blood is composed of two major parts: a liquid called plasma and a solid cellular portion known as blood cells (or corpuscles). The plasma suspends corpuscles, of which there are two major types: red blood cells (erythrocytes) and white blood cells (leukocytes). A third cellular component (really a cell fragment) is called platelets (thrombocytes). Blood circulates within the blood vessels (arteries, veins, and capillaries) and through the heart.	Lymphocyte / Basophil / Thrombocytes (platelets) / Monocyte / Erythrocytes / Eosinophil / Neutrophil
	2. Lymph— Transports tissue fluid, proteins, fats, and other materials from the tissues to the circulatory system. This occurs through a series of tubes called the lymphatic vessels.	Lymph is a fluid made up of water, glucose, protein, fats, and salt. The cellular components are lymphocytes and granulocytes. They flow in tubes called lymphatic vessels, which closely parallel the veins and bathe the tissue spaces between cells.	Lymph capillary / Red blood cells / White blood cell / Lymph / Cells / Blood capillary

III. MUSCLE

A. Cardiac
These cells help the heart contract to pump blood through and out of the heart.

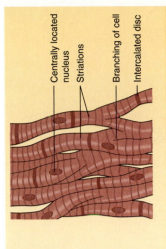

Centrally located nucleus
Striations
Branching of cell
Intercalated disc

Cardiac muscle is a striated (having a cross-banding pattern), involuntary (not under conscious control) muscle. It makes up the walls of the heart.

B. Skeletal (striated voluntary)
These muscles are attached to the movable parts of the skeleton. They are capable of rapid, powerful contractions and long states of partially sustained contractions, allowing for voluntary movement.

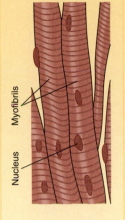

Myofibrils
Nucleus

Skeletal muscle is striated (having transverse bands that run down the length of muscle fiber); voluntary, because the muscle is under conscious control; and skeletal, because these muscles are attached to the skeleton (bones, tendons, and other muscles).

C. Smooth (nonstriated involuntary)
These provide for involuntary movement. Examples include the movement of materials along the digestive tract, controlling the diameter of blood vessels and the pupil of the eye.

Cells separated from each other
Spindle-shaped cell
Nucleus

Smooth muscle is called nonstriated because it lacks the striations (bands) of skeletal muscles; its movement is involuntary. It makes up the walls of the digestive, genitourinary, and respiratory tracts; blood vessels; and lymphatic vessels.

IV. NERVE

Neurons (nerve cells)
These cells have the ability to react to stimuli.

1. Irritability—
Ability of nerve tissue to respond to environmental changes.

2. Conductivity—
Ability to carry a nerve impulse (message).

Dendrites
Nucleus
Axon
Myelin
Terminal branches
Cell body

Nerve tissue is composed of neurons (nerve cells). Neurons have branches through which various parts of the body are connected and their activities coordinated. They are found in the brain, spinal cord, and nerves.

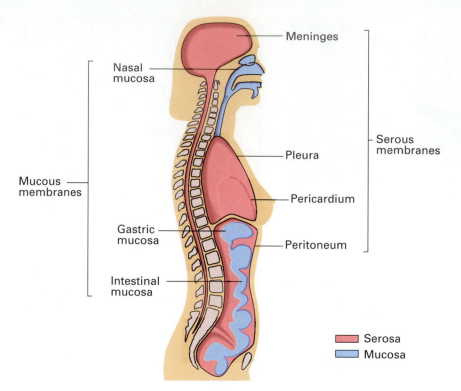

Nasal mucosa

Meninges

Mucous membranes

Serous membranes

Pleura

Pericardium

Gastric mucosa

Peritoneum

Intestinal mucosa

Serosa

Mucosa

● **FIGURE 4–1**   *Mucous and serous membranes.*

Connective Membranes

Connective membranes are made of two layers of connective tissue. In this classification is the **synovial membrane**, which lines joint cavities. Synovial membranes secrete synovial fluid, which prevents friction inside the joint cavity.

● ORGANS AND SYSTEMS

An organ is a structure made up of several tissues grouped together to perform a single function. For instance, the stomach is an organ composed of highly specialized vascular, connective, epithelial, muscular, and nerve tissues. All these tissues function together to enable the stomach to accomplish digestion and absorption.

The skin that covers our bodies is no mere simple tissue, but is a complex organ composed of connective, epithelial, muscular, and nervous tissue. These tissues enable the skin to protect the body and remove its wastes (water and inorganic salts), making us sensitive to our environment.

The various organs of the human body do not function separately. Instead, they coordinate their activities to form a complete, functional organism. A group of organs that act together to perform a specific, related function is called an **organ system**, see Figure 4-2.

The digestive system has the special function of processing solid food into liquid for absorption into the bloodstream. This organ system includes the mouth, salivary glands, esophagus, stomach, small intestine, liver, pancreas, gallbladder, and large intestine. The circulatory system transports materials to and from cells. It is composed of the heart, arteries, veins, capillaries, lymphatic vessels, and spleen.

Each of the 10 organ systems is highly specialized to perform a specific function; together they coordinate their functions to form a whole, live, functioning organism.

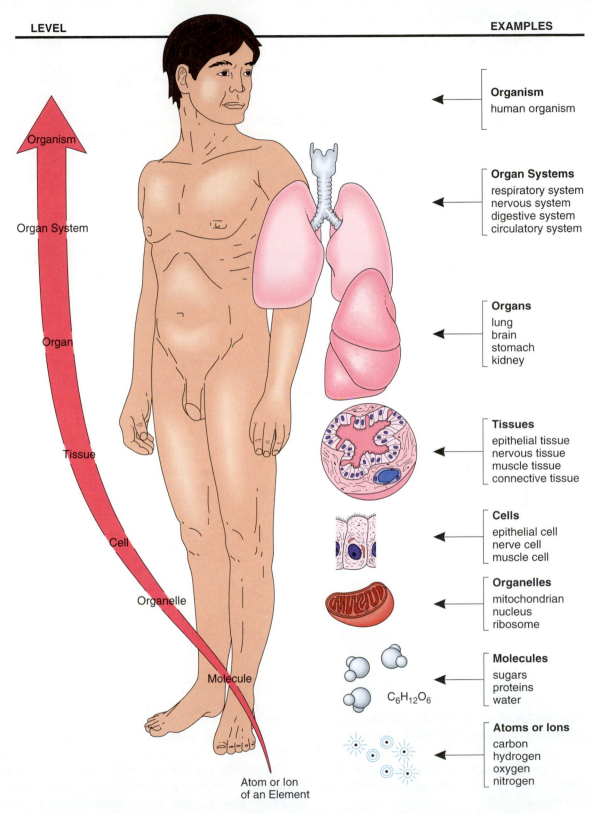

LEVEL   **EXAMPLES**

Organism

Organ System

Organ

Tissue

Cell

Organelle

Molecule

Atom or Ion
of an Element

Organism
human organism

Organ Systems
respiratory system
nervous system
digestive system
circulatory system

Organs
lung
brain
stomach
kidney

Tissues
epithelial tissue
nervous tissue
muscle tissue
connective tissue

Cells
epithelial cell
nerve cell
muscle cell

Organelles
mitochondrian
nucleus
ribosome

Molecules
sugars
proteins
water

$C_6H_{12}O_6$

Atoms or Ions
carbon
hydrogen
oxygen
nitrogen

● **FIGURE 4–2**   *The various organs of the human body function together. The formation of the human organism progresses from different levels of complexity.*

TABLE 4-2 *The Ten Body Systems*

SYSTEM	SYSTEM FUNCTIONS	ORGANS	
Skeletal	Gives shape to body; protects delicate parts of body; provides space for attaching muscles; is instrumental in forming blood; stores minerals.	Skull, spinal column, ribs and sternum, shoulder girdle, upper and lower extremities, pelvic girdle	
Muscular	Determines posture; produces body heat; provides for movement.	Striated voluntary muscles—skeletal striated involuntary—cardiac smooth—nonstriated	
Digestive	Prepares food for absorption and use by body cells through modification of chemical and physical states.	Mouth (salivary glands, teeth, tongue), pharynx, esophagus, stomach, intestines, liver, gallbladder, pancreas	
Respiratory	Acquires oxygen; rids body of carbon dioxide.	Nose, pharynx, larynx, trachea, bronchi, lungs	
Circulatory	Carries oxygen and nourishment to cells of body; carries waste from cells; body defense.	Heart, arteries, veins, capillaries, lymphatic vessels, lymph nodes, spleen	
Excretory	Removes waste products of metabolism from body.	Skin, lungs, kidneys, bladder, ureters, urethra	
Nervous	Communicates; controls body activity; coordinates body activity.	Brain, nerves, spinal cord, ganglia	
Endocrine	Manufactures hormones to regulate organ activity.	Glands (ductless): pituitary, thyroid, parathyroid, pancreas, adrenal, gonads (ovaries, testes)	
Reproductive	Reproduces human beings.	*Male* testes scrotum epididymis vas deferens seminal vesicles ejaculatory duct prostate gland Cowper's gland penis urethra	*Female* ovaries fallopian tubes uterus vagina Bartholin glands external genitals (vulva) breasts (mammary glands)
Integumentary	Helps regulate body temperature, establishes a barrier between the body and environment; eliminates waste; synthesizes Vitamin D; contains receptors for temperature, pressure, and pain.	Epidermis, dermis, sweat glands, oil glands	

The systems of the body are the skeletal, muscular, digestive, respiratory, circulatory, reproductive, excretory, endocrine, nervous, and integumentary systems. The functions and organs of each system are shown in Table 4-2.

DEGREE OF TISSUE REPAIR

Repair of damaged tissues occurs continually during the everyday activities of living. Depending on the type and location of injury, some tissue is quickly repaired. Muscle tissue heals slowly, and bone tissue repairs occur slowly because broken bone ends must be kept aligned and immobilized until the repair is complete. Heart muscle tissue does not repair itself, and nerve cell bodies destroyed by infection or injury do *not* grow back.

PROCESS OF EPITHELIAL TISSUE REPAIR

There are two types of epithelial tissue repair. One is called **primary repair** and the other is **secondary repair**.

Primary Repair

Primary repair takes place in "clean" wounds. A **clean wound** is a cut or incision on the skin where infection is not present. In a simple skin injury, the deep layer of stratified squamous epithelium divides. The new stratified squamous epithelial cells "push" themselves upward toward the surface of the skin. The damage or wound is quickly and completely restored to normal. However, if the damage is over a larger area, then the underlying connective tissue cells and fibroblasts are also involved.

Primary Repair over a Larger Skin Area

If a larger area of skin is damaged, fluid escapes from the broken capillaries. This capillary fluid dries and seals the wound, and typically a **scab** forms. Epithelial cells multiply at the edges of the scab and continue to grow over the damaged area until it is covered. If a much larger or deeper area of skin is destroyed, skin **grafts** are needed to promote wound healing.

Primary Repair of Deeper Tissues

When there is damage to deeper tissues, the edges of the wound must be brought (sewn) together with **sutures**. For example, in operative incisions or wounds, there is a tremendous amount of serous fluid that leaks out on to the wound. This helps to form a coagulation (clot) that seals the wound. The coagulum contains tissue fragments and white blood cells. In 24 to 36 hours the epithelial cells lining the capillaries (endothelium) and fibroblasts of connective tissue are rapidly regenerating. The newly formed cells remain along the edges of the wound. On the third day, new vascular tissue starts to form. These multiply across the wound along with connective tissue formation.

On the fourth or fifth day, fibroblast cells start to be very active. They help to make new collagen fibers. In addition, capillaries grow and "reach" across the wound, holding the edges firmly together. Toward the end of the healing process, the collagenous fibers shorten and scar tissue is reduced to a minimum.

Secondary Repair

A process called **granulation** occurs in a large open wound with small or large tissue loss. The granulation process forms new vertically upstanding blood vessels. These new blood vessels are surrounded by young connective tissue and wandering cells of different types. Granulation causes the surface area to have a pebbly texture. Fibroblasts are quite active in their production of new collagenous fibers. With all this activity going on, the wound eventually heals. In addition, as granulation occurs, a fluid is secreted. This fluid has strong **bactericidal** (bacterial destruction) properties. This is important to help reduce the risk of infection during wound healing.

As in any type of tissue repair, there is always some amount of scar tissue formed. The amount of scar (**cicatrix**) tissue formed depends on the extent of tissue damage. Careful attention must be given to patients, including burn victims, whose bodies are undergoing massive tissue repair. These areas *must* be kept in alignment and immobile at the beginning. However, active movement should be encouraged later so that as new tissue forms, pulling from scar tissue does not occur. It is the role of the health care professional to help prevent or minimize excessive scar tissue formation that can lead to disfigurement.

TABLE 4-3 *Vitamins Favorable to Tissue Repair*

VITAMIN	FUNCTION
Vitamin A	Repairs epithelial tissue, especially the epithelial cells lining the respiratory tract.
Vitamin B (thiamine, nicotinic acid, and riboflavin)	Helps to promote the general well-being of the individual. Specifically helps to promote appetite, metabolism, vigor, and pain relief in some cases.
Vitamin C	Helps in the normal production and maintenance of collagen fibers and other connective tissue substances.
Vitamin D	Needed for the normal absorption of calcium from the intestine. Possibly helps in the repair of bone fractures.
Vitamin K	Helps in the process of blood coagulation.
Vitamin E	Helps healing of tissues by acting as an antioxidant protector. It prevents important molecules and structures in the cell from reacting with oxygen. (When delicate components of living protoplasm are attacked by oxygen, they are literally "burnt.")

An EMS provider should also be mindful that proper nutrition plays an important part in the healing act. Newly growing tissues require lots of protein for repair; thus the need for protein-rich foods is great.

Vitamins also play an essential role in wound repair. They help the patient develop resistance to, as well as help prevent, infections. Table 4-3 lists some vitamins that are necessary to tissue repair.

● REVIEW QUESTIONS

Select the letter of the choice that best completes the statement.

1. Cells that are alike in size, shape, and function are called:
   a. elements
   b. tissues
   c. organs
   d. systems

2. The type of tissue found on the outer layer of skin is called:
   a. squamous epithelial
   b. stratified epithelial
   c. ciliated epithelial
   d. columnar epithelial

3. Collagen is a strong flexible protein found mainly in:
   a. adipose tissue
   b. cartilage tissue
   c. loose connective tissue
   d. bone tissue

4. Connective tissue structures that hold bones firmly together at joints are called:
   a. fascia
   b. tendons
   c. aponeuroses
   d. ligaments

5. The membrane that covers linings to the outside of the body is:
   a. cutaneous
   b. serous
   c. mucous
   d. synovial

6. The membrane that covers the lungs is called:
   a. parietal pleura
   b. visceral pleura
   c. parietal pericardial
   d. visceral pericardial

7. An inflammation of the lining of the abdominal cavity is called:
   a. pleurisy
   b. pericarditis
   c. peritonitis
   d. gastritis

8. The system that provides for movement of the body is the:
   a. skeletal
   b. nervous
   c. muscle
   d. circulatory

9. The type of repair that takes place in a clean wound is called:
   a. primary repair
   b. granulation
   c. secondary repair
   d. secretion of bactericidal fluid

10. The vitamin necessary to aid tissue repair as an antioxidant is:
    a. A
    b. D
    c. K
    d. E

● COMPLETION

Complete the following statements:

1. The tissue that has the ability to react to stimuli is _____.

2. The gastric mucosa is the mucous membrane lining of the _____ _____.

3. The secretion that prevents the bones in a joint from rubbing together is _____ _____.

4. The lining that protects the lung is the _____ membrane.

5. In secondary tissue repair, when there is a large open wound, the process of tissue repair is called _____.

●APPLYING THEORY TO PRACTICE

1. Feel your skin. What type of tissue is it? Is this tissue the same as the lining in your mouth?

2. Explain how mucous affects the air we breathe or the food we eat.

3. Name each organ system involved when you eat a slice of pizza.

4. You have fallen and scraped your knees. What type of healing will take place? Describe the process involved in the repair.

5. Describe the lunch you would prepare for a friend with severe injuries. The menu should include those vitamins necessary for tissue repair and those that help with pain relief.

Integumentary System

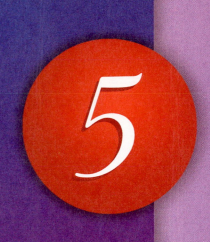

5

Objectives

- Describe the functions of the skin
- Describe the structures found in the two skin layers
- Explain how the skin serves as a channel of excretion
- Describe the action of the sweat glands
- Recognize some common skin disorders
- Define the key words that relate to this chapter

Key Words

abrasion
acne vulgaris
albinism
alopecia
arrector pili muscle
athlete's foot
avascular
boils
cortex
dermatitis
dermis
eczema
epidermis
full (third-degree) burn
genital herpes
hair follicle
herpes
impetigo
incision
integumentary system
keratin
laceration
liver spots

matrix
medulla
melanin
melanocytes
partial (second-degree) burn
psoriasis
puncture
ringworm
root
rule of nines
sebaceous gland
sebum
shaft
shingles (herpes zoster)
stratum corneum
stratum germinativum
sudoriferous gland
superficial (first-degree) burn
urticaria (hives)
wound

The skin is our protective covering and is called the integument or **integumentary system** or cutaneous membrane. It is tough, pliable, and multifunctional.

FUNCTIONS OF THE SKIN

The skin has seven functions.

1. Skin is a covering for the underlying, deeper tissues, protecting them from dehydration, injury, and germ invasion.

2. The skin also helps regulate body temperature by controlling the amount of heat loss. Evaporation of water from the skin, in the form of perspiration, helps rid the body of excess heat. Only a very small amount of waste is eliminated through the skin.

3. Skin helps to manufacture vitamin D. The ultraviolet light on the skin is necessary for the first stages of vitamin D formation.

4. The skin is the site of many nerve endings, Figure 5-1. A square inch of skin contains about 72 feet of nerves and hundreds of receptors.

5. The skin has tissues for the temporary storage of fat, glucose, water, and salts such as sodium chloride. Most of these substances are later absorbed by the blood and transported to other parts of the body.

6. The skin is designed to screen out any harmful ultraviolet radiation contained in sunlight.

7. The skin has special properties that allow it to absorb certain drugs and other chemical substances. We can apply drugs for localized treatment, as in the case of treating rashes, or we can apply medications that can be absorbed through the skin and have a general effect in the body. An example of this is Nitro-Bid paste, which is used to help dilate blood vessels in the treatment of angina pectoris (chest pain).

STRUCTURE OF THE SKIN

The skin consists of two basic layers:

1. The **epidermis**, or outermost covering, which is made of epithelial cells with no blood vessels present (**avascular**)

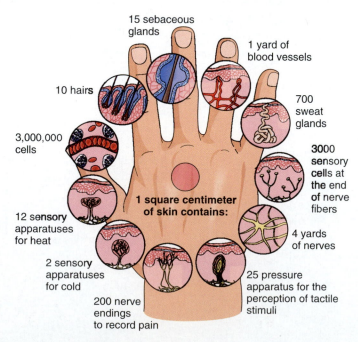

15 sebaceous glands

1 yard of blood vessels

10 hairs

3,000,000 cells

700 sweat glands

3000 **sensory cells** at the end of nerve fibers

1 square centimeter of skin contains:

12 sensory apparatuses for heat

4 yards of nerves

2 sensory apparatuses for cold

25 pressure apparatus for the perception of tactile stimuli

200 nerve endings to record pain

● **FIGURE 5–1**   *The skin is well supplied with nerves.*

2. The dermis, or true skin, which is made up of vascular connective tissue

Epidermis

The two most functionally important cellular layers of the epidermis are the stratum corneum and the stratum germinativum. The cytoplasm of the cells making up the stratum corneum is replaced by a hard, nonliving protein substance called keratin. This keratin layer acts as a waterproof covering. Cells making up the stratum corneum are flattened and scale-like. They flake off from the constant friction of clothing, rubbing, and washing. For this reason the stratum corneum is sometimes called the horny layer. As the cells of the horny layer are flaked off, they are replaced by new cells from the stratum germinativum.

The stratum corneum forms the body's first line of defense against invading bacteria. Because of the flaking action of the stratum corneum and because the oils on it are slightly acidic, many kinds of organisms that come in contact with the stratum corneum are unable to multiply and grow.

The thickness of the horny layer varies in different parts of the body. It is thickest on the palms of the hands and on the soles of the feet because of constant friction. Sometimes an overgrowth of tissue develops outwardly in a concentrated area, forming a callus. If the overgrowth grows inward, a corn may form.

The stratum germinativum is a very important epidermal layer. The replacement of cells in the epidermis depends on the division of cells in this layer. As new germinativum cells form, they push their way upward toward the epidermis. Eventually they become keratinized like the other epidermal cells within the horny layer.

Skin pigmentation is found in germinativum cells called melanocytes, which contain a skin pigment called melanin. Melanin can have a black, brown, or yellow tint, depending on racial origin. The amount of melanin (and other skin pigments such as carotene and hemoglobin) in the melanocytes determines the various shades of human skin color. Caucasians have a reduced amount of melanin in their melanocytes. If there are patches of melanin present, the skin is said to be freckled. In the elderly, melanin also collects in spots. These are referred to as "aging spots." Other races, on the other hand, possess a higher amount of melanin. Absence of pigments (other than hemoglobin) causes albinism. The skin of an albino has a pinkish tint because the red blood vessels can be seen through the skin. Basic skin coloring is inherited from our parents.

Environment is another factor that can modify skin coloring. For example, exposure to sunlight may result in a temporary increase in melanin within the melanocytes. This is the darkened or tanned effect with which we are all familiar. Tanning is produced by the melanocytes' reaction to ultraviolet (UV) rays of sunlight. It should be noted that prolonged exposure to sunlight is unwise because it may lead to the development of skin cancers.

As seen in Figure 5-2, the lower edge of the stratum germinativum is ridged. These ridges are known as the papillae of the skin. The papillae are raised from the dermal layer of the skin and push into the stratum germinativum of the epidermis. In the skin of the fingers, soles of the feet, and palms of the hands, these papillae are quite pronounced—so much so, in fact, that they raise the skin into permanent ridges. These ridges are arranged so that they provide maximum resistance to slipping when grasping and holding objects; thus they are also referred to as friction ridges. The ridges on the inner surfaces of the fingers create individual and characteristic fingerprint patterns used in identification. Newborn infants are also footprinted as a means of identification.

The many ridges, folds, and creases of the skin permit the skin to stretch and contract with the movement of the muscles underneath, thus preventing the skin from tearing. Across the entire body there are folds of skin that create tension lines, which help prevent injury to the skin. When an injury does occur along a tension line, it is slower to heal and may reduce movement of that extremity. For example, circumferential burns of the chest can prevent the chest from expanding, leading to suffocation.

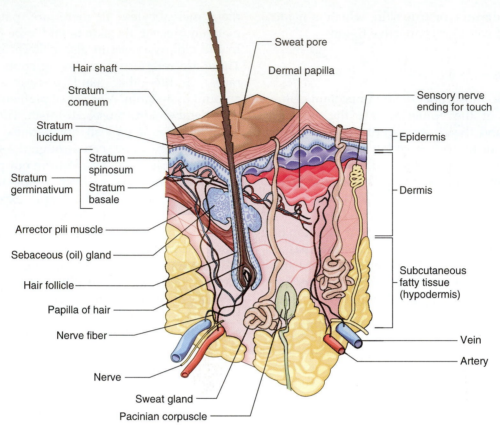

Hair shaft

Stratum corneum

Stratum lucidum

Stratum germinativum

Stratum spinosum

Stratum basale

Arrector pili muscle

Sebaceous (oil) gland

Hair follicle

Papilla of hair

Nerve fiber

Nerve

Sweat gland

Pacinian corpuscle

Sweat pore

Dermal papilla

Sensory nerve ending for touch

Epidermis

Dermis

Subcutaneous fatty tissue (hypodermis)

Vein

Artery

● **FIGURE 5–2**   *A cross-section of the skin.*

Dermis

The dermis, or corium, is the thicker, inner layer of the skin. It contains matted masses of connective tissue, collagen tissue bands, elastic fibers (through which pass numerous blood vessels), nerve endings, muscles, hair follicles, oil and sweat glands, and fat cells. The thickness of the dermis varies over different parts of the body. It is, for instance, thicker over the soles of the feet and the palms of the

STREET SMART

The depth of the skin, including the amount of fat underneath it, must be taken into account when deciding which needle to use for an injection. Generally speaking, a needle less than 1 inch long is used for a person weighing less than 100 pounds, a needle between 1 inch and 2 inches is used when a patient weighs between 100 and 200 pounds, and a needle longer than 2 inches is used if the patient weighs more than 200 pounds.

The location for the injection must also be taken into account. The skin over the shoulder, a common site for injections, is thinner than the skin over the buttocks, another common site for injections. ■

●APPLYING THEORY TO PRACTICE

1. If you get a cut on your skin, what may be the result?

2. Explain why you tan in the sun.

3. The skin helps to regulate body temperature by evaporation of water from the skin. Why do you feel uncomfortable on a hot, humid day?

4. A person is brought to the emergency room with full-thickness (third-degree) burns but is not complaining of pain. How is this possible?

5. The cosmetic industry sells many products that claim to remove or prevent wrinkles. If these claims are true, why do people who use these creams still wrinkle as they age?

6

Skeletal System

Objectives

- List the main function of the skeletal system
- Explain the formation of bone
- Name and locate the bones of the skeleton
- Name and define the main types of joint movement
- Identify common bone and joint disorders
- Define the key words that relate to this chapter

Key Words

abduction
adduction
amphiarthroses
appendicular skeleton
arthritis
articular cartilage
atlas
autonomic sniff box
axial skeleton
axis
ball-and-socket joint
blowout fracture
brachial pulse
bursa sacs
bursitis
calcaneus
carpal
cervical vertebrae
circumduction
clavicle
coccyx
diaphysis
diarthroses
diploë
dislocation

endosteum
epiphysis
ethmoid
extension
femur
fibula
flexion
fontanel
fracture
frontal
gliding joint
gout
growth plate
hangman's fracture
hinge joint
humerus
indirect force
inferior concha
intraosseous
joint
knee dislocation
kneecap dislocation
kyphosis
lacrimal
laryngoscope blade

(continues)

Key Words (continued)

lordosis	pulse
lumbar vertebrae	pulse points
magnum foramen	radius
mandible	rheumatoid arthritis
maxillae	rickets
medullary canal	rotation
metacarpal	sacrum
metatarsal	scapulae
nasal	scoliosis
navicular bone	skeletal system
occipital	slipped (herniated) disk
ossification	sphenoid
osteoarthritis	spongy bone
osteoblast	sprain
osteoclast	supination
osteocyte	suture
osteomyelitis	synarthroses
osteoporosis	synovial cavity
osteosarcoma	synovial fluid
palatine	synovial membrane
paralysis	tarsal
parietal	temporal
patella	thoracic vertebrae
periosteum	tibia
phalanges	traction device
phrenic nerve	true ribs
pivot joint	vomer
point tenderness	whiplash injury
pronation	zygomatic

If you have ever visited a beach, you may have seen a jellyfish floating lightly near the surface. The organs of the jellyfish are buoyed by the water. But if a wave should chance to deposit the jellyfish on the beach, it would collapse into a disorganized mass of tissue. This is because the jellyfish does not possess a supportive framework or skeleton. Fortunately, we humans do not suffer such a fate because we have a solid, bony skeleton to support body structures.

The **skeletal system** comprises the bony framework of the body. It is composed of 206 individual bones in the adult; some bones are hinged, whereas others are fused to one another.

FUNCTIONS

The skeletal system has five specific functions:

1. It *supports* body structures and provides shape to the body.

2. It *protects* the soft and delicate internal organs. For example, the cranium protects the brain, the inner ear, and parts of the eye. The ribs and breastbone protect the heart and lungs; the vertebral column encases and protects the spinal cord.

3. It allows *movement* and *anchorage* of muscles. Muscles that are attached to the skeleton are called skeletal muscles. Upon contraction, these muscles exert a pull on a bone and so move it. In this manner, bones play a vital part in body movement, serving as passively operated levers.

4. It provides *mineral storage.* Bones are a storage depot for minerals such as calcium and phosphorus. In case of inadequate nutrition, the body is able to draw on these reserves. For example, if the blood calcium dips below normal, the bone releases the necessary amount of stored calcium into the bloodstream. When calcium levels exceed normal, calcium release from the skeletal system is inhibited. In this way the skeletal system helps to maintain blood calcium homeostasis.

5. It supports *hematopoiesis,* the development of blood cells. The red marrow of the bone is the site of blood cell formation. Red marrow is found in long bones, sternum, and pelvis.

STRUCTURE AND FORMATION OF BONE

Bones are composed of microscopic cells called **osteocytes** (from the Greek word *osteon,* meaning "bone"). An osteocyte is a mature bone cell. Bone is made up of 35% organic material, 65% inorganic mineral salts, and water.

The organic part derives from a protein called bone collagen, a fibrous material. Between these collagenous fibers is a jellylike material. The organic substances of bone give it a certain degree of flexibility. The inorganic portion of bone is made from mineral salts such as calcium phosphate, calcium carbonate, calcium fluoride, magnesium phosphate, sodium oxide, and sodium chloride. These minerals give bone its hardness and durability.

A bony skeleton can be compared with steel-reinforced concrete. The collagenous fibers may be compared with flexible steel supports, and mineral salts with concrete. When pressure is applied to a bone, the flexible, organic material prevents bone damage, while the mineral elements resist crushing under pressure.

● BONE FORMATION

The embryonic skeleton is initially composed of collagenous protein fibers secreted by the osteoblasts (primitive embryonic cells). Later, during embryonic development, cartilage is deposited between the fibers. At this stage the embryo's skeleton consists of collagenous protein fibers and hyaline (clear) cartilage. During the eighth week of embryonic development, ossification begins. That is, mineral matter starts to replace previously formed cartilage, creating bone. Infant bones are soft and pliable because of incomplete ossification at birth. A familiar example is the soft spot on a baby's head, the fontanel. The bone has not yet been formed there, although it will become hardened later. Ossification as a result of mineral deposits continues through childhood. As bones ossify, they become hard and more capable of bearing weight.

● STRUCTURE OF LONG BONE

A typical long bone contains a shaft, or diaphysis. This is a hollow cylinder of hard, compact bone. It is what makes a long bone strong and hard, yet light enough for movement. At the ends (extremes) of the diaphysis are the epiphyses, Figure 6-1.

In the center of the shaft is the broad medullary canal. This is filled with yellow bone marrow, mostly made of fat cells. The marrow also contains many blood vessels and some cells that form white blood cells, called leukocytes. The yellow marrow functions as a fat storage center. The marrow canal is lined and the cavity kept intact by the endosteum.

The medullary canal is surrounded by compact or hard bone. Haversian canals branch into the compact bone. They carry blood vessels that nourish the osteocytes, or bone cells. Where less strength is needed in the bone, some of the hard bone is dissolved away, leaving spongy bone.

The ends of the long bones contain the red marrow, where some red blood cells, called erythrocytes, and some white blood cells are made. The outside of the bone is covered with the periosteum, a tough, fibrous tissue containing blood vessels, lymph vessels, and nerves. The periosteum is necessary for bone growth, repair, and nutrition.

Covering the epiphysis is a thin layer of articular cartilage, which acts as a shock absorber between two bones that meet to form a joint.

● GROWTH

Bones grow in length and ossify from the center of the diaphysis toward the epiphyseal ends. A long bone, for example, grows lengthwise in an area called the growth zone. Ossification occurs there, causing the bone to lengthen; this causes the epiphyses to grow away from the middle of the diaphysis. It is a sensible growth process, because it does not interfere with the articulation between two bones.

A bone increases its circumference by the osteoblasts' addition of more bone to the outer surface of the diaphysis. Osteoblasts are bone cells that deposit the new bone. As girth increases, bone material is dissolved from the central part of the diaphysis. This forms an internal cavity called the marrow cavity, or medullary canal. The medullary canal gets larger as the diameter of the bone increases.

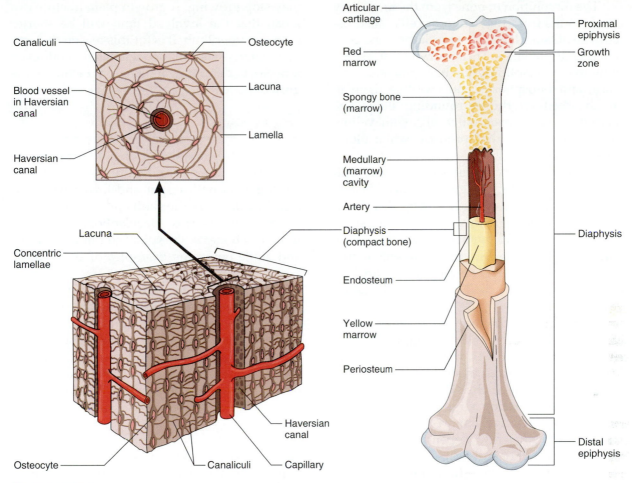

FIGURE 6–1   *Structure of a typical long bone.*

STREET SMART -

The medullary canal of the bone has a rich supply of blood vessels, such as arteries and veins. These blood vessels eventually return to the central circulation of the body. For this reason, any ability to inject medications or add fluids to the blood vessels in a bone means that the medication or fluid will eventually get into the rest of the body.

Physicians realized this fact years ago and developed a special bone needle called an **intraosseous** ("within the bone"; IO) needle. IO needles are now widely used by many emergency medical services (EMS) providers to provide life-saving medications and fluids when an intravenous (IV) line is not available. ■

The dissolution of bone from the medullary canal results from the action of cells called osteoclasts. **Osteoclasts** are very large bone cells that secrete enzymes. These enzymes digest the bony material, splitting the bone minerals, calcium, and phosphorus and enabling them to be absorbed by the surrounding fluid. The medullary canal eventually fills with yellow marrow and cells that produce white blood cells.

The bone shaft continues to lengthen until all the epiphyseal cartilage is ossified. At this point, bone growth stops. This fact is helpful in determining further growth in a child. First, an x-ray of the child's wrists is taken. If some epiphyseal cartilage remains, there will be further growth. If there is no epiphyseal cartilage left, the child has reached his or her full stature (height).

The average growth cycle in females continues to approximately 18 years; in males, to approximately 20 or 21 years, although new bone growth can occur in a broken bone at any time. Bone cells near the site of a fracture become active, secreting large amounts of new bone within a relatively short time. Bone healing proceeds efficiently, depending on the age and health of the individual. However, if a child's bone is broken (fractured) near the epiphyseal cartilage, or **growth plate**, the bone may stop growing. A growth plate fracture can mean that the involved limb will be shorter than the other limb. It is for this reason that any bone injury should be evaluated, and even x-rayed, to determine if there is a fracture of the growth plate.

● BONE TYPES

Bones are classified as one of four types on the basis of their form, Figure 6-2. *Long* bones are found in both upper and lower arms and legs. The bones of the skull are examples of *flat* bones, as are the ribs. *Irregular* bones are represented by bones of the spinal column. The wrist and ankle bones are examples of *short* bones, which appear cubelike in shape.

The bones in the hand are short, making flexible movement possible. The same is true of the irregular bones of the spinal column. The thigh bone is a long bone needed for support of the strong leg muscles and the weight of the body. The degree of movement at a joint is determined by bone shape and joint structure.

● PARTS OF THE SKELETAL SYSTEM

The skeletal system is composed of two main parts: the axial skeleton and the appendicular skeleton, Figure 6-3.

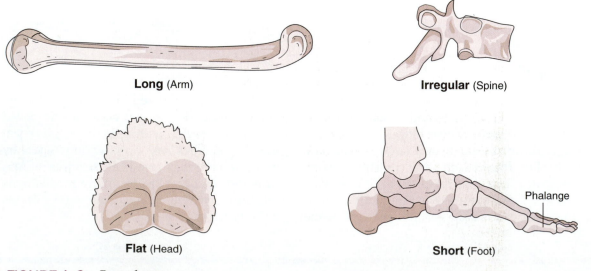

Long (Arm)

Irregular (Spine)

Flat (Head)

Short (Foot)

Phalange

● **FIGURE 6–2**   *Bone shapes.*

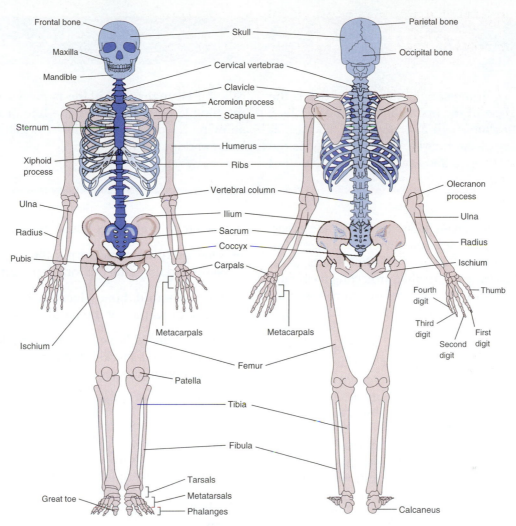

● **FIGURE 6–3**   *The axial skeleton* (blue) *and the appendicular skeleton.*

● AXIAL SKELETON

The **axial skeleton** consists of the skull, spinal column, ribs, sternum (breastbone), and hyoid bone. The hyoid bone is a U-shaped bone in the neck, to which the tongue is attached.

Skull

The skull is composed of the cranium and facial bones. The cranium houses and protects the delicate brain; the facial bones guard and support the sensory organs: the eyes, ears, nose, and mouth. Some of the facial bones, such as the nasal bones, are made of bone and cartilage. For example, the upper part of the

nose (bridge) is bone, whereas the lower part is cartilage.

Cranial bones are thin and slightly curved bones that form a sphere called the cranium. During infancy, these bones are held snugly together by an irregular band of connective tissue called a suture. These sutures allow the cranium to expand as the brain grows. As the child grows older and the brain stops growing, this connective tissue ossifies and turns into hard bone. Thus the cranium becomes a highly efficient, dome-shaped shield for the brain. The dome shape affords better protection than a flat surface, deflecting blows directed toward the head. The cranial bones of the cranium are actually not one bone

✳ STREET SMART -

Interestingly, the hyoid bone is the only bone in the body that does not contact, or articulate, with another bone. Located at the base of the tongue, the hyoid bone is the firm surface against which a special tool called a **laryngoscope blade** is placed to lift the tongue and jaw out of the line of sight, allowing direct visualization of the vocal cords and trachea. ◼

but two bones layered one on top of the other like a wafer. In between these two bones is a spongy tissue called **diploë**. Diploë acts as a shock-absorbing gel, further protecting the brain.

As a result of this organization, the cranium is able to withstand a great deal more force than other bones. If a swollen, painful deformity is noted on the skull, leading to a suspicion of a skull fracture, it can be assumed that a great deal of force must have been used to create the injury. The skull is not invulnerable, and a particularly hard blow may fracture it. This can lead to an injury of the brain as well. If the bone's surface is depressed, serious injury to underlying brain tissue may have resulted. A depressed skull fracture may require surgery to relieve the pressure from the brain.

There are 22 bones in the skull, Figure 6-4. There are eight bones in the cranium:

- One **frontal** bone forms the forehead

- Two **parietal** bones form the roof and sides of the skull

- Two **temporal** bones house the ears

- One **occipital** bone forms the base of the skull and contains the foramen magnum

- One **ethmoid** bone (located between the eyes) forms part of the nasal septum

- One **sphenoid** bone, which resembles a bat, is considered the key bone of the skull; all other bones connect to it

There are 14 facial bones:

- Five nasal bones (two are **nasal** bones that form the bridge of the nose [your glasses sit on this bone]; one is the **vomer** bone, which forms the lower part, or midline, of the nasal septum; and two are **inferior concha** bones, which make up the side walls of the nasal cavity)

- Two **maxillae** bones make up the upper jaw

- Two **lacrimal** bones (in the inner aspect of the eyes) contain the tear ducts

CHANGES OF AGING

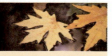

There are two gaps in the sutures of an infant, called the soft spots, or fontanels. Only a layer of strong connective tissue covers the fontanels and protects the soft brain underneath from injury. The anterior fontanel is located above the forehead; the posterior fontanel is at the base of the skull at the rear.

As a child grows, these fontanels become smaller and smaller; by approximately 9 months to 1 year, just as an infant starts to walk, they close. ◼

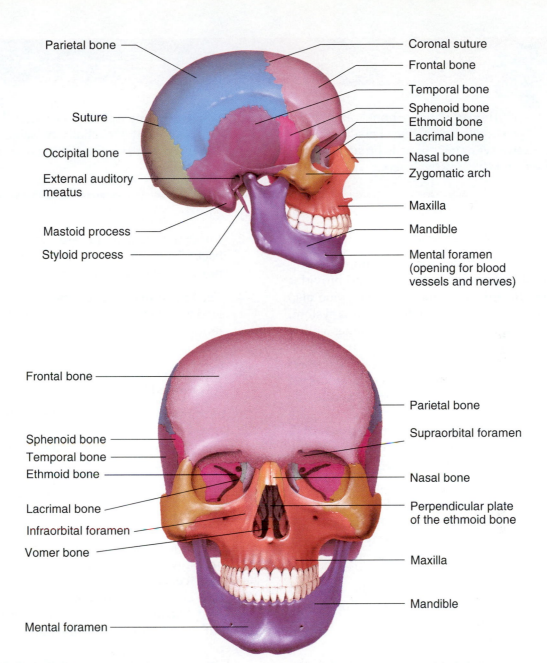

● **FIGURE 6–4**   *Bones of the skull.*

- Two **zygomatic** bones form the prominence of the cheek and the floor of the orbit that holds the eye in place

- Two **palatine** bones form the hard palate of the mouth

- One **mandible** bone is the lower jaw and the only movable bone in the face

The skull contains large spaces within the facial bones, referred to as paranasal sinuses. These sinuses are lined with mucous membranes. When a person suffers from a cold, flu, or hay fever, the membranes become inflamed and swollen, producing a copious amount of mucus. This may lead to sinus pain and a "stuffy" nasal sensation.

STREET SMART

The zygomatic bone, also called the cheekbone, holds the eyeball in place. When the zygomatic bone is broken, called a **blowout fracture**, the eyeball can fall forward and the retina can become detached from the rear of the eyeball. A detached retina is a cause of permanent blindness. ■

Spinal Column/Vertebrae

The spine, or vertebral column, is strong and flexible. It supports the head and provides for the attachment of the ribs. The spine also encloses the spinal cord of the nervous system.

The spine consists of small bones called vertebrae, which are separated from each other by pads of cartilage tissue called intervertebral disks, Figure 6-5. These disks serve as cushions between the vertebrae and act as shock absorbers.

The vertebral column is divided into five sections named according to the area of the body where they are located, see Figure 6-5 (A).

1. **Cervical vertebrae** (7) are located in the neck area. The **atlas**, see Figure 6-5 (B), is the first cervical vertebra that articulates, or is jointed, with the occipital bone of the skull. This permits us to nod our heads. On the **axis**, Figure 6-5 (C), the second cervical vertebra is the odontoid process, which forms a pivot on which the atlas rotates; this permits us to turn our heads.

2. **Thoracic vertebrae** (12) are located in the chest area. They articulate with the ribs.

3. **Lumbar vertebrae** (5) are located in the back. They have large bodies that bear most of the body's weight.

4. The **sacrum** is a wedge-shaped body created by five fused bones. It forms the posterior pelvic girdle and serves as an articulation point for the hips.

5. The **coccyx** is also known as the tailbone. It is formed by four fused bones.

The spinal nerves leave the brain through the largest opening in the skull, called the **magnum foramen**, and enter the spinal column. The spinal nerves enter and leave the spinal column through the openings (foramen) between the vertebrae. The spine is curved instead of straight. A curved spine has more strength than a straight spine. Before birth, the thoracic and sacral regions are convex curves. As the infant learns to hold up its head, the cervical region becomes concave. When the child learns to stand, the lumbar region also becomes concave. This completes the four curves of a normal adult human spine.

A typical vertebra, as seen in Figure 6-6, contains three basic parts: body, foramen, and

CHANGES OF AGING

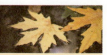

Vertebral disks become thinner throughout the life span, which accounts for a loss of height as persons age. ■

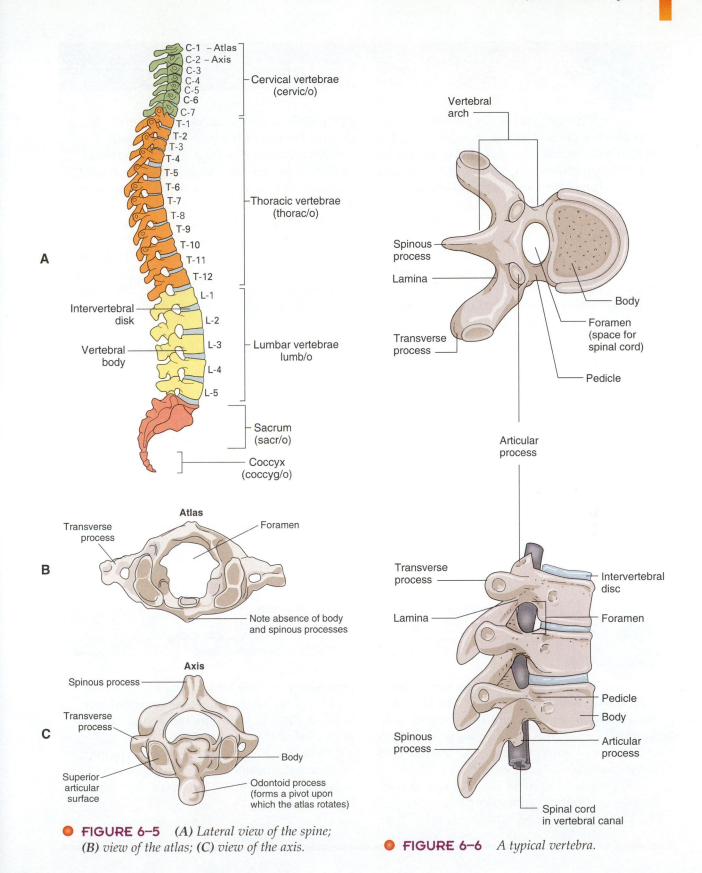

A

C-1 – Atlas
C-2 – Axis
C-3
C-4
C-5
C-6
C-7
} Cervical vertebrae (cervic/o)

T-1
T-2
T-3
T-4
T-5
T-6
T-7
T-8
T-9
T-10
T-11
T-12
} Thoracic vertebrae (thorac/o)

L-1
L-2
L-3
L-4
L-5
} Lumbar vertebrae lumb/o

Intervertebral disk

Vertebral body

Sacrum (sacr/o)

Coccyx (coccyg/o)

Vertebral arch

Spinous process

Lamina

Transverse process

Body

Foramen (space for spinal cord)

Pedicle

Articular process

Atlas

Transverse process

Foramen

Note absence of body and spinous processes

B

Axis

Spinous process

Transverse process

Body

Superior articular surface

Odontoid process (forms a pivot upon which the atlas rotates)

C

Transverse process

Intervertebral disc

Lamina

Foramen

Pedicle

Body

Spinous process

Articular process

Spinal cord in vertebral canal

● **FIGURE 6–5**   *(A) Lateral view of the spine; (B) view of the atlas; (C) view of the axis.*

● **FIGURE 6–6**   *A typical vertebra.*

STREET SMART -

The cervical spine is one of the most commonly injured portions of the spinal column. For this reason it is important for EMS providers to understand the unique relationship of the cervical spinal column and the nerves within it, called the spinal cord.

The first cervical spine, the atlas, is under and partially inside the skull. From that position it is relatively safe from injury. The second cervical spine, the axis, is found just at the base of the skull. A fracture of the second cervical vertebrae, axis, is called a **hangman's fracture**. A hangman's fracture is not usually compatible with life because the nerves that control the rest of the body are severed.

A fracture of the third and fourth cervical vertebrae can cut, or transect, the spinal cord, resulting in loss of motion, or **paralysis**, of all four extremities.

A fracture of the third, fourth, and fifth cervical vertebrae can also sever the nerve that controls the diaphragm, called the **phrenic nerve**, resulting in paralysis of the diaphragm. The diaphragm is the main muscle of breathing, and suffocation may result. ■

several bony outcroppings called processes. The large, solid, donut-shaped part of the vertebra is known as the body; the central opening within the body, made for the spinal cord, is called the foramen. Above and slightly in front of the foramen, two winglike bony structures protrude from the body of the vertebrae, called the transverse processes as well as the spinous process and the articular processes.

Ribs and Sternum

The thoracic area of the body is protected and supported by the thoracic vertebrae, ribs, and sternum.

The sternum (breastbone) is divided into three parts: the upper region (manubrium), the body of the sternum, and a lower cartilaginous part called the xiphoid process. Attached to each side of the upper region, or manubrium, of the sternum, by means of liga-

STREET SMART -

Occasionally a person with a back injury may believe that his or her back has been broken. An EMS provider immediately might associate the complications of paralysis that come with a spinal bone fracture and subsequent spinal cord injury.

Fortunately, in most cases of spinal fractures it is either the spinous process or one of the transverse processes that is broken. These processes protrude and can be felt down the middle of the back. The inner vertebral arch, being a ring, is very strong, and it takes a great deal of force to break it.

However, EMS providers treat all painful, swollen deformities down the spinal column as potential vertebral fractures that could lead to paralysis. ■

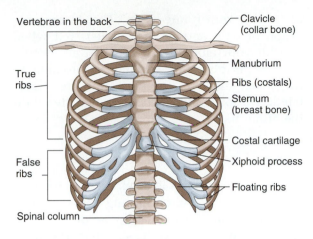

Vertebrae in the back

Clavicle (collar bone)

Manubrium

True ribs

Ribs (costals)

Sternum (breast bone)

Costal cartilage

Xiphoid process

False ribs

Floating ribs

Spinal column

● **FIGURE 6–7**   *Ribs and sternum.*

ments, are the two clavicles (collarbones). The juncture of the manubrium and the body of the sternum is called the sternal angle. The sternal angle is an important topographical landmark.

Seven pairs of costal cartilages join seven pairs of ribs directly to the sternum. These are known as **true ribs**, Figure 6-7. The human body contains 12 pairs of ribs. The first seven pairs are true ribs. The next three pairs are "false ribs" because their costal cartilages are attached to the seventh rib instead of directly to the sternum. Finally, the last two pairs of ribs, connected neither to the costal cartilages nor the sternum, are floating ribs.

● THE APPENDICULAR SKELETON

The **appendicular skeleton** includes the bones in the upper and lower extremities. There are 126 bones in the appendicular skeleton.

Shoulder Girdle

The shoulder girdle (also called the pectoral girdle) consists of four bones: two curved **clavicles** (collarbones) and two triangular **scapulae** (shoulder bones). Using a model of the human skeleton, we observe two broad, flat triangular surfaces (scapulae) on the upper posterior surface. They permit the attachment of muscles that assist in arm movement, while also serving as a place of attachment for the arms. The two clavicles, attached at one end to the scapulae and at the other to the sternum, help to brace the shoulders and prevent excessive forward motion.

Because of the attachment of the shoulder girdle bones to one another, any force that is applied to one bone can logically be assumed to possibly affect the other bones. This type of injury, injury of another bone not directly affected, is called **indirect force**.

Arm

The bones of the arm are the humerus, the radius, and the ulna. The humerus is located in the upper arm and the radius and ulna in the forearm.

✦ STREET SMART - - - - - - - - - - - - - - - - - -

Arteries, nerves, and veins lie directly next to bones that provide protection to these very important structures. Wherever a bone lies close to the skin, an artery can be felt, or palpated. When an artery is felt, the rhythmic flow of blood, called a **pulse**, can be felt. These locations along the bones are called **pulse points** and can be compressed to stop blood flow to the distal extremity.

The humerus has a pulse point, called the **brachial pulse**, that can be felt under the arm. The brachial pulse can be compressed to stop bleeding in the forearm or hand. ■

The **humerus**, the only bone in the upper arm, is the second largest bone in the body. The upper end of the humerus has a smooth, round surface called the head, which articulates with the scapula. The upper humerus is attached to the scapula socket (glenoid fossa) by muscles and ligaments. These muscles are the biceps and triceps brachii.

The forearm is composed of two bones: the radius and the ulna. The **radius** is the bone running up the thumb side of the forearm. Its name derives from the fact that it can rotate in a radius around the ulna. This is an important characteristic, permitting the hand to rotate freely and with greater flexibility. The ulna's range of motion, by contrast, is far more limited. The ulna is the largest bone in the forearm; at its upper end, it produces a projection called the olecranon process, forming the elbow, Figure 6-8. When you bang your elbow (the olecranon process), it is usually referred to

as "hitting your funny bone." The strange sensation of pain and tingling that is felt when you hit your elbow on a hard surface occurs because peripheral nerves that run proximal to the bones and over the olecranon are stimulated. The olecranon process articulates with the humerus.

Hand

The human hand is a remarkable piece of skeletal engineering, permitting vast ranges of motion resulting in exceptional dexterity. It contains more bones for its size than any other part of the body. Collectively, the hand has twenty-seven bones, Figure 6-9.

The wrist bone, or **carpals**, is composed of eight small bones arranged in two rows. They are held together by ligaments that permit sufficient movement to allow the wrist a great deal of mobility and flexion. However, there is very

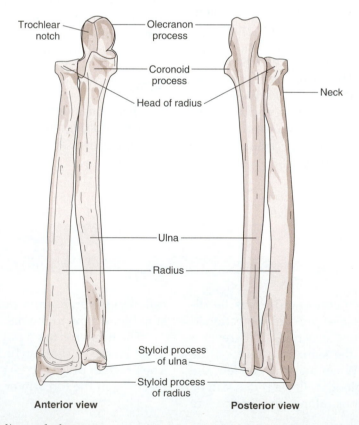

Trochlear notch
Olecranon process
Coronoid process
Head of radius
Neck
Ulna
Radius
Styloid process of ulna
Styloid process of radius

Anterior view   **Posterior view**

● **FIGURE 6–8**   *Radius and ulna.*

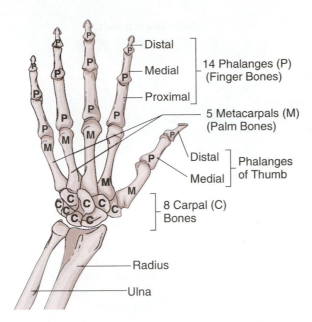

Distal
Medial
Proximal

14 Phalanges (P)
(Finger Bones)

5 Metacarpals (M)
(Palm Bones)

Distal
Medial

Phalanges
of Thumb

8 Carpal (C)
Bones

Radius

Ulna

● **FIGURE 6–9**   *The 27 bones of the left hand.*

little lateral (side) movement of these carpal bones. On the palm side of the hand are attached a number of short muscles that supply mobility to the little finger and thumb.

Falling onto an outstretched hand and landing on the thumb can cause a fracture of a small carpal bone next to the thumb called the **navicular bone**. The navicular bone is partially responsible for the movement of the thumb, particularly the pincer movement, which permits the hand to grasp objects. Acute pain at one spot, called **point tenderness**, in the hollow place behind the thumb (the **autonomic sniff box**), as well as an inability to move the thumb, should lead the EMS provider to suspect a navicular fracture.

The hand is composed of two parts: the palmar surface, with five **metacarpal** bones, and five fingers composed of fourteen **phalanges** (singular, phalanx). Each finger, except for the thumb, has three phalanges; the thumb has two. There are hinge joints between each phalanx, allowing the fingers to be bent easily. The thumb is the most flexible finger because the end of the metacarpal bone is rounded and there are muscles attached to it from the hand itself. Thus the thumb can be extended across the palm of the hand. Only

humans and other primates possess such a digit, known as an opposable thumb.

Pelvic Girdle

In youth the pelvic girdle (innominate bones) consists of three bones. Found on either side of the midline of the body, the innominate bones include the ilium, the ischium, and the pubis. These bones eventually fuse with the sacrum to form a bowl-shaped structure called the pelvic girdle. Eventually these two sets of innominate bones form a joint with the bones in front, called the symphysis pubis, and with the sacrum in back, as the sacroiliac joint.

The pelvic girdle serves as an area of attachment for the bones and muscles of the leg. It also provides support for the viscera (soft organs) of the lower abdominal region. There is an obvious anatomical difference between the male and female pelvis, Figure 6-10. The female pelvis is much wider than that of the male. This is necessary for childbearing (pregnancy) and childbirth. In addition, the pelvic inlet is wider in the female, and the pelvic bones are lighter and smoother than those of the male.

Upper Leg

The upper leg contains the longest and strongest bone in the body, the thigh bone, or **femur**. The upper part of the femur has a smooth, rounded head, Figure 6-11. It fits neatly into a cavity of the ilium known as the acetabulum, forming a ball-and-socket joint. The femur is an amazingly strong bone. A direct compression force applied to the top of the femur of from 15,000 to 19,000 pounds per square inch is required to break it.

Lower Leg

The lower leg consists of two bones: the **tibia** and the **fibula**. The tibia is the largest of the two lower leg bones. The **patella** (kneecap) is found in front of the knee joint. It is a flat, triangular, sesamoid bone, see Figure 6-3. The patella is formed in the tendons of the large

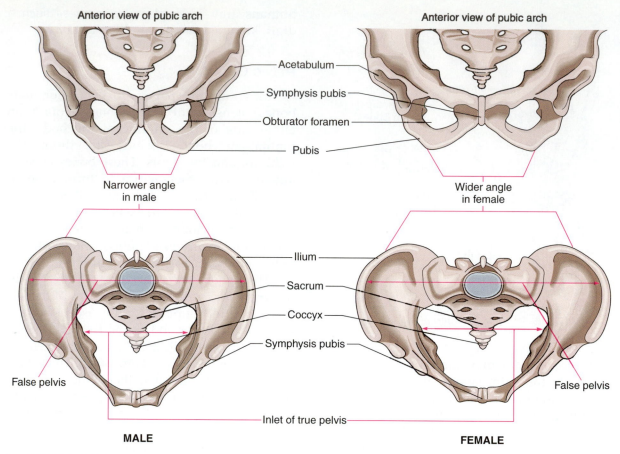

Anterior view of pubic arch

Anterior view of pubic arch

Acetabulum

Symphysis pubis

Obturator foramen

Pubis

Narrower angle
in male

Wider angle
in female

Ilium

Sacrum

Coccyx

Symphysis pubis

False pelvis

False pelvis

Inlet of true pelvis

MALE

FEMALE

● **FIGURE 6–10** *Comparison of the male and female pelvises.*

muscle in front of the femur (quadriceps femoris). In females it appears at approximately 2 to 3 years of age; in males, at about 6. The patella, attached to the tibia by a ligament, ossifies as early as puberty. Surrounding the patella are four bursae, which serve to cushion the knee joint.

The fibula is found deep in the calf muscle and is seldom broken, except by direct force to the back of the calf. Even if the fibula is fractured, it is seldom repaired, because it a non–weight-bearing bone.

Ankle

The ankle (tarsus) contains seven **tarsal** bones. These bones provide a connection between the foot and leg bones. The largest ankle bone is the heel bone, or **calcaneus**. The tibia

and fibula articulate with a broad tarsal bone called the talus. Ankle movement is a sliding motion, allowing the foot to extend and flex when walking.

Foot

The foot has five **metatarsal** bones, which are somewhat comparable with the metacarpals of the hand. However, there is an important difference between the metatarsals and the metacarpals within the palm of the hand. The metatarsal and tarsal bones are arranged to form two distinct arches, which of course are not found in the palm of the hand. One arch runs longitudinally from the calcaneus to the heads of the metatarsals; it is called the longitudinal arch. The other, which lies perpendicular to the longitudinal arch in the metatarsal re-

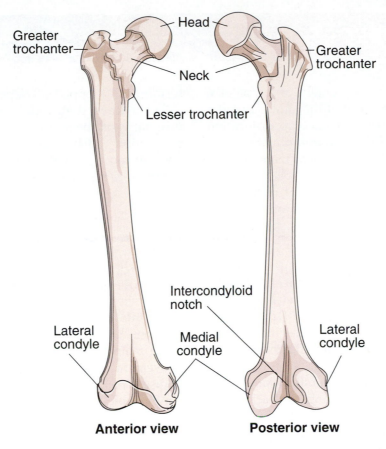

Head
Greater trochanter
Greater trochanter
Neck
Lesser trochanter
Intercondyloid notch
Lateral condyle
Medial condyle
Lateral condyle
Anterior view
Posterior view

● **FIGURE 6–11** *Anterior/posterior view of the femur.*

gion, is known as the transverse arch. Strong ligaments and leg muscle tendons help to hold the foot bones in place to form those two arches. In turn, arches strengthen the foot and provide flexibility and spring to the stride. In certain cases these arches may "fall" as a result of weakened foot ligaments and tendons. Then downward pressure by weight of the body

STREET SMART

Hip fractures are common bony injuries in the elderly. Although called hip fractures, these are actually fractures of the femur, usually at the neck of the femur.

During aging, bones become brittle as a result of a process called osteoporosis, explained later in the chapter. Therefore bones break more easily. Hip fractures can occur as a result of a sudden twist or turn, after which the patient falls to the ground, instead of the more traditional mechanism of injury in which the patient falls and then breaks a bone. Carefully listening to the patient's story may reveal that the patient first heard the crack of the bone breaking before the fall. ■

STREET SMART

A lateral movement of the patella, as a result of force, out of the joint is called a **kneecap dislocation**. A kneecap dislocation is usually treated with a minimum of complications because there are no proximal nerves or blood vessels.

When there is a movement of the tibia and fibula off the femur and out of joint, forming a stepped-off appearance, it is called a **knee dislocation**. Because of the proximity of the popliteal arteries, a knee dislocation can be a surgical emergency. A knee dislocation, with a loss of peripheral pulses, can result in amputation of the leg below the knee. ■

slowly flattens them, causing "flatfeet." Flatfeet cause a good deal of stress and strain on the foot muscles, leading to pain and fatigue. Factors that may lead to chronic flatfeet include excessive weight, poor posture, and improperly fitting shoes.

The toes are similar in composition to the fingers. There are three phalanges in each, with the exception of the big toe which has only two. Because the big toe is not opposable like the thumb, it cannot be brought across the sole. There are a total of fourteen phalanges in each foot, Figure 6-12.

JOINTS AND RELATED STRUCTURES

Joints, or articulations, are points of contact between two bones. Joints are classified into three main types according to their degree of movement: diarthroses (movable), amphiarthroses (partially movable), and synarthroses (immovable), Figure 6-13.

Most of the joints in the body are **diarthroses**. They tend to have the same structure. These movable joints consist of three main parts: articular cartilage, a bursa (joint capsule), and a synovial (joint) cavity.

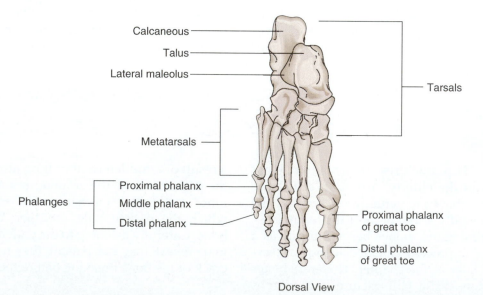

Calcaneous
Talus
Lateral maleolus
Tarsals
Metatarsals
Phalanges
Proximal phalanx
Middle phalanx
Distal phalanx
Proximal phalanx of great toe
Distal phalanx of great toe

Dorsal View

● **FIGURE 6-12**   *The foot—dorsal view.*

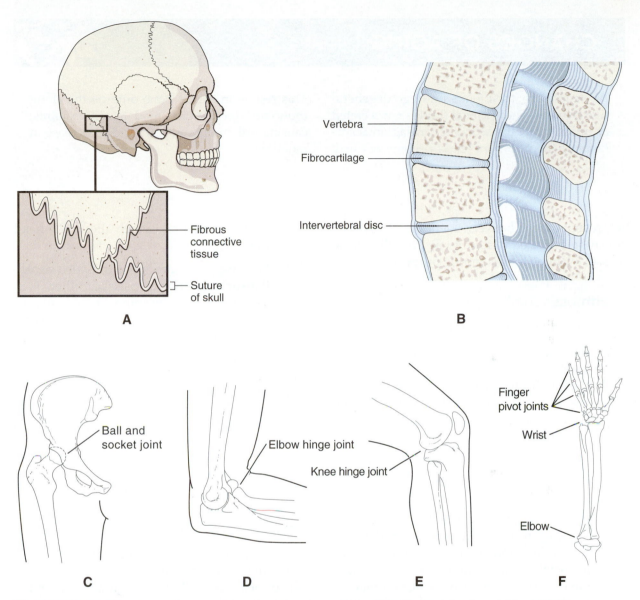

● FIGURE 6–13   *Types of joints: **(A)** a synarthrosis, an immovable fibrous joint (cranial bones); **(B)** an amphiarthrosis, a slightly movable cartilaginous joint (ribs or vertebrae); **(C–F)** diarthroses, freely movable hinge of ball-and-socket joints.*

When two movable bones meet at a joint, their surfaces do not touch. The two articular (joint) surfaces are covered with a smooth, slippery cap known as **articular cartilage**. This articular cartilage helps to absorb shocks and prevent friction between parts.

Enclosing two articular surfaces of the bone is a tough, fibrous connective tissue called an articular capsule. Lining the articular capsule is a **synovial membrane**, which secretes **synovial fluid** (a lubricating substance) into the **synovial cavity** (an area between the two articular cartilages). The synovial fluid reduces the friction of joint movement.

The clefts in connective tissue between muscles, tendons, ligaments, and bones contain **bursa sacs**. An inflammation of this area is called **bursitis**. The synovial fluid serves as a lubricant

CHANGES OF AGING

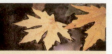

As people age, their joints undergo degenerative changes. The synovial fluid is not secreted as quickly, and the articular cartilaginous surfaces of the two bone ends become ossified. This results in excess bone outgrowths along the joint edges, which tend to stiffen joints, causing inflammation, pain, and a decrease in mobility. ■

to prevent friction between a tendon and a bone. It can be aspirated (withdrawn) from the bursa sacs to examine for diagnostic purposes.

Diarthroses Joints

There are four types of diarthroses joints:

1. **Ball-and-socket joints** allow the greatest freedom of movement. In these joints, one bone has a ball-shaped head, which nestles into a concave socket of the second bone. Shoulders and hips have ball-and-socket joints.

2. **Hinge joints** move in one direction or plane, as in the knees, elbows, and outer joints of the fingers.

3. **Pivot joints** are those with an extension rotating in a second, arch-shaped bone. The radius and ulna (long bones of the forearm) are pivot joints. Another example is the joint between the atlas (first cervical vertebra in the neck), which supports the head, and the axis (second cervical vertebra), which allows the head to rotate.

4. **Gliding joints** are those in which nearly flat surfaces glide across each other, as in the vertebrae of the spine. These joints enable the torso to bend forward, backward, and sideways, as well as rotate.

Between each body of the vertebrae are fibrous disks. At the center of each fibrous disk is a pulpy, elastic material, which loses its resiliency with increased usage and age. Disks can be compressed by sudden and forceful jolts to the spine. This may cause a disk to protrude from the vertebrae and impinge on the spinal nerves, resulting in extreme pain. Such a condition is known as a herniated or slipped disk.

Amphiarthroses Joints

Amphiarthroses are partially movable joints that have cartilage between their articular surfaces. Examples are the attachment of the ribs to the spine and the symphysis pubis, the joint between the two pubic bones.

STREET SMART

On-the-job back injuries are the single greatest cause of disability among EMS providers. Recognizing this fact, many EMS employers have established back care programs that teach EMS providers how to properly lift, carry, and exercise their back to prevent injury. Every EMS provider should make the effort to lift correctly, possibly preventing a debilitating back injury from prematurely ending a career in EMS. ■

Synarthroses Joints

Synarthroses are immovable joints linked by tough, fibrous connective tissue. They are found in the adult cranium. The bones are fused together in cranial joints, commonly called **sutures**, that form a heavy protective cover for the brain.

Ligaments are fibrous bands that connect bones and cartilages and serve as support for muscles. Joints are also bound together by ligaments. Tendons are fibrous cords that connect muscles to bones.

● TYPES OF MOTION

Joints can move in many directions, Figure 6-14. **Flexion** is the act of bringing two

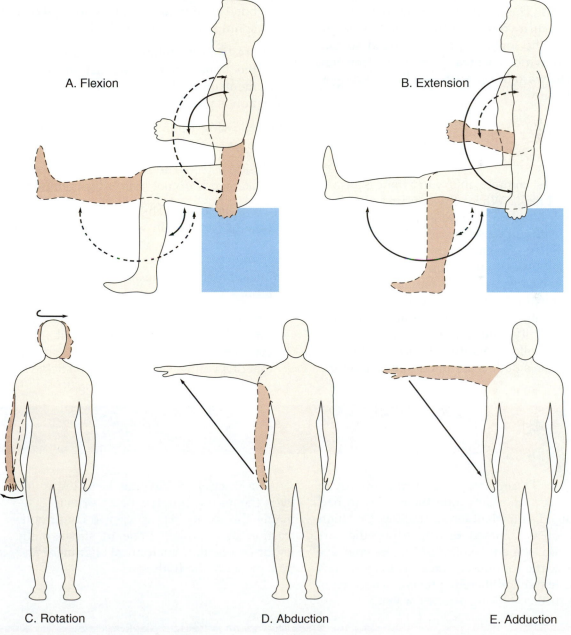

A. Flexion

B. Extension

C. Rotation

D. Abduction

E. Adduction

● **FIGURE 6–14**   *Joint movements.*

bones closer together, decreasing the angle between the bones.

Extension is the act of increasing the angle between two bones, which results in a straightening motion. Abduction is the movement of an extremity away from the midline (an imaginary line that divides the body from head to toe). Adduction is movement toward the midline. Circumduction includes flexion, extension, abduction, and adduction.

Rotation allows a bone to move around a central axis. This type of pivot motion occurs when you turn your head from side to side. In pronation the forearm turns the hand so the palm is down or backward. In supination the palm is forward or up, such as when cradling a bowl of soup.

● DISORDERS OF THE BONES AND JOINTS

The most common injury to a bone is a fracture, or break. When this occurs, there is swelling caused by bleeding into the tissues. Persons with a fracture, in addition to general pain, experience a sharp pain when the fracture site is compressed, called point tenderness.

In some cases the bones remain in line and no deformity of the bone can be appreciated externally. In other cases the bones are out of line and a deformity, a bump, can be felt.

Any swollen, painful deformity that is along a bone's path is assumed to be a fracture until proven otherwise by medical imaging (x-ray).

There are three primary methods used to restore bone:

1. *Closed reduction*—the bony fragments are brought into alignment by manipulation, and a cast or splint is applied.

2. *Open reduction*—through surgical intervention, devices such as wires, metal plates, or screws are used to hold the bone in alignment, and an external cast or splint may then be applied as well.

3. *Traction*—a pulling force is used to hold the bones in neutral anatomical alignment until either open or closed reduction is possible.

The following outline identifies the common types of fractures, Figure 6-15:

- *Closed/simple*—The bone is broken, but the broken ends do not pierce through the skin.

- *Open/compound*—This is the most serious type of fracture, in which the broken bone ends pierce and protrude through the skin, leaving an external wound. This can cause infection of the bone and of the neighboring tissues.

- *Greenstick*—This is the simplest type of fracture. The bone is partly bent, but it never completely separates. The break is similar to that of a young, sap-filled wood stick whose

STREET SMART

During the first World War there was a 50% mortality rate for men who had sustained a midshaft femur fracture. Dr. Hugh O. Thomas, a noted British orthopedic surgeon, developed a splinting device that applied gentle continuous traction along the axis of the femur and thereby prevented bone ends from further injuring arteries or veins.

The traction device has been improved over the years, but the basic principle remains the same: Apply gentle continuous traction to a broken bone to stabilize the femur in a neutral anatomical alignment and thus preserve the limb. ■

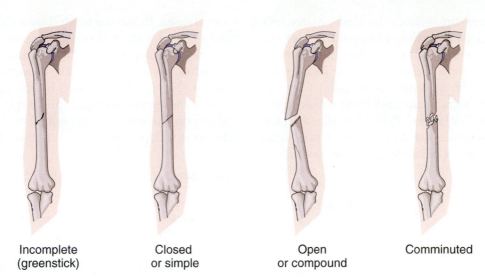

| Incomplete (greenstick) | Closed or simple | Open or compound | Comminuted |

● **FIGURE 6–15**   *Types of fractures.*

fibers separate lengthwise when bent. Such fractures are common among children because their bones contain flexible cartilage.

- *Comminuted*—The bone is splintered or broken into many pieces, which can become embedded in the surrounding tissue.

Bone and Joint Injuries

A **dislocation** occurs when a bone is displaced from its proper position in a joint. This may result in the tearing and stretching of the ligaments. Reduction, or return of the bone to its proper position, is necessary, along with rest to allow the ligaments to heal.

A **sprain** is an injury to a joint caused by any sudden or unusual motion, such as "turning" the ankle. The ligaments are either torn from their attachments to the bones or torn across, but the joint is not dislocated. A sprain is accompanied by rapid swelling and acute pain in the area and is treated with nonsteroidal anti-inflammatory drugs (NSAIDs).

● DISEASES OF THE BONES

Arthritis is an inflammatory condition of one or more joints, accompanied by pain and often by changes in bone position. There are at least twenty different types, the most common being rheumatoid arthritis and osteoarthritis:

- **Rheumatoid arthritis** (RA) is a chronic, autoimmune (the body's immune system attacks the tissue) disease that affects the connective tissue and joints. There is acute inflammation of the connective tissue, thickening of the synovial membrane, and ankylosis, or fusing, of joints. The joints are badly swollen and painful. The pain, in turn, causes muscle spasms, which may lead to deformities in the joints. In addition, the cartilage that separates the joints degenerates and hard calcium fills the spaces. When the joints become stiff and immobile, muscles attached to these joints slowly atrophy (shrink in size). This disease affects approximately three times more women than men. Its cause is unknown, although everything from emotional factors to endocrine and metabolic disorders has been cited.

- **Osteoarthritis** (OA) is known as degenerative joint disease. It occurs with aging; about 80% of all U.S. residents are affected. In this disease the articular cartilage degenerates and a bony spur forms at the joint. The joints may enlarge; there is pain and swelling, especially after activity.

Treatment for arthritis includes many folk remedies such as wearing a copper bracelet, using special tonic mixtures, and eating vitamins and certain foods. There is no known cure for arthritis. Treatment with NSAIDs may alleviate pain and swelling. Hip and knee replacement (arthroplasty) may be done for the affected joints. Researchers are working on a new class of arthritic drugs, because they now have a better understanding of how the body produces inflammation.

Gout is an increase of uric acid in the bloodstream. Uric acid crystals are deposited in joint cavities and kidneys; the site most commonly affected is the great toe. There is severe pain. More males are affected than females.

Rickets is usually found in children; it is caused by a lack of vitamin D. Bones become soft because of a lack of calcification, causing such deformities as bowlegs and pigeon breast. The disease may be prevented with sufficient quantities of calcium, vitamin D, and exposure to sunshine. Rickets is rare in developed countries.

Slipped (herniated) disk is a condition in which a cartilage disk (one of which is between each vertebra and acts as a shock absorber for the spine) ruptures, or protrudes out of place, and places pressure on the spinal nerve. This usually occurs in the lower back (lumbar-sacral) area. It may be treated by a chiropractor or with bed rest, traction, or surgery.

Whiplash injury is trauma to the cervical vertebra, usually the result of an automobile accident. The force generated by the car's speed whips the head backward, putting tremendous strain on the cervical spine and neck muscles. Treatment depends on the extent of the injury.

Abnormal Curvatures of the Spine

Kyphosis ("hunchback") is a humped curvature in the thoracic area of the spine, Figure 6-16.

Lordosis ("swayback") is an exaggerated inward curvature in the lumbar region of the spine just above the sacrum.

Scoliosis is a side-to-side or lateral curvature of the spine.

● OTHER MEDICALLY RELATED DISORDERS

Osteoporosis is a disease that affects 25 million persons in the United States; according to the National Osteoporosis Foundation, 80% are women. In osteoporosis the mineral density of the bone is reduced from 65% to 35%. By age 55, the average woman has lost approximately 30% of her bone mass. This loss of bone mass leaves

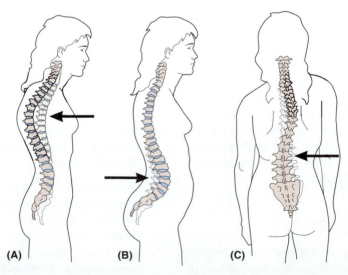

(A)   (B)   (C)

● **FIGURE 6–16**   *Abnormal curvatures of the spine:* **(A)** *kyphosis,* **(B)** *lordosis,* **(C)** *scoliosis.*

the bone thinner, more porous, and susceptible to fracture. An x-ray of the bone is said to resemble Swiss cheese. Treatment is aimed at preventing or slowing down osteoporosis. Average intake of calcium in the diet and regular exercise help to build bone mass and prevent osteoporosis. Postmenopausal women may take estrogen to help maintain bone mass. Diets that are too high in sodium and potassium contribute to the loss of calcium from the body. Women are encouraged to have bone density studies done to detect early onset of osteoporosis.

Osteomyelitis is an infection that may involve all parts of the bone. It may result from injury or systemic infection and most commonly occurs in children between the ages of 5 and 14 years.

Osteosarcoma, or bone cancer, may occur in younger people. The most common site of affliction is just above the knee.

MEDICAL HIGHLIGHTS

Arthroscopy is the examination of a joint using an arthroscope, a small fiberoptic viewing instrument made up of a tiny lens, a light source, and a video camera. Through an incision approximately a quarter of an inch long, a physician may examine, diagnose, and treat injuries of joint areas. Most knee injuries are treated through arthroscopic technique.

Microdiskectomy is an operation to remove a prolapsed or damaged intervertebral disk through a tiny incision. To replace the damaged disk, the surgeon uses a bone plug, which can be a graft from the patient's hip bone or from a bone bank. Another option is to fill the space with coralline, which is obtained from sea coral. The patient may be out of bed the next day. ■

● REVIEW QUESTIONS

Select the letter of the choice that best completes the statement.

1. Supination is one type of:
   a. extension
   b. abduction
   c. adduction
   d. rotation

2. The bones found in the skull are:
   a. irregular bones
   b. flat bones
   c. short bones
   d. long bones

3. The cranium protects the:
   a. lungs
   b. brain
   c. heart
   d. stomach

4. Pivot joints may be found in the:
   a. vertebral column
   b. skull
   c. wrist
   d. shoulder

5. Bones are a storage place for minerals such as:
   a. calcium and sodium
   b. calcium and potassium
   c. sodium and potassium
   d. calcium and phosphorous

6. The site of blood cell formation is:
   a. yellow marrow
   b. periosteum
   c. articular cartilage
   d. red marrow

7. Immovable joints are found in the:
   a. infant's skull
   b. adult's cranium
   c. adult's spinal column
   d. child's spinal column

8. *Flexion* means:
   a. bending
   b. rotating
   c. extending
   d. abducting

9. The degree of motion at a joint is determined by:
   a. the amount of synovial fluid
   b. the number of bursae
   c. an unusual amount of exercise
   d. bone shape and joint structure

10. The bone that forms the base of the skull is the:
    a. parietal
    b. temporal
    c. occipital
    d. frontal

11. The key bone of the skull is the:
    a. ethmoid
    b. frontal
    c. parietal
    d. sphenoid

12. The only moveable bone of the face is the:
    a. lacrimal
    b. mandible
    c. maxilla
    d. palatine

13. The central opening on the vertebrae for passage of the spinal cord is the:
    a. transverse process
    b. intervertebral disk
    c. foramen
    d. spinous process

14. The shoulder girdle is composed of two bones:
    a. radius and ulna
    b. clavicle and scapula
    c. tibia and fibula
    d. metatarsal and tarsal

15. The ribs that are attached directly to the sternum are called:
    a. floating
    b. true
    c. false
    d. humerus

16. The arm bone located on the thumb side is called:
    a. ulna
    b. radius
    c. humerus
    d. carpal

17. The bones of the wrist are called:
    a. tarsal
    b. metatarsal
    c. carpal
    d. metacarpal

18. The longest, strongest bone in the body is the:
    a. humerus
    b. tibia
    c. femur
    d. fibula

19. The heel bone is known as the:
    a. calcaneus
    b. patella
    c. fibula
    d. talus

20. An inflammation of the bone is known as:
    a. arthritis
    b. bursitis
    c. osteomyelitis
    d. osteoarthritis

MATCHING

Match each term in Column A with its correct description in Column B.

Column A	Column B
_____ 1. osteoarthritis	a. first cervical vertebra
_____ 2. closed fracture	b. shock absorbers
_____ 3. fontanel	c. moveable joint
_____ 4. endosteum	d. degeneration of articular cartilage
_____ 5. bursa	e. bone broken, skin intact
_____ 6. epiphysis	f. joint capsule
_____ 7. periosteum	g. area in infant skull where bone is not yet formed
_____ 8. atlas	h. lining of the marrow cavity
_____ 9. intervertebral disk	i. calcium and phosphorous
_____ 10. diarthrosis joint	j. end structure of long bone
	k. bone cells or osteocytes
	l. bone covering that contains blood vessels

●APPLYING THEORY TO PRACTICE

1. What type of joint movement is used:
   - to shut off a light?
   - to comb your hair?

2. If someone you know has broken the long bone of his leg skiing, what type of treatment should be used?

3. You are running and have "turned" your ankle. Name the bones involved. What is the best way to treat a sprain?

4. Your grandmother tells you her bones are stiff. Explain what causes this condition.

5. More Americans are living longer, which means more people will be susceptible to osteoporosis. Define this condition and its treatment. How will this condition affect Medicare costs?

● LABELING

1. Label the parts of the skeleton.

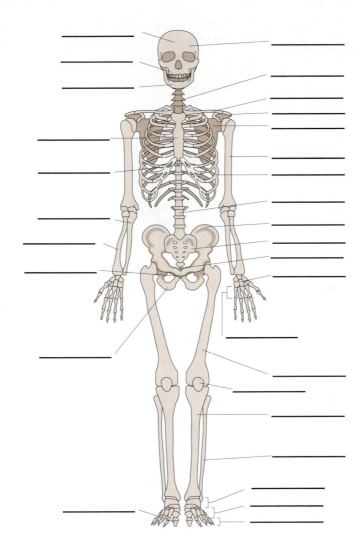

2. Label the parts of the long bone.

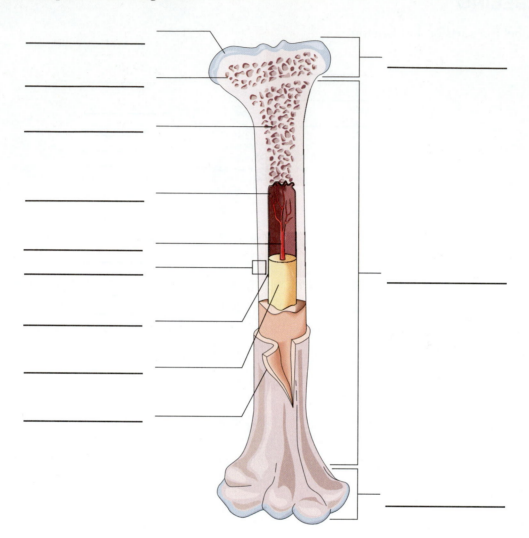

Muscular System

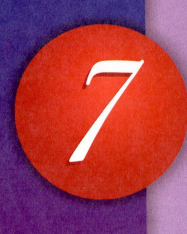

Objectives

- Describe the function of muscle
- Describe each of the muscle groups
- List the characteristics of muscle
- Describe how pairs of muscles work together
- Explain origin and insertion of muscle
- Locate the important skeletal body muscles
- Describe the function of these muscles
- Discuss how sports training affects these muscles
- Identify some common muscle disorders
- Define the key words that relate to this chapter

Key Words

abdominal hernia
acetylcholine
antagonist
atrophy
belly
biceps
cardiac muscle
compartment syndrome
contractility
deltoid
elasticity
ergonomics
excitability
extensibility
fascia
fasciotomy
fibromyalgia
flatfeet (talipes)
hernia
hiatal hernia
hypertrophy
inguinal hernia
insertion
intramuscular
isometric

isotonic
motor unit
muscle fatigue
muscle spasm
muscle tone
muscular dystrophy
myalgia
myasthenia gravis
neuromuscular junction
origin
paresthesia
paralysis
prime mover
pulselessness
rehabilitation
rotator cuff disease
sarcolemma
sarcoplasm
shin splints
skeletal muscle
smooth (visceral) muscle
sphincter (dilator) muscle
strain
strength
synergists

(continues)

The ability to move is an essential activity of the living human body; it is made possible by the unique function of contractility in muscles. Muscles compose a large part of the human body: nearly half our body weight comes from muscle tissue. If you weigh 140 pounds, about 60 pounds of it comes from the muscles attached to your bones. Collectively there are more than 650 different muscles in the human body. Muscles are responsible for all body movement. They allow us to move from place to place, as well as perform involuntary functions such as maintaining a heartbeat and breathing. Muscles give our bodies form and shape; just think what you would look like if all your muscles "collapsed." Muscles are responsible for producing most of our body heat.

There are three main functions of the muscle system:

1. Body movement

2. Body form and shape (maintaining posture)

3. Body heat (maintaining body temperature)

● TYPES OF MUSCLES

All body movements are determined by three principal types of muscles: skeletal, smooth, and cardiac muscle. These muscles are also described as striated, spindle-shaped, and nonstriated because of the way their cells look under an ordinary compound light microscope.

Skeletal muscles are attached to the bone of the skeleton. They are called striped or striated because they have cross-bands (striations) of alternating light and dark bands running perpendicular to the length of the muscle, Figure 7-1. Skeletal muscle is also called voluntary muscle, because it contains nerves under voluntary control. Skeletal muscle is composed of bundles of muscle cells. Each muscle cell, known as a muscle fiber, is multinucleate (containing many nuclei). The cell membrane is sarcolemma and the cytoplasm is sarcoplasm (refer to p. 112 for further explanation of sarcolemma).

The fleshy body parts are made of skeletal muscles. They provide movement to the limbs but contract quickly, fatigue easily, and lack the ability to remain contracted for prolonged periods. Blinking the eye, talking, breathing, dancing, eating, and writing are all actions produced by the motion of these muscles. This chapter focuses on skeletal muscle.

Smooth (visceral) muscle cells are small and spindle shaped. There is only one nucleus, located at the center of the cell. They are called smooth muscles because they are unmarked by any distinctive striations. Unattached to bones, they act slowly, do not tire easily, and can remain contracted for a long time, Figure 7-2.

Smooth muscles are not under conscious control; for this reason they are also called

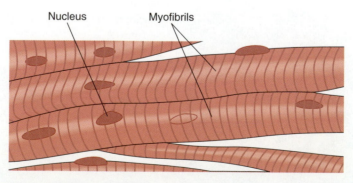

Nucleus   Myofibrils

● **FIGURE 7–1** *Voluntary or striated (skeletal) muscle cells.*

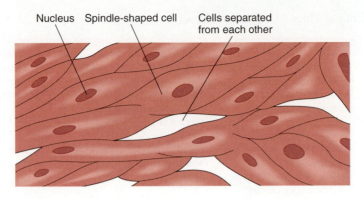

Nucleus   Spindle-shaped cell   Cells separated
from each other

● **FIGURE 7–2**   *Involuntary or smooth muscle cells.*

involuntary muscles. Their actions are controlled by the autonomic (automatic) nervous system. Smooth muscles are found in the walls of the internal organs, including the stomach, intestines, uterus, and blood vessels. They help push food along the length of the alimentary canal, contract the uterus during labor and childbirth, and control the diameter of blood vessels as blood circulates throughout the body.

Cardiac muscle is found only in the heart. Cardiac muscle cells are striated and branched, and they are involuntary, Figure 7-3. Cardiac cells are joined in a continuous network without a sheath separation. The membranes of adjacent cells are fused at places called intercalated disks. A communication system at the fused area does not permit independent cell contraction. When one cell receives a signal to contract, all neighboring cells are stimulated and contract together to produce the heartbeat. Healthy cardiac muscle contracts rapidly and is very strong. When the heart beats normally, it holds a rhythm of approximately 72 beats per minute. However, the activity of various nerves leading to the heart can increase or decrease its rate. Cardiac muscle requires a continuous supply of oxygen to function.

Sphincter (dilator) muscles are special circular muscles in the openings between the esophagus and stomach and the stomach and small intestine. They are also found in the walls of the anus, urethra, and mouth. They open and close to control the passage of substances.

Table 7-1 summarizes the characteristics of the three major muscle types.

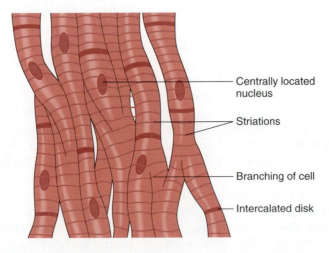

Centrally located
nucleus

Striations

Branching of cell

Intercalated disk

● **FIGURE 7–3**   *Cardiac muscle cells.*

TABLE 7-1 *Characteristics of Three Major Muscle Types*

MUSCLE TYPE	LOCATION	STRUCTURE	FUNCTION
Skeletal muscle (striated voluntary)	Attached to the skeleton; also located in the wall of the pharynx and esophagus.	Skeletal muscle fiber is long, cylindrical, multinucleated, and contains alternating light and dark striations. Nuclei are located at edge of fiber.	Contractions occur voluntarily and may be rapid and forceful. Contractions stabilize the joints.
Smooth muscle (nonstriated, involuntary)	Located in the walls of tubular structures and hollow organs, such as in digestive tract, urinary bladder, and blood vessels.	Smooth muscle fiber is long and spindle-shaped, with no striations.	Contractions occur involuntarily and are rhythmic and slow.
Cardiac (heart) muscle	Located in the heart.	Cardiac muscle fibers are short and branching, with a centrally located nucleus; striations are not distinct.	Contractions occur involuntarily and are rhythmic and automatic.

CHARACTERISTICS OF MUSCLES

All muscles, whether skeletal, smooth or cardiac, have four common characteristics. One is contractility, a quality possessed by no other body tissue. When a muscle shortens, or contracts, it reduces the distance between the parts of its contents or the space it surrounds. The contraction of skeletal muscles that connect a pair of bones brings the attachment points closer together. This causes the bone to move. When cardiac muscles contract, they reduce the area in the heart chambers, pumping blood from the heart into the blood vessels. Likewise, smooth muscles surround blood vessels and the intestines, causing the diameter of these tubes to decrease upon contraction.

Excitability (irritability), another characteristic of both muscle and nerve cells (neurons), is the ability to respond to certain stimuli by producing electric signals called action potentials (impulses), discussed later in the text.

Another property of muscles is extensibility (the ability to be stretched). When we bend our forearm, the muscles on the back of it are extended or stretched. Finally, muscles exhibit elasticity (ability of a muscle to return to its original length when relaxing). Collectively these four properties of muscles—contractility, excitability, extensibility, and elasticity—produce a veritable mechanical device capable of complex, intricate movements.

MUSCLE ATTACHMENTS AND FUNCTIONS

There are more than 600 different muscles in the body. For one of these muscles to produce movement in any part of the body, it must be able to exert its force on a movable object. Muscles must be attached to bones for leverage to have something to pull against. Muscles only pull, never push.

Muscles are attached to the bones of the skeleton by nonelastic cords called tendons. Bones are connected to each other by joints. Skeletal muscles are attached in such a way as to bridge these joints. When a skeletal muscle contracts, the bone to which it is attached moves.

Muscles are attached at both ends to bones, cartilage, ligaments, tendons, skin, and sometimes each other. The origin is the part of a skeletal muscle that is attached to a fixed structure or bone; it moves least during muscle contraction. The insertion is the other end, attached to a movable part; it is the part that moves most during a muscle contraction. The belly is the central body of the muscle, Figure 7-4.

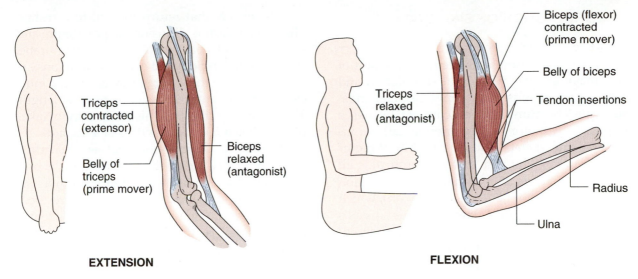

Triceps contracted (extensor)

Belly of triceps (prime mover)

Biceps relaxed (antagonist)

EXTENSION

Biceps (flexor) contracted (prime mover)

Belly of biceps

Tendon insertions

Triceps relaxed (antagonist)

Radius

Ulna

FLEXION

● **FIGURE 7–4**   *Coordination of prime mover and antagonist muscles.*

The muscles of the body are arranged in pairs. The **prime mover** produces movement in a single direction; the **antagonist** produces movement in the opposite direction. This arrangement of muscles with opposite actions is known as an antagonist pair.

For example, upper arm muscles are arranged in antagonist pairs, see Figure 7-4. The muscle located on the front part of the upper arm is the **biceps.** One end of the biceps is attached to the scapula and humerus (its origin). When the biceps contracts, these two bones remain stationary. The opposite end of the biceps is attached to the radius of the lower arm (its insertion); this bone moves during contraction of the biceps.

The muscle on the back of the upper arm is the **triceps.** Try this simple demonstration: Bend your elbow. With your other hand, feel the contraction of the belly of the biceps. At the same time, stretch your fingers out around the arm to touch your triceps; it will be in a relaxed state. Now extend your forearm; feel the simultaneous contraction of the triceps and relaxation of the biceps. Now bend the forearm halfway and contract the biceps and triceps. They cannot move, because both sets of muscles are contracting at the same time. In some muscle activity the role of prime mover and antagonist may be reversed. When you flex your

arm, the biceps brachii is the prime mover and triceps is the antagonist. When you extend your arm, the triceps is the prime mover and the biceps is the antagonist.

There is also another group of muscles called the **synergists**, which help steady a movement or stabilize joint activity.

● **SOURCES OF ENERGY AND HEAT**

When muscles do their work, they not only move the body but also produce the heat our bodies need. To get warm on a cold day, you shiver. Human beings must maintain their body temperatures within a narrow range (98.6° F to 99.8° F). For muscles to contract and do their work, they need energy. The major source of this energy is adenosine triphosphate (ATP), a compound found in the muscle cell. To make ATP, the cell requires oxygen, glucose, and other material that is brought to the cell by the circulating blood. Extra glucose can be stored in the cell in the form of glycogen. When a muscle is stimulated, the ATP is released, producing the heat the body needs and the energy the muscle needs to contract. During this process, lactic acid, which is a byproduct of cell metabolism, builds up.

CONTRACTION OF SKELETAL MUSCLE

Movement of muscles occurs as a result of two major events: myoneural stimulation and contraction of muscle proteins. Skeletal muscles must be stimulated to contract by nerve impulses. A motor neuron (nerve cell) stimulates all the skeletal muscles within a **motor unit**. A motor unit is a motor neuron plus all the muscle fibers it stimulates. The junction between the motor neuron's fiber (axon), which transmits the impulse, and the muscle cell's sarcolemma (muscle cell membrane) is the **neuromuscular junction**. The gap between the axon and the muscle cell is known as the synaptic cleft.

When the nerve impulses reach the end of the axon, the chemical neurotransmitter **acetylcholine** is released. Acetylcholine diffuses across the synaptic cleft and attaches to receptors on the sarcolemma. The sarcolemma then becomes temporarily permeable to sodium ions (Na+), which rush into the muscle cell. This gives the muscle cell excessive positive ions, which upset and change the electrical condition of the sarcolemma. This electrical upset causes an action potential (an electric current).

Skeletal muscle contraction begins with the action potential, which travels along the length of the muscle fiber. The basic source of energy is from glucose, and the energy derived is stored in the form of ATP and phosphocreatine. The latter serves as a trigger mechanism by allowing energy transfer to the protein molecules, actin and myosin, within the muscle fibers. Once begun, the action potential travels over the entire surface of the sarcolemma, conducting the electric impulse from one end of the cell to the other. This results in the contraction of the muscle cell. The movement of electrical current along the sarcolemma causes calcium ions (Ca^{++}) to be released from storage areas inside the muscle cell. When calcium ions attach to the action myofilaments (contractile elements of skeletal muscle), the sliding of the myofilaments is triggered and the whole cell shortens. The sliding of the myofilaments is energized by ATP.

The events that return the cell to a resting phase include the diffusion of potassium and sodium ion cells back across the cell membrane. When the action potential ends, calcium ions are reabsorbed into their storage areas and the muscle cell relaxes and returns to its original length. The amazing part is that this entire activity takes place in just a few thousandths of a second.

While the action potential is occurring, acetylcholine (which began the process) is broken down by enzymes on the sarcolemma. For this reason, a single nerve impulse produces only one contraction at a time. The muscle cell relaxes until it is stimulated by the next release of acetylcholine, Figure 7-5.

MUSCLE FATIGUE

Muscle fatigue is caused by an accumulation of lactic acid in the muscles. During periods of vigorous exercise, the blood is unable to transport enough oxygen for the complete oxidation of glucose in the muscles. This causes the muscles to contract anaerobically (without oxygen).

The lactic acid normally leaves the muscle, passing into the bloodstream. But if vigorous exercise continues, the lactic acid level in the blood rises sharply. In such cases, lactic acid accumulates within the muscle. This impedes muscular contraction, causing muscle fatigue and cramps. After exercise, a person must stop, rest, and take in enough oxygen to change the lactic acid back to glucose and other substances to be used by the muscle cells. The amount of oxygen needed is called the oxygen debt. When the debt is paid back, respirations resume at a normal rate.

MUSCLE TONE

To function, muscles should always be slightly contracted and ready to pull. This is **muscle tone**. Muscle tone can be achieved through proper nutrition and regular exercise. Muscle contractions may be **isotonic** or **isometric**. When muscles contract and shorten, it is called an isotonic contraction. This occurs when we walk, talk, and so on. When the tension in a muscle increases but the muscle does

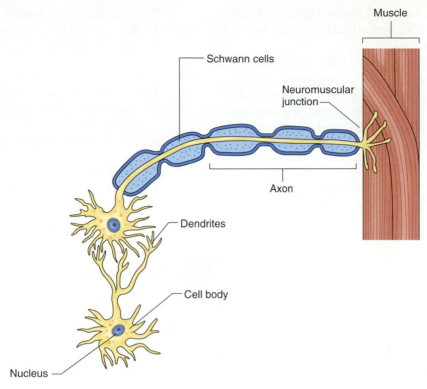

● **FIGURE 7–5** *A neuron-stimulating muscle.*

not shorten, it is called an isometric contraction. This occurs with exercises such as tensing the abdominal muscles. If we fail to exercise, our muscles become weak and flaccid. Muscles may also **atrophy**, or shrink from disuse. If we overexercise, the size of the muscle fiber (cell) enlarges. This is known as **hypertrophy**.

● PRINCIPAL SKELETAL MUSCLES

The skeletal or voluntary muscles are made up of all the muscles that are attached to and help move the skeleton. These muscles line the walls of the oral, abdominal, and pelvic cavities. Skeletal muscles also control the movement of the eyeballs, eyelids, lips, tongue, and skin.

Naming of Skeletal Muscles

Muscles are named by location, size, direction, number of origins, location of origin and insertion, and action; however, not all muscles are named in this manner.

- Location   frontalis—forehead
- Size   gluteus maximus—largest muscle in buttock
- Direction of fibers   external abdominal oblique—edge of the lower rib cage
- Number of origins   biceps—two-headed muscle in humerus
- Location of origin and insertion   sternocleidomastoid—origin in sternum
- Action
  flexor   flexor carpi ulnaris—flexes the wrist
  extensor   extensor carpi ulnaris—extends the wrist
  levator and depressor   raises or lowers body parts; depressor anguli oris—depresses the corner of the mouth

Figures 7-6 and 7-7 show other muscles named by location, size, direction, number of origins, and action.

There are 656 muscles in the human body. This breaks down to 327 antagonistic muscle pairs and two unpaired muscles. These two unpaired muscles are the orbicularis oris and the diaphragm. The 656 muscles can be divided and subdivided into the following muscle regions:

A. *Head muscles*
   1. Muscles of expression
   2. Muscles of mastication (chewing)
   3. Muscles of the tongue
   4. Muscles of the pharynx
   5. Muscles of the soft palate

B. *Neck muscles*
   1. Muscles moving the head
   2. Muscles moving the hyoid bone and the larynx
   3. Muscles moving the upper ribs

C. *Trunk and extremity muscles*
   1. Muscles that move the vertebral column

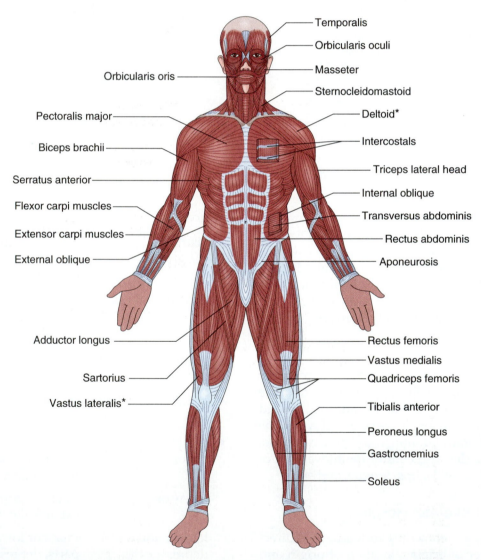

● **FIGURE 7–6** *Principal skeletal muscles of the body—anterior view.*
Intramuscular medication injection sites.

2. Muscles that move the scapula
3. Muscles of breathing
4. Muscles that move the humerus
5. Muscles that move the forearm
6. Muscles that move the wrist, hand, and finger digits
7. Muscles that act on the pelvis
8. Muscles that move the femur
9. Muscles the move the leg
10. Muscles that move the ankle, foot, and toe digits

Tables 7-2 through 7-7 on the following pages give a listing of some representative skeletal muscles that are involved in various types of bodily movements.

MUSCLES OF THE HEAD AND NECK

The muscles of the head and neck, shown in Figure 7-8, control human facial expressions such as anger, fear, grief, joy, pleasure, and pain (refer to Table 7-2). They also include the muscles of mastication, which control the mandible (lower jaw), raising it to close the jaw and lowering it to open the jaw (refer to Table 7-3). Neck muscles that move the head allow extension, flexion, and rotation (refer to Table 7-4).

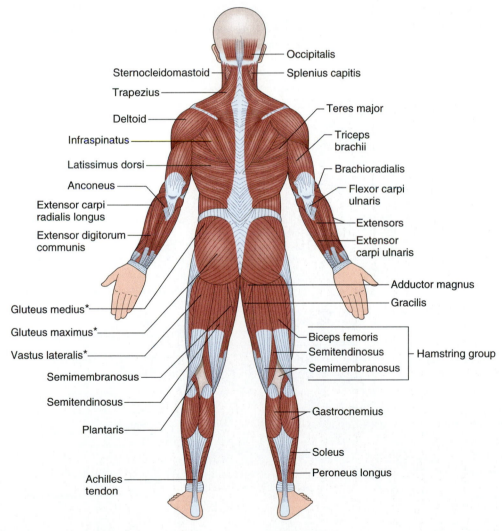

FIGURE 7–7 *Principal skeletal muscles of the body—posterior view.*
Intramuscular medication injection sites.

TABLE 7-2 *Representative Muscles of Facial Expression*

MUSCLE	EXPRESSION	LOCATION	FUNCTION
Frontalis	Surprise	On either side of the forehead.	Raises eyebrow and wrinkles forehead.
Depressor anguli oris	Doubt, disdain, contempt	Along the side of the chin.	Depresses corner of mouth.
Orbicularis oris	Doubt, disdain, contempt	Ring-shaped muscle around the mouth.	Compresses and closes the lips.
Platysma (broad sheet muscle)	Horror	Broad, thin muscular sheet covering the side of the neck and lower jaw.	Draws corners of mouth down and backward.
Zygomaticus major	Laughing or smiling	Extends diagonally upward from corner of mouth.	Raises corner of mouth.
Nasalis	Fear, pain	Over the nasal bones.	Closes and opens the nasal openings.
Orbicularis oculi	Sadness	Surrounds the eye orbit underlying the eyebrows.	Closes the eyelid and tightens the skin on the forehead.

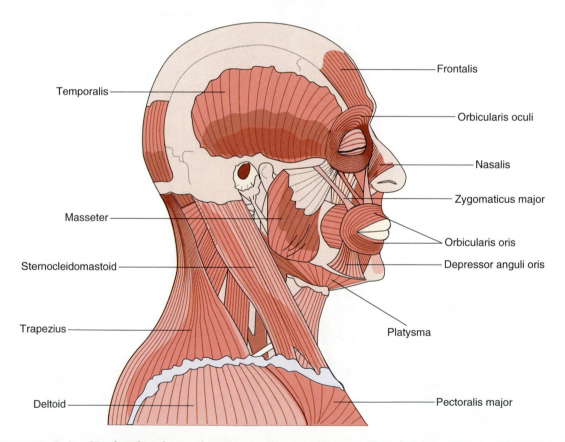

● **FIGURE 7–8**   *Head and neck muscle arrangement: muscles controlling facial expression, mastication, and movement of the head.*

TABLE 7-3 *Representative Muscles of Mastication*

MUSCLE	LOCATION	FUNCTION
Masseter	Covers the lateral surface of the ramus angle) of the mandible.	Closes the jaw.
Temporalis	Located on the temporal fossa of the skull.	Raises the jaw, closes the mouth, and draws the jaw backward.

TABLE 7-4 *Representative Muscles of the Neck*

MUSCLE	LOCATION	FUNCTION
Sternocleidomastoid (two heads)	Large muscles extending diagonally down sides of neck.	Flexes head; rotates the head toward opposite side from muscle.

● MUSCLES OF THE UPPER EXTREMITIES

The muscles of the upper extremities help to move the shoulder (scapula) and arm (humerus), including the forearm, wrist, hand, and fingers. Refer to Table 7-5 and Figure 7-9.

TABLE 7-5 *Representative Muscles of the Upper Extremities*

MUSCLE	LOCATION	FUNCTION
*Trapezius	A large triangular muscle located on the upper surface of back.	Moves the shoulder; extends the head.
*Deltoid	A thick triangular muscle that covers the shoulder joint.	Abducts the upper arm.
*Pectoralis major	Anterior chest.	Flexes the upper arm and helps to abduct the upper arm.
Serratus	Anterior chest.	Moves scapula forward and helps to raise the arm.
*Biceps brachii	Upper arm to radius.	Flexes the lower arm.
*Triceps brachii	Posterior arm to ulna.	Extends the lower arm.
Extensor and flexor carpi muscle groups	Extends from the anterior and posterior forearm to the hand.	Moves the hand.
Extensor and flexor digitorum muscle groups	Extends from the anterior and posterior forearm to the fingers.	Moves the fingers.
*Major prime movers		

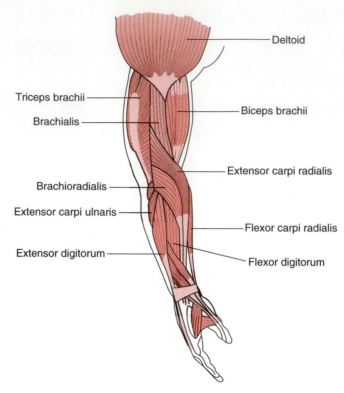

- Deltoid
- Triceps brachii
- Biceps brachii
- Brachialis
- Extensor carpi radialis
- Brachioradialis
- Extensor carpi ulnaris
- Flexor carpi radialis
- Extensor digitorum
- Flexor digitorum

● **FIGURE 7–9**   *Muscles of the upper extremity.*

● MUSCLES OF THE TRUNK

The trunk muscles control breathing and the movements of the abdomen and the pelvis. Refer to Table 7-6 and Figure 7-10, p. 119.

● MUSCLES OF THE LOWER EXTREMITIES

The muscles of the lower extremities, Figure 7-11, p. 119, assist in the movement of the

TABLE 7-6 *Representative Muscles of the Trunk*

MUSCLE	LOCATION	FUNCTION
External intercostals	Between the ribs.	Raises the ribs to help in breathing.
Diaphragm	A dome-shaped muscle separating the thoracic and abdominal cavities.	Helps to control breathing.
Rectus abdominis	From the ribs to the pelvis.	Compresses the abdomen.
External oblique	Anterior inferior edge of the last eight ribs.	Depresses ribs, flexes the spinal column, and compresses the abdominal cavity.
Internal oblique	Directly beneath the external oblique, its fibers running in the opposite direction.	Depresses ribs, flexes the spinal column, and compresses the abdominal cavity.

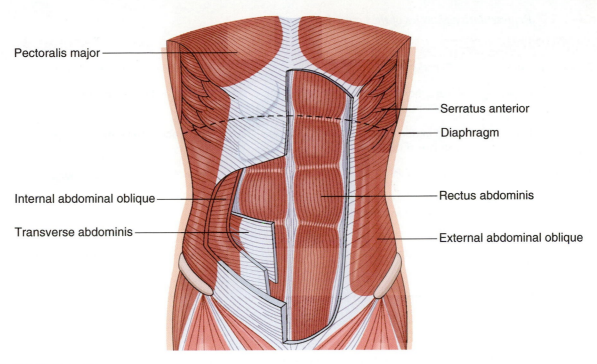

● **FIGURE 7–10**   *Muscles of the trunk.*

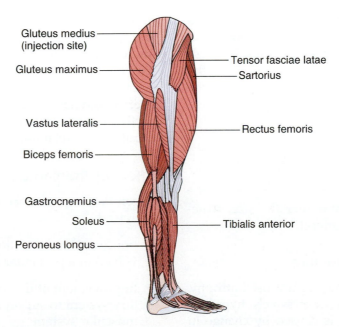

● **FIGURE 7–11**   *Muscles of the lower extremity.*

TABLE 7-7 *Representative Muscles of the Lower Extremities*

MUSCLE	LOCATION	FUNCTION
*Gluteus maximus	Buttocks.	Extends femur and rotates it outward.
Gluteus medius	From the deep femur to the buttocks; injection site.	Abducts and rotates the thigh.
Tensor fasciae latae	Flat muscle found along the upper lateral surface of the thigh.	Flexes, abducts, and medially rotates the thigh.
*Rectus femoris	Anterior thigh.	Flexes thigh and extends the lower leg.
*Sartorius (Tailor's muscle)	Long, straplike muscle that runs diagonally across the anterior and medial surface of the thigh.	Flexes and rotates the thigh and leg.
*Tibialis anterior	In front of the tibia bone.	Dorsiflexes the foot; permits walking on the heels.
*Gastrocnemius	Calf muscle.	Points toes and flexes the lower leg.
*Soleus	Broad, flat muscle found beneath the gastrocnemius.	Extends foot.
Peroneus longus	Superficial muscle found on the lateral side of the leg.	Extends and everts the foot and supports arches.
*Major prime movers		

thigh (femur), leg, ankle, foot, and toes. Refer to Table 7-7. Athletes often pull what is known as the hamstring. The group of muscles that make up the hamstring are the semitendinosus, biceps femoris, and semimembranosus. The tendons of these muscles attach posteriorly to the tibia and fibula. They can be felt behind the knee. The hamstring muscle group is responsible for flexing the knee.

● HOW EXERCISE AND TRAINING CHANGE MUSCLES

Exercise and training alter the size, structure, and strength of a muscle.

Size and Muscle Structure

Skeletal muscles that are not used atrophy, and those that are used excessively hypertrophy. The hypertrophy is caused by change in the sarcoplasm (cytoplasm found in the individual skeletal muscle fibers), *not* to an increase in the number of muscle fibers (cells). Muscles that have been injured can regenerate only to a limited degree. If the muscle damage is extensive, the muscle tissue is replaced by connective (scar) tissue. Muscles that are overexercised or overworked have a tremendous increase of connective tissue between the muscle fibers. This causes the skeletal muscle to become tougher.

Effect of Training on Muscle Efficiency

The following will occur when muscles are exercised:

- Improved coordination of all muscles involved in a particular activity

- Improvement of the respiratory and circulatory system to supply the needs of an active muscular system

- Elimination or reduction of excess fat
- Improved joint movement involved with that particular muscle activity

Effect of Training on Muscle Strength

Strength (capacity to do work) is increased by proper training. Training can have the following effects on skeletal muscles:

- Increased muscle size
- Improved antagonistic muscle coordination, in which antagonist muscles are relaxed at the right moment and do not interfere with the functioning of the working muscle
- Improved functioning in the cortical brain region, where the nerve impulses start muscular contraction

● INTRAMUSCULAR INJECTIONS

An EMS provider occasionally has to administer an **intramuscular** (into the muscle) injection into the patient. Therefore a working knowledge of the major skeletal muscles and the underlying anatomy of the injection area is needed. The most common sites for an intramuscular injection are the **deltoid** muscle of the upper arm, vastus lateralis (anterior thigh), and gluteus medius (buttocks).

● MUSCULOSKELETAL DISORDERS

Muscle and skeletal systems work as a team to move the body. Muscular coordination is very important if a person is to perform his or her daily functions efficiently. Injuries and diseases that affect the musculoskeletal system sometimes interfere with these functions. The retraining of injured or unused muscles is a type of **rehabilitation** called therapeutic exercise.

Muscle atrophy can occur in infrequently used muscles; they shrink and lose muscle strength, such as occurs in a stroke (cerebrovascular accident). The muscles are understimulated and gradually waste away. Muscle atrophy caused by nerve paralysis may reduce a muscle by up to 25% of its normal size. Muscle atrophy can also be caused by prolonged bed rest or the immobilization of a limb in a cast. Muscle atrophy can be minimized by massage or special exercise.

A muscle **strain** is a muscle tear resulting from excessive use. Limited bleeding inside the muscle can cause pain and swelling. Ice packs help to stop bleeding and reduce swelling.

Muscle spasm, or cramp, is a sustained contraction of the muscle. These contractions may occur because of overuse of the muscle.

Myalgia is a term used to describe muscle pain. **Fibromyalgia** is a disease characterized by a collection of symptoms (syndrome). In fibromyalgia the most definite symptom is chronic muscle pain lasting three or more months in specific muscle points. Other symptoms may include fatigue, headache, feelings of numbness and tingling, and feelings of joint pain. Treatment is directed at pain relief and counseling.

Hernia occurs when an organ protrudes through a weak muscle. **Abdominal hernia** occurs when organs protrude through the abdominal wall. **Inguinal hernia** occurs in the inguinal area (see Figure 1-4, Chapter 1), and **hiatal hernia** occurs when the stomach pushes through the diaphragm.

Flatfeet (talipes) result from a weakening of the leg muscles that support the arch. The downward pressure on the foot eventually flattens out the arches. The condition can be helped by exercise, massage, and corrective shoes.

Tetanus (lockjaw) is an infectious disease characterized by continuous spasms of the voluntary muscles. It is caused by a toxin from the bacillus *Clostridium tetani*, a bacterium that can enter the body through a puncture wound. This disease can be prevented by a tetanus antitoxoid vaccine.

Torticollis, or wry neck, may be due to an inflammation of the trapezius or sternocleidomastoid muscle.

Muscular dystrophy is a group of diseases in which the muscle cells deteriorate. The most common type is Duchenne muscular dystrophy, caused by a genetic defect. At birth the child appears normal; as growth occurs and muscle cells die, the child becomes weak. The child loses the ability to walk by the ages of 9 to 11. There is progressive deterioration of muscle, and death occurs in the late teens or early twenties unless mechanical breathing is instituted.

Myasthenia gravis leads to progressive muscular weakness and paralysis, sometimes even death. The cause is still unknown, but many researchers believe it may be due to a defect in the immune system, affecting myoneural function. In extreme cases it can be fatal because of the paralysis of the respiratory muscles.

Recreation Injuries

Exercise can sometimes lead to excessive stress on the tendons, which are cords of connective tissue that attach the muscles to bone. They are not able to contract and return to their original place; therefore they are more susceptible to straining and tearing. For example, a sudden severe muscle contraction needed for playing tennis can cause the tendons to tear.

Tennis elbow, or lateral epicondylitis, occurs at the bony prominence (lateral epicondyle) on the sides of the elbow. The tendon that connects the arm muscle to elbow becomes inflamed because of repetitive use of the arm and underconditioning, Figure 7-12. This can occur from carrying luggage, playing tennis, swinging a golf club, or pounding a hammer. Treatment consists of relief of pain and ice packs to reduce the inflammation. Sleeping on the affected arm should be avoided. Surgery is used as a last resort.

Shin splints occur when there is injury to the muscle tendon in the front of the shin, such as is caused by jogging. Shin splints can be prevented by choosing the correct running shoe—one that is comfortable and has proper arch support.

Rotator cuff disease is an inflammation of a group of tendons that fuse together and surround the shoulder joint. This injury can occur because of repetitive overhead swinging, such as swinging a tennis racquet or pitching a ball. The most common complaint is aching in the top and front of the shoulder. Pain increases when the arm is lifted overhead. Treatment includes rest and physical therapy.

STREET SMART

Muscles are enclosed and divided by thin sheets of fibrous tissue, called **fascia**, into individual compartments. If a limb is crushed under a large weight for a prolonged period, such as may occur in a cave-in, swelling results within these muscular compartments. As the swelling steadily worsens, the pressure within these compartments increases and compresses nerves and blood vessels. The result of compressed nerves and blood vessels is a loss of feeling (**paresthesia**), a loss of motion (**paralysis**), and a loss of circulation (**pulselessness**). Together these three signs indicate that the patient may be experiencing **compartment syndrome**.

Compartment syndrome is a true surgical emergency. Treatment includes cutting through the skin and into the fascia to relieve the pressure. This surgical procedure is called a **fasciotomy**. ■

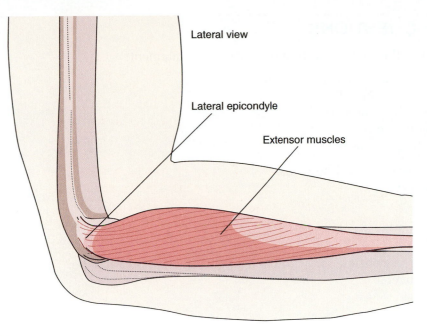

Lateral view

Lateral epicondyle

Extensor muscles

● **FIGURE 7–12**   *Tennis elbow.*

MEDICAL HIGHLIGHTS

Computerization of the workplace has not only created a new way of life for many workers, but has also contributed to one of the fastest growing occupational disorders. Cumulative trauma disorder (CTD), or repetitive motion disorder, is characterized by tissue inflammation and pain that results from the repeated muscle use required for an activity such as using a computer keyboard.

A United States Bureau of Labor Statistics report shows that CTD accounted for more than half of all occupational illnesses in the United States. This disorder has given rise to a new area of expertise called ergonomics, which is the study of the application of biology and engineering to the relationship between workers and their environment.

Workers must be educated in the causes and symptoms of CTD, as well as in the proper use of tools and lifting techniques to prevent this disorder. For example, wrist disorders may be prevented by making changes in the computer work station, such as adjusting the height of the keyboard and monitor, and making sure that chairs are well suited to both the job and the individual worker. ■

● REVIEW QUESTIONS

Select the letter of the choice that best completes the statement.

1. The muscle system is responsible for:
   a. producing red blood cells
   b. providing a framework
   c. moving the body
   d. conducting impulses

2. Skeletal muscle is also known as:
   a. involuntary
   b. voluntary
   c. cardiac
   d. smooth

3. The muscle responsible for action in a single direction is called the:
   a. prime mover
   b. antagonist
   c. synergist
   d. adduction

4. Muscles are always in a state of partial contraction called:
   a. muscle atrophy
   b. muscle tone
   c. tetanus
   d. muscle hypertrophy

5. The muscle you use to turn your head is the:
   a. trapezius
   b. sternocleidomastoid
   c. orbicularis
   d. temporalis

6. The upper arm muscle that is used as an injection site is the:
   a. triceps
   b. biceps
   c. trapezius
   d. deltoid

7. The muscle used in breathing is the:
   a. oblique
   b. diaphragm
   c. rectus abdominis
   d. serratus

8. A muscle located on the chest wall is the:
   a. trapezius
   b. frontalis
   c. pectoralis major
   d. rectus abdominis

9. Muscle fatigue is caused by a buildup of:
   a. glycogen
   b. oxygen
   c. lactic acid
   d. ATP

10. The muscle on the calf portion of the leg is the:
    a. gastrocnemius
    b. sartorius
    c. rectus femoris
    d. tibialis anterior

●APPLYING THEORY TO PRACTICE

1. Your body feels very warm after exercising. What has happened?

2. After running up a hill, you are out of breath and have a cramp in your leg. What caused the cramp? How can you relieve it? When will your breathing get back to normal?

3. While looking at yourself in the mirror, look surprised. Name and locate the muscle you used. Place your fingers on the muscle and feel it contract. Do the same exercise making a frown and a smile.

4. Name the leg muscles that you would use to kick a soccer ball.

5. A friend has had an accident and his leg is in a cast. Describe the condition that will occur without exercise. How can you prevent this condition?

6. A patient comes to the office and explains that she is on the school all-star tennis team; her right shoulder and arm is hurting all over. The doctor states that her condition is known as rotator cuff disease. Explain rotator cuff disease and recreation injuries to the patient.

8 Brain and Central Nervous System

Objectives

- Describe the functions of the central nervous system
- List the main divisions of the central nervous system
- Identify the parts of the brain
- Describe the structure of the brain and spinal cord
- Describe the functions of the parts of the brain
- Describe the functions of the spinal cord
- Describe disorders of the brain and spinal cord
- Define the key words that relate to this chapter

Key Words

absence seizure
action potential
Alzheimer's disease
anticonvulsant
aphasia
arachnoid (mater)
associative neuron
  (interneuron)
aura
autonomic nervous
  system
axons
blood-brain barrier
bradycardia
brainstem
brain tumor
Broca's area
cauda equina
central nervous system
cerebellum
cerebral aqueduct
cerebral cortex
cerebral edema
cerebral palsy
cerebral ventricles
cerebrospinal fluid

cerebrum
choroid plexus
clonic phase
complex partial seizure
corpus callosum
cranium
Cushing's triad
delirium
dementia
dendrites
diencephalon
dura mater
emboli
embolic stroke
encephalitis
epidural space
epilepsy
expressive aphasia
fibers
fibrinolytics
fissure
fontanels
fourth ventricle
frontal lobe
generalized seizure
gyri (convolutions)

(continues)

Key Words (continued)

hematoma	poliomyelitis
hemorrhage	pons
hemorrhagic stroke	postictal phase
hydrocephalus	preictal
hypertension	receptive aphasia
hypothalamus	seizure
interventricular foramen	sensory neuron
intracranial pressure	(afferent)
lateral ventricles	simple partial seizure
lumbar puncture	spastic quadriplegia
medulla oblongata	spinal cord
membrane excitability	status epilepticus
memory	stroke
meninges	subarachnoid space
meningitis	subdural space
motor aphasia	sulci
motor neuron (efferent)	synapse
multiple sclerosis	synaptic cleft
myelin sheath	temporal lobe
(neurilemma)	thalamus
neuroglia	third ventricle
neuron	thrombotic stroke
nystagmus	thrombus
occipital lobe	tic
occlusive stroke	tonic phase
parietal lobe	tonic-clonic generalized
Parkinson's disease	seizure
partial seizure	transient ischemic
peripheral nervous	attacks
system	vagus nerve
pia mater	Wernicke's area

● INTRODUCTION TO THE CENTRAL NERVOUS SYSTEM

The study of body functions reveals that the body is made up of millions of small structures that perform a multitude of different activities; these are coordinated and integrated into one harmonious whole. The two main communications systems are the endocrine system and the nervous system. They send chemical messengers and nerve impulses to all the structures. The endocrine system and hormonal regulation are discussed in other chapters. Hormonal regulation is slow, whereas neural regulation is comparatively rapid.

Functions of the central nervous system include the following:

1. It is the body's communication and coordination system.
   - It receives messages from stimuli all over the body.
   - The brain interprets the message.
   - The brain responds to the message and carries out an activity.

2. The brain is the seat of intellect and reasoning.

The central nervous system is the most highly organized system of the body, consisting of the brain, spinal cord, and nerves. The nerve cell, or **neuron**, is specially constructed to carry out its function: transmitting a message from one cell to the next. In addition to the nucleus, cytoplasm, and cell membrane, the neuron has extensions of cytoplasm from the cell body. These extensions, or processes, are called **dendrites** and **axons**. There may be several dendrites, but only one axon. These processes, or **fibers**, as they are often called, are paths along which nerve impulses travel. The axon has a specialized covering called **neurilemma** or **myelin sheath**, Figure 8-1. This covering speeds up the nerve impulse as it travels along the axon. The myelin sheath produces a fatty substance called myelin, which protects the axon; this substance is also called "white matter." The nodes of Ranvier have no myelin present. This is important in the conduction of a nerve impulse. Axons carry messages away from the cell body. Dendrites carry messages to the cell body.

Nervous Tissue

Nerve tissue is made up of two major types of nerve cells: **neuroglia** and neurons. Neuroglia are cells that insulate, support, and protect the neurons. They are sometimes referred to as "nerve glue."

All neurons possess the characteristics of being able to react when stimulated and of being able to pass on to other neurons the nerve impulse generated when that stimulation occurs. These reactions are irritability (the ability to react when stimulated) and conductivity (the ability to

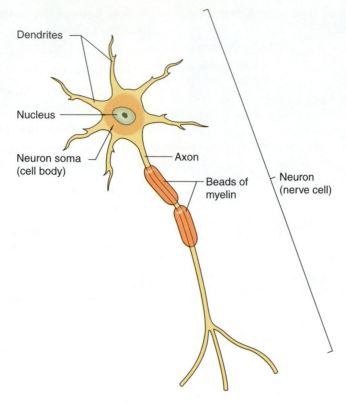

Dendrites

Nucleus

Neuron soma
(cell body)

Axon

Beads of
myelin

Neuron
(nerve cell)

● **FIGURE 8–1**   *A neuron.*

transmit a disturbance to distant points). The dendrites receive the impulse and transmit it to the cell body and then to the axon, where it is passed on to another neuron or to a muscle or gland. There are three types of neurons:

1. **Sensory neurons** or **afferent** neurons, which emerge from the skin or sense organs and carry messages, or impulses, toward the spinal cord and brain

2. **Motor neurons** or **efferent** neurons, which carry messages from the brain and spinal cord to the muscles and glands

3. **Associative neurons** or **interneurons**, which carry impulses from the sensory neuron to the motor neuron

Function of the Nerve Cell/Membrane Excitability

Nerves carry impulses by creating electric charges in a process known as **membrane ex-citability**. Neurons have a membrane that separates the cytoplasm inside from the extracellular fluids outside the cell, thereby creating two chemically different areas. Each area has differing amounts of potassium and sodium ions and some other charged substances, with the inside being the more negatively charged. When a neuron is stimulated, ions move across the membrane, creating a current that, if large enough, briefly changes the inside of the neuron to be more positive than the outside area. This state is known as **action potential**. Neurons and other cells that produce action potentials are said to have membrane excitability.

To understand how impulses are carried along nerves or throughout a muscle when it contracts, we need to learn a little more about membrane excitability. Ions cross a membrane through channels, some of which are open and allow ions to "leak" (diffuse) continuously. Other channels are called "gated" and open only during action potential. Another membrane opening is a sodium-potassium pump, which, by active transport, maintains the flow of ions from higher to lower concentration levels across the membrane and restores the cytoplasm and extracellular fluid to their original value after an action potential occurs. This action is in response to an imbalance between the cytoplasm and the extracellular fluid. When diffusion takes place, particles move from an area of greater concentration to an area of lesser concentration.

The following simplified description explains how this whole process works:

1. A neuron membrane is at rest. There are large amounts of potassium (K^+) ions inside the cells but not many sodium (NA^+) ions. The reverse is true outside the cell in the extracellular fluid. Most of the open channels are for potassium to pass through, so it leaks out of the cell.

2. As the K^+ ions leave, the inside becomes relatively more negative until some K^+ ions are attracted back in, the electrical force balances the diffusion force, and

movement stops. The inside is still more negative and the amount of energy between the two differently charged areas is ready to work (carry an impulse). This state is called the resting membrane potential, Figure 8-2 (A). The membrane is now polarized. The sodium ions are not able to move in, because their channels are closed during the resting state; however, if a few leak in, the membrane pump sends an equal number out.

3. Now suppose a sensory neuron receptor is stimulated by something—a sound, for instance. This causes a change in the membrane potential. The stimulus energy is converted to an electrical signal, and if it is strong enough, it depolarizes a portion of the membrane and allows the gated sodium ion channels to open, initiating an action potential, Figure 8-2 (A).

4. The sodium ions move through the gated channels into the cytoplasm and the inside becomes more positive, until the

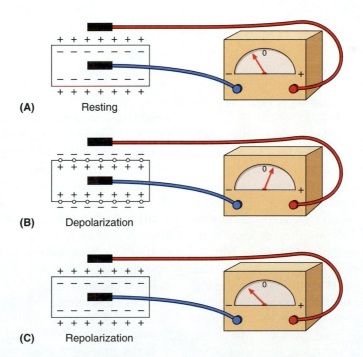

(A)   Resting

(B)   Depolarization

(C)   Repolarization

● **FIGURE 8–2** *Sequence of events in membrane potential and relative positive and negative states: (A) Normal resting potential (negative inside/positive outside); (B) depolarization (positive inside/negative outside); (C) repolarization (negative inside/positive outside).*

membrane potential is reversed and the gates close to sodium ions, Figure 8-2 (B).

5. Next the potassium gates open and large amounts of potassium leave the cytoplasm, resulting in the repolarization of the membrane, Figure 8-2 (C). After repolarization, the sodium-potassium pump restores the initial concentrations of sodium and potassium ions inside and outside the neuron.

This whole process occurs in a few milliseconds. When this action occurs in one part of the cell membrane, it spreads to adjacent membrane regions, continuing away from the original site of stimulation, sending "messages" over the nerve. This cycle is completed millions of times a minute throughout the body, day after day, year after year.

Synapse

A synapse is the means by which messages go from one cell to the next. The nerve cell has both an axon and a dendrite. Messages go from the axon of one cell to the dendrite of another; they never actually touch. The space between them is known as the synaptic cleft. The conduction is accomplished through neurotransmitters (special chemicals, namely norepinephrine, and acetylcholine) at the end of each axon.

An impulse travels along the axon to the end, where the neurotransmitter is released. This helps the impulse to "jump" the space between and the impulse is sent to the dendrite of the next nerve cell. The neurotransmitter between muscle cells and the nervous system is acetylcholine.

MEDICAL HIGHLIGHTS

Scientists have unraveled the secret of how a nerve communicates with a muscle. Dr. George Yancopoulos and another team working independently have produced the most detailed picture of this incredibly complex system. Their reports were published in the journal *Cell.*

Nerve cells communicate with each other, as well as give orders to muscles, by sending messages across gaps called synapses. Nerves and muscles create chemically intricate synapses in just the right places. The secret is two proteins: one is called agrin and another is known as muscle-specific receptor kinase, or MuSK. Working with mice, the researchers found that both proteins were necessary during embryonic development to make working connections between nerves and muscles. If either protein was missing, the mice were unable to breathe and died soon after birth.

During development it appears that nerve cells grow toward muscles and release agrin. On the muscle side of the gap, the agrin is received by MuSK, which works in combination with another protein called muscle-associated specificity component. This connection starts a complicated chain reaction that eventually results in changes in both the nerve and the muscle, which add up to a working synapse. The nerve cells talk to the muscle cells by releasing the neurotransmitter acetylcholine. Agrin is the first step; it signals the muscle to pull together the chemicals it needs to construct acetylcholine receptors so that it can receive these messages.

This discovery may offer insight into how cell-to-cell communication goes on inside the brain, and it could also lead to new treatments for nerve injuries and a variety of diseases. ■

DIVISIONS OF THE NERVOUS SYSTEM

The nervous system can be divided into three divisions: the central, peripheral, and autonomic nervous systems.

1. The **central nervous system** consists of the brain and spinal cord.

2. The **peripheral nervous system** is made up of the nerves of the body, consisting of 12 pairs of cranial nerves extending out from the brain and 31 pairs of spinal nerves extending out from the spinal cord.

3. The **autonomic nervous system** includes peripheral nerves and ganglia (a group of cell bodies outside the central nervous system that carry impulses to involuntary muscles and glands).

When decision is called for and action must be considered, the central and peripheral nervous systems are involved. They carry information to the brain, where it is interpreted, organized, and stored. An appropriate command is sent to organs or muscles. The autonomic nervous system supplies heart muscle, smooth muscle, and secretory glands with nervous impulses as needed. It is usually involuntary in action.

THE BRAIN

The adult human brain is a highly developed, complex, and intricate mass of soft nervous tissue. It weighs approximately 1400 grams (3 pounds) and is composed of 100 billion neurons. The brain is protected by the bony cranial cavity; further protection is afforded by three membranous coverings, called **meninges**, and the cerebrospinal fluid. The brain is composed of white and gray matter. The outer cortex, known as the **cerebral cortex**, is gray. This is the highest center of reasoning and intellect. You may have heard people say when trying to resolve a problem, "I need to use my gray matter." The deeper part of the cerebral cortex is composed of myelinated nerve tracts; it is called the white matter. An adequate blood supply to the brain is critical. Without oxygen, brain damage occurs within 4 to 8 minutes. The brain is divided into four major parts: the cerebrum, diencephalon, cerebellum, and brainstem, see Figure 8-3.

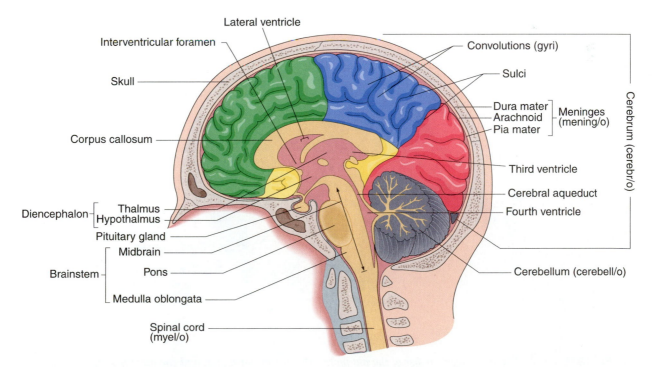

● **FIGURE 8–3**   *Cross-section of the brain.*

Memory

The brain is our warehouse, packaging and storing information. We call this process **memory**. To create a memory, it is believed that nerve cells form new interconnections. No one area of the brain stores all memories; the storage site depends on the type of memory. For example, the knowledge of how to swim is held in the motor area of the brain, whereas visual memories are stored in the visual area of the brain. Scientists believe that the hippocampus of the limbic system acts like a receptionist, deciding the significance of the event and determining in which part of the brain the information should be stored.

Memory may be short term or long term. It depends on how much attention we paid to an event, how many times we repeated an activity, and what the memory is associated with. People frequently recall what took place during a traumatic event, such as their first day at school. Compare that with how many times you have to see a commercial before you can remember it.

Coverings of the Brain

The three meninges are the dura mater, arachnoid, and pia mater, Figure 8-4. The **dura mater**, which literally translated means "tough mother," is the outer brain covering, which lines the skull on the inside. This is a tough, dense membrane of fibrous connective tissue containing an abundance of blood vessels. The **arachnoid (mater)** is the middle layer. It resembles a fine cobweb with fluid-filled spaces. Covering the brain surface itself is the **pia mater**, composed of blood vessels held together by fine areolar connective tissue. The space between the arachnoid and pia mater is filled with cerebrospinal fluid, produced within the ventricles of the brain. This fluid acts both as a shock absorber and a source of nutrients for the brain.

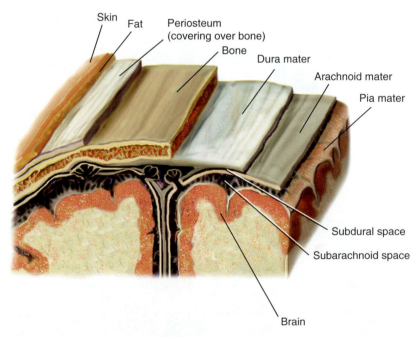

● **FIGURE 8–4** *The meninges consist of the pia mater, the arachnoid mater, and the dura mater.*

STREET SMART

Between each membrane are blood vessels that nourish the cerebral cortex. Just above the dura mater, in the epidural space, are cerebral arteries. Just below the dura mater, in the subdural space, are cerebral veins. Finally, below the arachnoid, in the subarachnoid space, there is a network of thin capillaries.

A head injury can create injury to one, two, or all three of these blood vessels. An injury to a cerebral artery can create an epidural bleed. Epidural bleeds can accumulate blood rapidly and cause the brain to be crushed within the rigid walls of the skull, causing coma and death.

An injury to the veins in the subdural space can create subdural bleeds (subdural hematoma, Figure 8-5). Venous bleeds are slow bleeds by nature and it can take up to 24 hours before the patient exhibits overt clinical symptoms. Subdural bleeds present with a classic constellation of symptoms, including headache, projectile vomiting, hypertension, bradycardia, and unconsciousness.

Injury to the delicate capillaries within the subarachnoid space results in a cerebral contusion (brain bruise) and leads to headaches, nausea, and drowsiness. The amount of associated cerebral edema (swelling) is a function of how much of the brain's surface was affected.

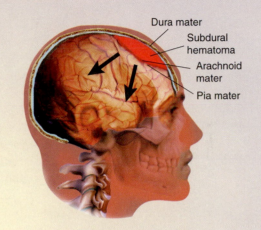

Dura mater
Subdural hematoma
Arachnoid mater
Pia mater

● **FIGURE 8–5** *A subdural hematoma is usually the result of the tearing of small veins under the dura mater.*

Occasionally a congenital (present since birth) intracranial aneurysm spontaneously ruptures, resulting in bleeding. A subarachnoid hemorrhage usually occurs at the bifurcation (division) of a cerebral artery at the base of the brain when the artery ruptures and bleeds into the subarachnoid space.

After rupture there is an acute headache, followed by rapid decline within 24 hours. A subarachnoid hemorrhage has about a 35% mortality rate. ■

STREET SMART

The only thing between the outside world and the brain at a fontanel is a layer of skin and membranes, Figure 8-6. EMS providers often assess the fontanels, particularly the anterior fontanel, which remains open until about the sixth month of life, for bulges or depressions. A bulging fontanel may indicate increased pressure inside the skull, whereas a depressed fontanel may indicate dehydration. ■

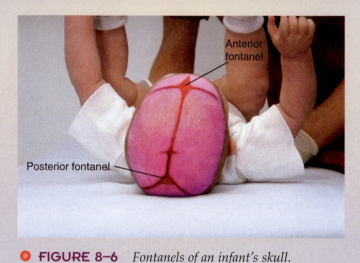

Anterior fontanel

Posterior fontanel

● **FIGURE 8–6** *Fontanels of an infant's skull.*

VENTRICLES OF THE BRAIN

The brain contains four lined cavities filled with cerebrospinal fluid. These cavities are called **cerebral ventricles**, Figure 8-7. The ventricles lie deep within the brain. The two largest, located within the cerebral hemispheres, are known as the right and left **lateral ventricles**.

The **third ventricle** is placed behind and below the lateral ventricles. It is connected to the two lateral ventricles via the **interventricular foramen**. The **fourth ventricle** is situated below the third, in front of the cerebellum, and behind the pons and the medulla oblongata. The third and fourth ventricles are interconnected via a narrow canal called the **cerebral aqueduct**.

Each of the four ventricles contains a rich network of blood vessels of the pia mater, referred to as the **choroid plexus**. The choroid plexus is in contact with the cells lining the ventricles, which helps in the formation of cerebrospinal fluid.

Cerebrospinal Fluid and its Circulation

Cerebrospinal fluid is a substance that forms inside the four brain ventricles from the blood vessels of the choroid plexuses. This fluid serves as a liquid shock absorber protecting the delicate brain and spinal cord. It is formed by filtration from the intricate capillary network of the choroid plexuses. The fluid transports nutrients to and removes metabolic waste products from the brain cells.

Choroid plexus capillaries differ significantly in their selective permeability from capillaries in other areas of the body. As a result, drugs carried in the bloodstream may not effec-

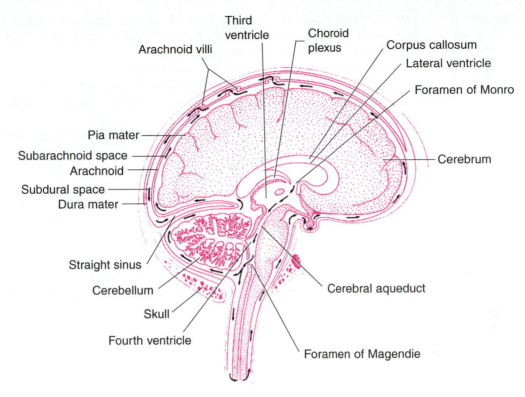

● **FIGURE 8–7**   *Circulation of the cerebrospinal fluid.*

tively penetrate brain tissue, rendering infections (such as meningitis) difficult to cure. This phenomenon is commonly referred to as the **blood-brain barrier**.

After filling the two lateral ventricles of the cerebral hemispheres, the cerebrospinal fluid seeps into the third ventricle through the interventricular foramen (opening). From there it flows through the cerebral aqueduct into the fourth ventricle. The fluid then passes through the fourth ventricle into the small, tubelike central canal of the spinal cord, which bathes the spinal cord in cerebrospinal fluid. Three openings in the walls of the fourth ventricle connect to the subarachnoid spaces. The subarachnoid spaces are thus filled with cerebrospinal fluid which bathes the brain. Ultimately the cerebrospinal fluid returns to the bloodstream via the venous structures in the brain, called arachnoid villi.

The diagnostic tests of cerebrospinal fluid is used by members of the health team to detect some defects or diseases of the brain. For example, inflammation of the cranial meninges quickly spreads to the meninges of the spinal cord. This leads to an increased secretion of cerebrospinal fluid, which collects in the confined bony cavity of the brain and spinal column. The accumulation of excess fluid causes headaches, reduced pulse rate, slow breathing, and unconsciousness.

Removal of cerebrospinal fluid for diagnostic purposes is accomplished with a **lumbar puncture**. The needle used to withdraw the cerebrospinal fluid is inserted between the third and fourth lumbar vertebrae. The fluid, or exudate, withdrawn contains byproducts of the inflammation and organisms causing it. Therefore a lumbar puncture is helpful in diagnosing such diseases as cerebral hemorrhage, increased pressure, intracranial tumors, meningitis, and syphilis. It also serves to alleviate the pressure caused by meningitis and especially hydrocephalus.

A needle can be inserted into the spinal cavity without risk of spinal cord injury because the spinal cord in an adult ends at about the level of the first lumbar vertebra. Below the first lumbar vertebra is a tail-like appendage called the cauda equina, literally "horse's tail."

CEREBRUM

The cerebrum is the largest and highest part of the brain. It occupies the whole upper part of the skull and weighs about 2 pounds. Covering the upper and lower surfaces of the cerebrum is a layer of gray matter called the cerebral cortex; *cortex* means "back" in Latin.

The cerebrum is divided into two hemispheres, right and left, by a deep groove known as the longitudinal fissure. The cerebral surface is completely covered with furrows and ridges. The deeper furrows, or grooves, are referred to as fissures, and the shallower ones, sulci.

The elevated ridges between the sulci are the gyri, also known as convolutions, Figure 8-8. These convolutions serve to increase the surface area of the brain, resulting in a proportionately larger amount of gray matter. The

arrangement of the gyri and sulci on the brain's surface varies from one brain to another. Certain fissures, however, are constant and represent important demarcations. They help to localize specific functional areas of the cerebrum and to divide each hemisphere into four lobes.

Each cerebral hemisphere is divided into a frontal, parietal, occipital, and temporal lobe. These lobes correspond to the cranial bones by which they are overlaid, see Figure 8-8.

The five major fissures dividing the cerebral hemispheres include the following:

1. *Longitudinal fissure*—a deep groove divides the cerebrum into two hemispheres. The middle region of the two hemispheres is held together by a wide band of axonal fibers called the corpus callosum.

2. *Transverse fissure*—divides the cerebrum from the cerebellum.

3. *Central fissure* or *fissure of Rolando*—located beneath the coronal suture of the skull, dividing the frontal lobe from the parietal lobe.

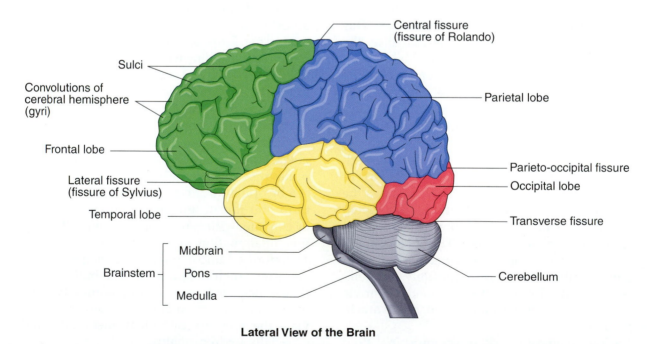

Lateral View of the Brain

● **FIGURE 8–8** *Lateral view of the brain.*

4. *Lateral fissure* or *fissure of Sylvius*—situated on the side of the cerebral hemispheres, dividing the frontal and temporal lobes.

5. *Parieto-occipital fissure*—the least obvious of all the fissures, serves to separate the occipital lobe from the parietal and temporal lobes. There is, however, no definite demarcation between these two lobes.

Cerebral Functions

Each lobe of the cerebral hemispheres controls different types of functions, Figure 8-9.

1. **Frontal lobe**—The cerebral cortex of the frontal lobe controls the motor functions of humans. The motor area occupies a long band of cortex, just in front of the central fissure in the posterior part of the frontal lobe. This motor area controls the voluntary muscles. Cells in the right hemisphere activate voluntary movements that occur in the left side of the body; the left hemisphere controls voluntary movements of the right side. The frontal lobe also includes two areas that

control speech. The speech area, located anterior to the central fissure, usually in the left hemisphere, is also called Broca's area. This area is associated with our ability to speak. Damage to this area means that you may know what to say, but you cannot vocalize the words.

A loss of language function, the ability to understand the spoken word or to express words, is called **aphasia**. Because language is a function of the brain, it follows that any damage to the brain could lead to aphasia.

Injury to an area of the temporal lobe called **Wernicke's area**, caused by a stroke or trauma, may result in **receptive aphasia**, sometimes called sensory aphasia. Receptive aphasia is the inability to understand the printed or spoken word.

Injury to the inferior portion of the frontal lobe, in **Broca's area**, can produce an **expressive aphasia**. When the patient knows what he or she wants to say but cannot say it because of an inability to coordinate the muscles of speech, it is

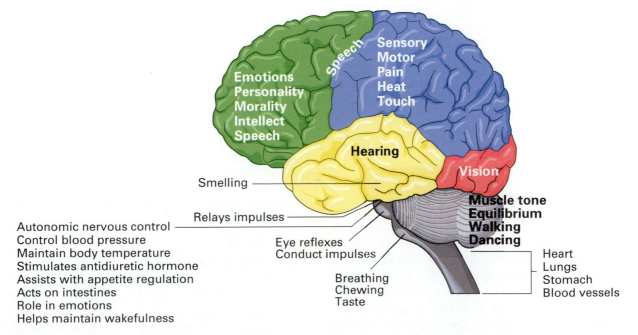

Autonomic nervous control
Control blood pressure
Maintain body temperature
Stimulates antidiuretic hormone
Assists with appetite regulation
Acts on intestines
Role in emotions
Helps maintain wakefulness

Emotions
Personality
Morality
Intellect
Speech

Speech

Sensory
Motor
Pain
Heat
Touch

Hearing

Smelling

Relays impulses

Eye reflexes
Conduct impulses

Breathing
Chewing
Taste

Vision

Muscle tone
Equilibrium
Walking
Dancing

Heart
Lungs
Stomach
Blood vessels

● **FIGURE 8–9** *Cerebral functions.*

called a **motor aphasia**. The person with motor aphasia makes incomprehensible sounds.

It should be emphasized that aphasia can be a sign of an injury or disease of the brain and should not be thought of as being caused by mental illness until a complete medical evaluation is performed.

The speech area that allows us to recognize words and to interpret the meaning, spoken or read, is located at the junction of the temporal, parietal, and occipital lobes, right behind the ear.

2. **Parietal lobe**—the parietal lobe contains the sensory (somesthetic) area. It is found behind the fissure of Rolando, in front of the parietal lobe. This area receives and interprets nerve impulses from the sensory receptors for pain, touch, heat, and cold. It further helps in the determination of distances, sizes, and shapes.

3. **Occipital lobe**—The occipital lobe, located over the cerebellum, houses the visual area, controlling eyesight.

4. **Temporal lobe**—The upper part of the temporal lobe contains the auditory area (including specific tones); the anterior part of the lobe is occupied by the olfactory (smell) area.

The cerebral cortex also controls conscious thought, judgment, memory, reasoning, and will power. This high degree of development makes the human the most intelligent of all animals.

● DIENCEPHALON

The **diencephalon** is located between the cerebrum and the midbrain. It is composed of two major structures, the **thalamus** and the hypothalamus. The thalamus is a spherical mass of gray matter. It is found deep inside each of the cerebral hemispheres, lateral to the third ventricle. The thalamus acts as a relay station for incoming and outgoing nerve impulses. It receives direct or indirect nerve impulses from

the various sense organs of the body (with the exception of olfactory sensations). These nerve impulses are then relayed to the cerebral cortex. The thalamus also receives nerve impulses from the cerebral cortex, cerebellum, and other areas of the brain. Damage to the thalamus may result in increased sensibility to pain or total loss of consciousness.

The **hypothalamus** lies below the thalamus. It forms part of the lateral walls and floor of the third ventricle. A bundle of nerve fibers connects the hypothalamus to the posterior pituitary gland, the thalamus, and the midbrain. The limbic system is the part of the brain associated with emotional control. The hippocampal gyri of the limbic system helps to store and retain short-term memory. The hypothalamus is part of the limbic system and is considered to be the "brain" of the brain. Through the use of feedback, the hypothalamus stimulates the pituitary to release its hormones. Nine vital functions are performed by the hypothalamus:

1. *Autonomic nervous control*—Regulates the parasympathetic and sympathetic systems of the autonomic nervous system.

2. *Cardiovascular control*—Controls blood pressure, regulating the constriction and dilation of blood vessels and the beating of the heart.

3. *Temperature control*—Helps maintain normal body temperature (37° C or 98.6° F).

4. *Appetite control*—Assists in regulating the amount of food we ingest. The "feeding center," found in the lateral hypothalamus, is stimulated by hunger "pangs," which prompt us to eat. In turn, the "satiety center" in the medial hypothalamus becomes stimulated when we have eaten enough.

5. *Water balance*—Within the hypothalamus, certain cells respond to the osmotic pressure of the blood. When osmotic pressure is high because of water deficiency, the antidiuretic hormone (ADH) is secreted. A "thirst area" is found near the satiety area, becoming stimulated when the

MEDICAL HIGHLIGHTS

The limbic system relates to the primitive behavior of mankind. It influences unconscious, instinctive behaviors that relate to survival. This behavior is modified by the action of the cerebral cortex. Our primitive brain says, "I want it now"; our higher functioning brain says, "You can't have it now. You have to wait until later."

The limbic system encircles the top of the brainstem almost like a covering (the word *limbic* means "border"), linking the cerebral cortex and the midbrain areas with the lower centers that control the automatic functions of the body.

The limbic system plays a role in the expression of instincts, drives, and emotions; mediates the effects of the moods on external behavior; and influences internal changes in bodily functions. The association of feelings with sensations such as sight and smell and the formation of memories are influenced by the limbic system.

Parts of the limbic system include:

- *Septum pellucidum*—Connects the fornix to the corpus callosum.

- *Mammillary body*—This nucleus transmits messages between the fornix and thalamus.

- *Olfactory bulbs*—This connection may explain why the sense of smell evokes forgotten memories (think of good smells from your childhood).

- *Amygdala*—This structure influences behavior appropriate to meet the body's needs, which include feeding, sexual interest, and emotional reactions such as anger.

- *Parahippocampal gyrus*—Helps to modify strong emotions such as rage and fright.

- *Hippocampus*—Involved with learning and memory, recognizes new information, and recalls spatial relationships.

- *Fornix*—Pathway of nerve fibers transmits information from the hippocampus to the mammillary body.

- *Cingulate gyrus*—This area, with others, composes the limbic cortex, which modifies behavior and emotion. ■

blood's osmolality is high. This causes us to consume more liquids.

6. *Manufacture of oxytocin*—Contracts the uterus during labor.

7. *Gastrointestinal control*—Increases intestinal peristalsis and secretion from the intestinal glands.

8. *Emotional state*—Plays a role in the display of emotions such as fear and pleasure.

9. *Sleep control*—Helps keep us awake when necessary.

CEREBELLUM

The **cerebellum** is located behind the pons and below the cerebrum, see Figure 8-8. It is composed of two hemispheres, or wings: the right cerebellar hemisphere and the left cerebellar hemisphere. These two hemispheres are connected to a central portion called the vermis. The cerebellum consists of gray matter on the outside and white matter on the inside. The white matter on the inside of the cerebellum is marked with a treelike pattern. This pattern is called arbor vitae ("tree of life").

The cerebellum communicates with the rest of the central nervous system by three pairs of tracts called peduncles. These three peduncles are composed of "incoming" axons that carry nerve messages into the cerebellum and "outgoing" axons that transmit messages out of the cerebellum. The incoming axons carry messages to the cerebellum regarding movement within joints, muscle tone, position of the body, and tightness of ligaments and tendons. Any and all information relating to skeletal muscle activity is carried to the cerebellum. This information reaches the cerebellum directly from sensory receptors, including the inner ear, the eye, and the proprioceptors of the skeletal muscle. The outgoing axons carry nerve messages to the different parts of the brain that control skeletal muscles.

Cerebellar Function

The cerebellum controls all body functions that have to do with skeletal muscles.

- *Maintenance of balance*—If the body is imbalanced, sensory receptors in the inner ear send nerve messages to the cerebellum. Then the cerebellum carries impulses to the motor controlling areas of the brain. These brain areas in turn stimulate muscle contraction that restores balance.

- *Maintenance of muscle tone*—The cerebellum transmits nerve impulses to the red nucleus

that in turn relays them to the spinal cord and then to the skeletal muscles.

- *Coordination of muscle movements*—Any voluntary movement is initiated in the cerebral cortex. However, once the movement is started, its smooth execution is the role of the cerebellum. The cerebellum allows each muscle to contract at the right time, with the right strength, and for the right amount of time, so that the overall movement is smooth and flowing. This is important when doing complex or skilled movements such as speaking, walking, and writing; even simple movements need the coordinating abilities of the cerebellum. A simple action such as raising the hand to the face to avoid a blow requires the synchronized action of 50 or more muscles. These muscles then act on 30 separate bones of the arm and hand.

The removal of or injury to the cerebellum results in motor impairment.

● BRAINSTEM

The **brainstem** is made up of three parts: the midbrain, pons, and medulla. The brainstem provides a pathway for the ascending and descending tracts (messages going to the cerebrum and messages coming back from the cerebrum). The gray matter of the reticular formation system extends the length of the brain-

STREET SMART

The cerebellum is sometimes called the athletic brain because it controls balance and coordination of muscle movements, such as dribbling a basketball or swinging a bat.

When a law enforcement officer (LEO) stops a motorist and asks him or her to perform a series of intricate maneuvers, such as

walking toe-to-heel, the LEO is testing the motorist's cerebellar functions. Inability to perform these "street sobriety tests" may indicate that the driver is intoxicated. These tests are reasonable when it is understood that a driver must perform many intricate physical maneuvers to operate a motor vehicle safely. ■

STREET SMART

Foramen magnum literally means "big hole" and is the point in the skull where the base of the brain exits the skull. When increased **intracranial pressure** (ICP) occurs because of a space-occupying lesion, like an accumulation of blood or a brain tumor, the pressure compresses the medulla oblongata, the pons, and several cranial nerves.

The pons controls respiration, and compression of the pons results in irregular breathing. Compression of the cranial nerves also has a dramatic effect. The tenth cranial nerve, the **vagus nerve**, controls the heart's rate; when compressed it slows the heart (**bradycardia**). The medulla oblongata controls, among its many other functions, the blood pressure; when the medulla oblongata is compressed, blood pressure elevates to dangerous levels (**hypertension**).

These three symptoms, irregular breathing, bradycardia, and profound hypertension, are referred to as **Cushing's triad**. Cushing's triad is indicative of high ICP, which can lead to coma and death. Forceful vomiting, called projectile vomiting, is also indicative of increasing ICP. ∎

stem. The gray matter are the neurons that are involved in the sleep-wake cycle. If there is damage to this area, coma results. The **pons** is located in front of the cerebellum, between the midbrain and the medulla oblongata. It contains interlaced transverse and longitudinal myelinated, white nerve fibers mixed with gray matter. The pons serves as a two-way conductive pathway for nerve impulses among the cerebrum, cerebellum, and other areas of the nervous system. The pons is also the site of the emergence of four pairs of cranial nerves, and it contains a center that controls respiration.

The midbrain extends from mammillary bodies to the pons. The cerebral aqueduct travels through the midbrain. It contains the nuclei for reflex centers involved with vision and hearing.

The **medulla oblongata** is a bulb-shaped structure found between the pons and the spinal cord. It lies inside the cranium and above the foramen magnum of the occipital bone. The medulla is white on the outside, just like the pons, because of the myelinated nerve fibers that serve as a passageway for nerve impulses between the brain and spinal cord. It contains the nuclei for vital functions such as the heart rate; the rate and the depth of respiration; the vasoconstrictor center, which affects blood pressure; and the center for swallowing and vomiting.

SPINAL CORD

The **spinal cord** continues down from the brain. It begins at the foramen magnum of the occipital bone and continues to the second lumbar vertebra. It is white and soft and lies within the vertebrae of the spinal column. Like the brain, the spinal cord is submerged in cerebrospinal fluid and is surrounded by the three meninges. The gray matter in the spinal cord is located in the internal section; the white matter comprises the outer part, Figure 8-10. In the gray matter of the cord, connections can be made between incoming and outgoing nerve fibers, which provide the basis for reflex action. The spinal cord functions as a reflex center and as a conduction pathway to and from the brain.

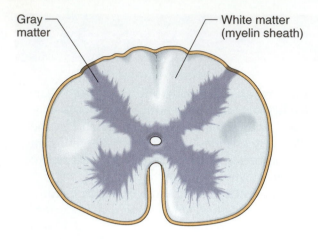

Gray matter

White matter (myelin sheath)

● **FIGURE 8–10** *Cross-section of the spinal cord.*

● DISORDERS OF THE CENTRAL NERVOUS SYSTEM

Meningitis is an inflammation of the linings of the brain and spinal cord. The cause may be bacterial or viral. Communities experience periodic outbreaks of meningitis, usually in high school or college-age students. Symptoms include headache, fever, and stiff neck. In severe form it may lead to paralysis, coma, and death. If the cause is bacterial, it may be treated with antibiotics.

Encephalitis is an inflammation of the brain. The disease may be caused by a virus; in certain conditions, the cause may be chemical. The symptoms of this disorder usually are fever, lethargy, extreme weakness, and visual disturbance.

Epilepsy is a seizure disorder of the brain characterized by a recurring and excessive discharge from neurons. Approximately one person out of 200 in the United States suffers from some form of epilepsy. Epileptic seizures are believed to be a result of spontaneous, uncontrolled cycles of electrical activity in the neurons of the brain. The cause is uncertain. One portion of the brain stimulates another, setting off a cycle of activity that accelerates and runs its course until the neurons become fatigued. The person may suffer hallucinations, a seizure (convulsion), and a loss of consciousness.

A **seizure** is a disruption of brain function that may be due to a number of causes, including low blood sugar (hypoglycemia) or a low percentage of oxygen in the blood (hypoxia).

Some people have seizures without any known reason; a disease or illness with no known cause is referred to as an idiopathic condition. *Epilepsy* is a term used to describe people who have idiopathic seizures or who have seizures for reasons that would not cause most people to have a seizure.

In the past, inaccurate terms such as *grand mal* ("great sickness") or *petit mal* ("little sickness") were used to describe seizures. Those terms have been dropped in favor of a new, more precise classification of seizure disorders.

Not all seizures involve the entire brain. Some seizures involve only a portion of the brain and thus are called **partial seizures**. Some of these seizures affect a small portion of the brain and only cause movement in one part of the body. These seizures are called **simple partial seizures**. **Tics**, uncontrollable rhythmic contractions of facial muscles, are examples of simple partial seizures.

Some partial seizures are more complex, involving an entire lobe of the brain; these are labeled **complex partial seizures**. A person experiencing a complex partial seizure may have an **aura** before the seizure. An aura is a sensation, often a flash of light or a strange metallic taste in the mouth, that occurs just before the seizure. These complex partial seizures are characterized by confusion, unintelligible sounds, or purposeless movements that last for just a minute or two. Afterward the patient may not understand that he or she just had a seizure.

When a seizure involves the entire brain and causes an extensive disruption in brain function, it is called a **generalized seizure**. Generalized seizures usually start at one point in the brain, called a focus, and then spread over the entire brain.

Some generalized seizures are brief, lasting only 10 to 30 seconds. These seizures, formerly called petit mal, are now called **absence seizures**. Absence seizures typically involve a loss of consciousness but may not involve loss of muscle tone. The result is that the patient remains sitting or standing and appears to be staring off into space, oblivious to his or her surroundings.

A seizure that results in the rhythmic jerking of the entire body is called a **tonic-clonic generalized seizure**; these can be divided into three phases.

The **preictal phase** begins when the patient experiences an aura and then loses consciousness. Not all patients experience an aura, but for those who do there is not enough time to react and to sit or lie down before the next phase.

In the next phase, the **tonic phase**, all the muscles in the body contract. This sudden contraction of the muscles of the body causes the entire body to stiffen.

After the tonic phase, there is a repetitive contraction and then relaxation of the muscles, which is referred to as the **clonic phase**. During this phase, the patient cannot breath effectively or control his or her airway. The bladder, a muscular organ, also contracts, and the patient may soil him or herself, called **incontinence**.

The period after the seizure subsides is called the **postictal phase**. A patient who is postictal is usually tired and may continue to be confused for up to 30 minutes.

Medications used to control seizures are referred to as **anticonvulsants**. Examples are phenobarbital (Phenobarbital), phenytoin (Dilantin), and carbamazepine (Tegretol).

Cerebral palsy is a disturbance in voluntary muscular action resulting from brain damage. Definite causes are unknown; it may be due to birth injury or abnormal brain development. The most pronounced characteristic is **spastic quadriplegia**, or spastic paralysis of all four limbs. The person with cerebral palsy frequently exhibits head rolling, grimacing, and difficulty in speech and swallowing. In cerebral palsy there is usually no impairment of the intellect; the person frequently has normal or above normal intelligence.

Poliomyelitis is a disease of the nerve pathways of the spinal cord, which causes paralysis. Because the Sabin and Salk vaccines are now used, this disease has been almost eliminated in the United States; however, it still occurs in other countries.

Hydrocephalus is a condition in which there is an increased volume of cerebrospinal fluid within the ventricles of the brain. The usual cause is a blockage somewhere in the third or fourth ventricle. There is an enlargement of the head; this condition is usually noted at birth. A bypass or shunt operation is performed that diverts the cerebrospinal fluid around the blocked area. This operation prevents a buildup of pressure on brain tissue.

Parkinson's disease is characterized by tremors, a shuffling gait, pill-rolling (movement of the thumb and index finger), and muscular rigidity. The patient with Parkinson's has difficulty initiating movement. The

STREET SMART

Some patients have a long history of a seizure disorder and take medications. These people are said to be *controlled*. A person who suffers a seizure for the first time should be evaluated immediately by a physician. New-onset seizure may result from a head injury; infections of the covering of the brain, the meninges (meningitis); or a brain tumor.

If untreated, these seizures can increase in frequency until the patient experiences one prolonged seizure or a series of seizures without an intervening period of consciousness. This condition, called **status epilepticus**, is a true medical emergency. Untreated, status epilepticus can lead to brain injury and death. ■

cause may be a decrease of the neurotransmitter dopamine. Persons with Parkinson's disease are treated with the drug L-dopa and other drugs that help to control the symptoms of the disease.

Multiple sclerosis (MS) is a chronic inflammatory disease of the central nervous system in which immune cells attack the myelin sheath of nerve cell axons. The myelin sheaths are destroyed, leaving scar tissue on the nerve cells. This destruction delays or completely blocks the transmission of nerve impulses in the affected areas. The cause is unknown. There is no definitive test for MS. The diagnosis of multiple sclerosis is made through symptoms and signs of impairment to more than one area of the central nervous system occurring at more than one time.

Symptoms include weakness of extremities, numbness, double vision, **nystagmus** (tremorous movement of the eye), speech problems, loss of coordination, and possible paralysis. It typically strikes young adults between the ages of 20 and 40; about two thirds of these are women. With MS there are outbreaks of the symptoms and then the disease may go into remission for a long period. This disease is classified in the autoimmune category; the drug interferon has been used as a treatment. In May 1996 the Food and Drug Administration (FDA) approved the use of a drug called interferon beta-1a (Avonex), which, tests have shown, can slow progression of multiple sclerosis and decrease the number of flare-ups. Adequate rest, exercise, and minimal stress may also lessen the effects of multiple sclerosis.

Dementia is a general term that includes specific disorders such as Alzheimer's disease, vascular dementia, and others. Dementia is defined as a loss in at least two areas of complex behavior, such as language, memory, visual, spatial abilities, or judgment, that significantly interferes with a person's daily life.

Alzheimer's disease is a progressive disease in which the initial symptom is usually difficulty remembering recently learned information. In Alzheimer's disease, the nerve endings in the cortex of the brain degenerate and block the signals that pass between nerve cells. These areas of degeneration have a unique appearance; they are called plaques. The nerve cells undergo further change and abnormal fibers build up, creating neurofibrillary tangles, like a group of telephone lines getting tangled.

The cause of Alzheimer's is unknown. The cells that produce the neurotransmitter acetylcholine are sometimes destroyed in this disease. The cause of the disease may be virus related, environmental factors may play a role, or it may be associated with a gene defect on chromosome 21, which is also involved with Down syndrome.

Alzheimer's disease usually has three stages. The first may last from 2 to 4 years and

STREET SMART

EMS providers must distinguish between when a confused person is experiencing dementia or **delirium**. Delirium is a state of mental confusion, often associated with excitement or frenzy, which can be the result of intoxication, fever, or drug overdose (intentional or unintentional).

Fortunately the onset of delirium is abrupt, whereas the onset of dementia is progressive and involves irreversible deterioration of mental functions. Any abrupt changes in behavior—that is, delirium—should be evaluated and treated by a physician before permanent brain injury can occur. ■

involves confusion, short-term memory loss, anxiety, and poor judgment. In the second stage, which may last from 2 to 10 years, there is an increase in memory loss, difficulty in recognizing people, motor problems, logic problems, and loss of social skills. The third stage includes the inability to recognize oneself, weight loss, seizures, mood swings, and aphasia (loss of speech). This stage may last from 1 to 3 years.

Factors that may help prevent Alzheimer's disease include continued education; cardiovascular exercise; estrogen replacement therapy; antioxidants such as vitamins C and E and betacarotene; and the use of antiinflammatory agents.

Brain tumors may develop in any area of the brain. The symptoms depend on which area of the brain is involved. Early detection, surgery, and chemotherapy may lead to successful treatment of some brain tumors.

Hematoma is a localized mass of blood collection and may occur in the spaces between the meninges. The cause may be a blow to the head; the person may have a subdural hematoma (located between the dura mater and arachnoid layer).

A **stroke**, also called a brain attack, is a loss of function in a portion of the brain as a result of loss of oxygen-rich blood to that portion of the brain. The loss of blood can be due to a rupture of a cerebral blood vessel, which leads to bleeding, or **hemorrhage**. This type of stroke is called a **hemorrhagic stroke**. Hemorrhagic strokes are often preceded by years of high blood pressure (hypertension), which strains and weakens the blood vessels.

A stroke can also be the result of a blockage or occlusion of a cerebral blood vessel. This occlusion stops blood flow distal to the blockage, causing injury or death of brain tissue. This mechanism creates what is called an **occlusive stroke**. The occlusion is frequently caused by a blood clot (**thrombus**) that is formed in the brain; thus these are called **thrombotic strokes**. New drugs called **fibrinolytics** (formerly called thrombolytics), which break up those clots very early in their creation, offer hope of recovery to these stroke victims. Therefore a patient with stroke-like symptoms should be immediately seen in an emergency department for evaluation and treatment.

Sometimes the occlusion is caused by another substance that arrives from somewhere else in the body. This substance is called an **emboli**; it can block a cerebral blood vessel and cause an **embolic stroke**. Common sources of emboli include blood clots that migrate from the heart or legs to the brain; pieces of fat from a broken bone; and amniotic fluid from a pregnant uterus postpartum. Regardless of the source, the effect is the same; a cerebral blood vessel is blocked and an occlusive stroke occurs.

Symptoms of a stroke include confusion, drop attacks (falling without a loss of consciousness), slurred speech (dysarthria), one-sided blindness, facial droop, and hemiparesis (one-sided weakness of the extremities).

Some strokes start as a weakness in one arm and progress to one entire side of the body. The patient gets progressively worse as the area of injury enlarges. This is called a stroke in evolution. The symptoms of a stroke depend on the area of ischemia and damage.

Sometimes stroke symptoms spontaneously resolve. These short-lived strokes, sometimes called mini-strokes, are actually **transient ischemic attacks (TIA)**. Untreated, a patient who experiences a TIA has a 50% chance of having another episode, which may result in a stroke and permanent brain injury, within a year.

● REVIEW QUESTIONS

Select the letter of the choice that best completes the statement.

1. Each nerve cell has only one:
   a. axon
   b. neurilemma
   c. dendrite
   d. myelin

2. The fatty substance that helps to protect the axon is called:
   a. neurotransmitter
   b. myelin
   c. dendrite
   d. nodes of Ranvier

3. The junction between the axon of one cell and the dendrite of another is called:
   a. neurilemma
   b. myelin
   c. synaptic cleft
   d. nodes of Ranvier

4. The neurons that carry messages to the brain are called:
   a. motor
   b. associate
   c. connective
   d. sensory

5. The nervous system, which is composed of 12 pairs of cranial nerves and 31 pairs of spinal nerves, is called:
   a. central
   b. peripheral
   c. sympathetic
   d. parasympathetic

6. The outermost covering of the meninges is the:
   a. arachnoid
   b. arachnoid villa
   c. dura mater
   d. pia mater

7. The lumbar puncture must be done below the:
   a. first lumbar vertebra
   b. second lumbar vertebra
   c. third lumbar vertebra
   d. sacrum

8. The front, parietal, temporal, and occipital lobes make up the:
   a. cerebrum
   b. cerebellum
   c. midbrain
   d. brainstem

9. The part of the brain associated with muscle movement is the:
   a. midbrain
   b. thalamus
   c. cerebrum
   d. medulla

10. The thalamus and hypothalamus are parts of the:
    a. cerebrum
    b. cerebellum
    c. diencephalon
    d. brainstem

● MATCHING

Match each term in Column A with its correct description in Column B.

Column A	Column B
_____ 1. frontal lobe—cerebrum	a. auditory
_____ 2. occipital lobe—cerebrum	b. receptor for pain, touch, etc.
_____ 3. hypothalamus	c. reflex center
_____ 4. temporal lobe	d. speech area
_____ 5. parietal lobe	e. maintains balance
_____ 6. cerebellum	f. eyesight
_____ 7. thalamus	g. respiratory center
_____ 8. spinal cord	h. appetite control
_____ 9. medulla	i. site for four pairs of cranial nerves
_____ 10. pons	j. relay station for nerve impulses

●APPLYING THEORY TO PRACTICE

1. The central nervous system serves as the communication center of our bodies. Explain how your hand touches something cold and you know it; refer to a sensory neuron and the correct lobe of the cerebrum.

2. A blow to the head can cause a loss of consciousness. What centers in the brain are associated with alertness?

3. You frequently hear the expression "I have early Alzheimer's"; explain what this means. Do you think this illness will have an impact on the cost of health care? Explain your answer.

9 Peripheral and Autonomic Nervous System

Objectives

- Describe a mixed nerve
- Describe the functions of the cranial and spinal nerves
- Relate the functions of the sympathetic and parasympathetic nervous systems
- Explain the simple reflex arc pattern
- Describe common disorders of the peripheral nervous system
- Define the key words that relate to this chapter

Key Words

acetylcholine
adrenergic receptors (alpha and beta)
analgesic
ascending tract
Bell's palsy
blown pupil
carpal tunnel syndrome
central canal
cholinergic receptors
cranial nerves
descending tract
effector
electromyograph
femoral nerve
hypoperfusion
mixed nerve
motor (efferent) nerve
muscarinic receptor
neuralgia
neuritis
neuromuscular blocking agent
neurotransmitter
nicotinic receptor
norepinephrine

paresthesia
paralysis
paraplegia
parasympathetic system
paresis
paresthesia
phrenic nerve
plexus
priapism
pruritus
quadriplegia
radial nerve
receptor
referred pain
reflex
reflex arc
relative hypovolemia
sciatica
sciatic nerve
sensory (afferent) nerve
shingles (herpes zoster)
shock
somatic pain
spinal canal
spinal nerves

(continues)

Key Words (continued)

spinal (neurogenic)
   shock
stimulus
sympathetic system

transection
trigeminal neuralgia
visceral pain

specialized part of the peripheral system; it controls the involuntary, or automatic, activities of the vital internal organs.

Functions of the peripheral nervous system include the following:

1. Control the automatic (involuntary) activities of the body

2. Act as the reflex center of the body

● PERIPHERAL NERVOUS SYSTEM

The peripheral nervous system includes all the nerves of the body and the ganglia (groups of cell bodies), see Figure 9-1. It connects the central nervous system to the various body structures. The autonomic nervous system is a

● NERVES

A nerve is composed of bundles of nerve fibers enclosed by connective tissue. If the nerve is composed of fibers that carry impulses

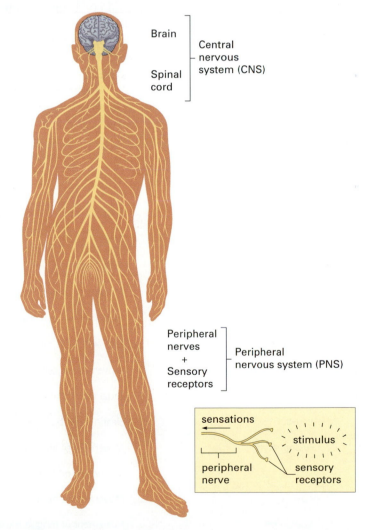

● **FIGURE 9–1**   *Peripheral nervous system. This connects the central nervous system to the structures of the body.*

from the sense organs to the brain or spinal cord, it is called a **sensory**, or **afferent**, nerve; if it is composed of fibers carrying impulses from the brain or spinal cord to muscles or glands, it is known as a **motor**, or **efferent**, nerve; and if it contains both sensory and motor fibers, it is referred to as a **mixed nerve**.

In short, afferent nerves carry impulses regarding how we feel, or affect, whereas efferent nerves carry impulses that cause us to react; that is, they effect movement of our muscles.

● CRANIAL AND SPINAL NERVES

Cranial and spinal nerves are part of the peripheral nervous system.

There are 12 pairs of **cranial nerves**, which begin in different areas of the brain. The cranial nerves are designated by number and name; the name may give a clue to its function, Table 9-1. For example, the olfactory nerve, cranial nerve I, is responsible for the sense of smell. The optic nerve, cranial nerve II, is responsible for vision. The functions of the cranial nerves are concerned mainly with the activities of the head

and neck, with the exception of the vagus nerve. The vagus nerve, cranial nerve X, is responsible for activities involving the throat, as well as regulating the heart rate; it also affects the smooth muscle of the digestive tract. Most of the cranial nerves are mixed: They carry both sensory and motor fibers. However, the olfactory, optic, and acoustic nerves carry only the sensory fibers. They only pick up the stimuli.

The **spinal nerves** originate at the spinal cord and go through openings in the vertebrae. There are 31 pairs of spinal nerves, all of which are mixed nerves. The spinal nerves are named in relation to their location on the spinal cord. Because spinal nerves carry messages to and from the spinal cord, when there is a spinal cord injury there is no sensation or movement. The spinal nerves carry messages to and from the spinal cord and brain and to all parts of the body. Each of these spinal nerves divides and branches. They go either directly to a particular body segment or they form a network with adjacent spinal nerves and veins, called a plexus, Figure 9-2 and Table 9-2.

TABLE 9-1 *Cranial Nerves*

NUMBER	NAME	FUNCTION
I	Olfactory	Smell
II	Optic	Vision, eyesight
III	Oculomotor	Movement of eye muscle
IV	Trochlear	Movement of eye muscle
V	Trigeminal	Face and teeth muscles, chewing
VI	Abducens	Movement of eye muscle
VII	Facial	Facial expressions, taste
VIII	Acoustic	Hearing and balance
IX	Glossopharyngeal	Movement of throat muscle, taste
X	Vagus	Movement of throat; affects heart, digestive system
XI	Accessory	Movement of neck muscles
XII	Hypoglossal	Movement of tongue muscles

STREET SMART

Some of the cranial nerves exit from the base of the skull at the same place as the spinal cord. When pressure increases inside the skull because of sudden bleeding or a growing tumor, pressure is exerted downward. This pressure, in turn, compresses the cranial nerves as well.

Two nerves that are particularly affected are the vagus nerve (CN X) and the oculomotor nerve (CN III). The vagus nerve helps to regulate the heart; pressure on the vagus nerve causes the heart to slow, called bradycardia.

The oculomotor nerve helps to control the iris (a muscle of the eye), resulting in changes in pupil size (the black opening of the eye). Pressure on the oculomotor nerve results in extreme pupil dilation, called a **blown pupil**.

Bradycardia and a blown pupil are both signs of increasing intracranial pressure. ■

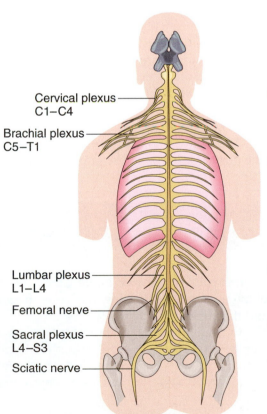

Cervical plexus
C1–C4

Brachial plexus
C5–T1

Lumbar plexus
L1–L4

Femoral nerve

Sacral plexus
L4–S3

Sciatic nerve

Cervical plexus
Nerve supply to muscles of neck and shoulder
Includes phrenic nerve, which stimulates the
  diaphragm

Brachial plexus
Includes axillary, radial, median, musculocutaneous,
  ulnar

Lumbar plexus
Includes femoral, obturator

Sacral plexus
Includes sciatic (largest nerve in the body),
  commonpuoneal, tibeal

● **FIGURE 9–2** *Spinal nerve plexus and important nerves.*

TABLE 9-2 *Spinal Nerve Plexus*

NAME	LOCATION	FUNCTION
Cervical plexus	C1—C4	Supplies motor movement to muscles of the neck and shoulders and receives messages from these areas.
		The **phrenic nerve** is part of this group and stimulates the diaphragm.
Brachial plexus	C5—C8, T1	Supplies motor movement to the shoulder, wrist, and hand and receives messages from these areas.
		The **radial nerve** is part of this group and stimulates the wrist and hand.
Lumbar plexus	T12, L1—L4	Supplies motor movement to the buttocks, anterior leg, and thighs and receives messages from these areas.
		The **femoral nerve** is part of this group and stimulates the hip and leg.
Sacral plexus	L4—L5, S1—S2	Supplies motor movement to the posterior of the leg and thighs and receives messages from these areas.
		The **sciatic nerve** is the largest nerve in the body and is part of this group. It passes through the gluteus maximus and down the back of the thigh and leg. It extends the hip and flexes the knee. (This nerve must be avoided when giving an intramuscular injection.)

● THE SPINAL CORD

The spinal cord is a long column of nerves that runs from the base of the brain, at the foramen magnum, to the small of the back through the middle of the spinal column in a space called the spinal canal. These nerves branch off, exit the spinal column, and form 31 pair of spinal nerves.

The spinal cord has two layers of tissue, like the brain. There is an outer layer, the white matter, and an inner layer, where gray matter is found. The shape of the gray matter of the inner layer can be roughly compared with the shape of a butterfly.

The upper wings of the butterfly are called the posterior horns of the gray matter, whereas

✳ STREET SMART

An injury to the cervical spine caused by a motor vehicle collision or a fall can result in injury to the nerves within the cervical plexus. The most important of these spinal nerves is the phrenic nerve. The phrenic nerve exits the cervical spine at the third, fourth, and fifth cervical vertebrae and controls the movement of the diaphragm, which is the largest muscle of breathing.

If the phrenic nerve is injured, the patient's diaphragm stops working (becomes frozen) and the patient has difficulty breathing.

To remember this important relationship between the spinal column, the phrenic nerve, and the diaphragm, EMS providers have learned this rhyme: "3-4-5 keeps a man alive." ■

the lower wings are called the lateral and anterior horns. In the middle, where the body of the butterfly would be, is the gray commissure. The gray commissure connects the two sides, or the wings of the butterfly.

In the middle of the commissure there is a thin channel, called the **central canal**, that contains cerebrospinal fluid. The central canal runs the entire length of the spine and shares cerebrospinal fluid with the brain. Thus if the cerebrospinal fluid in the outer layer of the brain, the meninges, becomes infected (meningitis), the infection can travel down the length of the spinal cord.

The spinal cord can be thought of as the main line of a complex communications system. The job of the spinal cord is to transmit messages from the body, via the spinal nerves, to the brain and to relay messages from the brain, via the spinal nerves, to the muscles and organs of the body.

Naturally those spinal nerve bundles within the spinal cord that carry sensory messages *to* the brain are called **ascending tracts**. The spinal nerves that carry impulses to the brain, impulses that are interpreted as touch, pressure, pain, and temperature, run from the spine to the thalamus (spinothalamic tracts) and are located in the anterior and lateral horns.

The spinal nerves that carry impulses from the muscles of the legs and abdomen *to* the cerebellum of the brain, which allow the brain to sense position, are part of the spinocerebellar tract and can be found in the lateral horns.

Just as there are ascending tracts, there are also **descending tracts**. The most important of the descending tracts is the corticospinal tract, also located in the anterior and lateral horns. The spinal nerves of the corticospinal tract run from the cortex of the brain to the muscles of the body via the spinal cord. The spinal nerves that branch off from the corticospinal tract control voluntary muscle movement in the body.

The Reflex Arc

The simplest type of nervous response is the **reflex** arc, which is unconscious and involuntary. Blinking an eye when a particle of dust touches

it, removing a finger from a hot object, secreting saliva at the sight or smell of food, are all examples of reflexive actions caused by a reflex arc.

Every reflex is preceded by a **stimulus**, which is a change in the environment. Examples of stimuli are sound waves, light waves, heat energy, and odors. Specialized nerve cells called **receptors** pick up these stimuli. For example, the retina of the eye is the receptor for light; special cells in the inner ear are receptors for sound waves; and special structures in the skin are the receptors for heat and cold.

A simple reflex is one in which there is only a sensory nerve and a motor nerve involved. The classic example is the "knee-jerk" reflex. The knee is tapped and the leg extends, Figure 9-3. This is used by physicians to test both the muscle and the nervous system.

Response is the reaction to a stimulus. The response may be in the form of movement, in which case the muscular contraction is the **effector**. If the response is in the form of a secretion, the glands are the effectors. Reflex actions involving the skeletal muscles are controlled by the spinal cord; these are also known as autonomic or somatic reflexes.

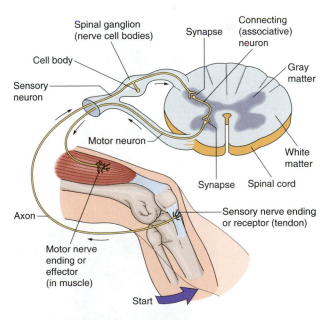

● **FIGURE 9–3** *In this example, tapping the knee (patellar tendon) results in extension of the leg, producing the knee-jerk reflex.*

AUTONOMIC NERVOUS SYSTEM

The autonomic nervous system includes nerves, ganglia, and plexuses that carry impulses to all smooth muscle, secretory glands, and heart muscle, Figure 9-4. It regulates the activities of the visceral organs (heart and blood vessels, respiratory organs, alimentary canal, kidneys and urinary bladder, and reproductive organs). The activities of these organs are usually automatic and are not subject to conscious control.

The autonomic system is composed of two divisions: the sympathetic and the parasympathetic. These two divisions may be antagonistic in their action. The sympathetic system may accelerate the heartbeat in response to fear, whereas the parasympathetic system

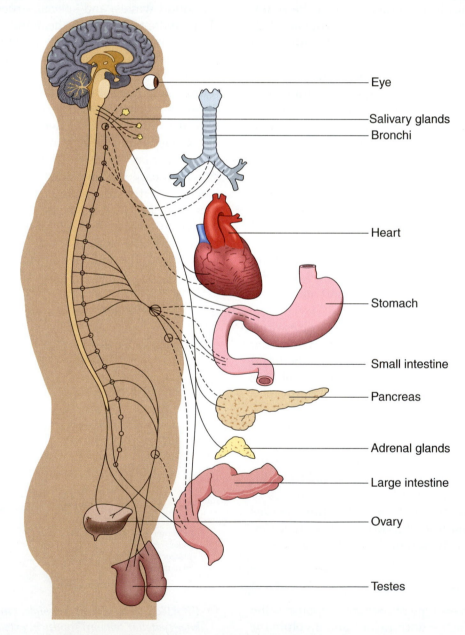

Eye
Salivary glands
Bronchi
Heart
Stomach
Small intestine
Pancreas
Adrenal glands
Large intestine
Ovary
Testes

● **FIGURE 9–4** *Autonomic nervous system and target organs.*

slows it down. Normally the two divisions are in balance; the activity of one or the other becomes dominant as dictated by the needs of the organism.

The sympathetic system consists primarily of two cords that begin at the base of the brain and proceed down both sides of the spinal column. These are made up of nerve fibers and ganglia of nerve cell bodies. The cord between the ganglia is a cable of nerve fibers closely associated with the spinal cord. Sympathetic nerves extend to all the vital internal organs, including the liver and pancreas, heart, stomach, intestines, blood vessels, iris of the eye, sweat glands, and bladder. The sympathetic nervous system is often referred to as the "fight or flight system." When the body perceives it is in danger or under stress, it prepares to run away or stand and fight, Figure 9-5. The sympathetic nervous system sends the message to the adrenal medulla, which secretes its hormones to prepare the body for this action. Think about how you feel when you are facing a major exam, or think about the patient waiting in the doctor's office for test results. You can feel your heart beating faster and your mouth going dry—all results of the automatic response to danger. When the danger passes, the parasympathetic nervous system helps restore balance to the body system. If our body experiences too much stress, health problems may result. Learning to live with stress is the key to being a healthier person.

The parasympathetic system is primarily composed of two important nerves: the vagus nerve and the pelvic nerves. The vagus nerve, which extends from the medulla and proceeds down the neck, sends branches to the chest and neck. The pelvic nerve, emerging from the spinal cord around the hip region, sends branches to the organs in the lower part of the body.

Both the sympathetic and parasympathetic systems are strongly influenced by emotion. During periods of fear, anger, or stress, the sympathetic division prepares the body for action. The effects of the parasympathetic system generally counteract the effects of the sympathetic system. For example, the sympathetic nervous system increases the rate of heart mus-

cle contraction, and the parasympathetic decreases the rate. The two systems operate as a pair, striking a nearly perfect balance when the body is functioning properly.

Neurotransmitters

The body's use of chemical energy, or its conservation of its available energy stores, is a function of the external environment. The ever-changing external environment requires the body to constantly adjust to maintain the internal environment so that cells can function properly. The nervous system helps to maintain that balance.

The sympathetic nervous system is primarily interested in energy-expending activities, such as increasing the heart rate. The parasympathetic nervous system is primarily interested in energy-conserving activities, such as slowing the heart rate. These two portions of the autonomic nervous system are constantly fluctuating—one is dominant one minute and the other is dominant the next.

Most organs of the body have both sympathetic and parasympathetic nerves that affect the way that organ functions. For example, the upper portion of the heart has both sympathetic and parasympathetic nerve fibers, whereas the lower portion of the heart, which is the main pumping portion of the heart, has only sympathetic nerves. Nerves that affect organs are called visceral effectors. That means that these nerves determine how that target organ functions.

These nervous system messages are transmitted across the synapse to the target organ by a chemical messenger called a neurotransmitter. In the case of sympathetic nerves, the neurotransmitter is norepinephrine.

On the other side of the synapse, on the target organ, are receptors. In the case of the sympathetic nervous system, they are called sympathetic receptors. There are several different types of sympathetic receptors.

The first type of sympathetic receptors is called the adrenergic receptors. The adrenergic receptors are broken down into alpha or beta receptors. The alpha- or beta-adrenergic

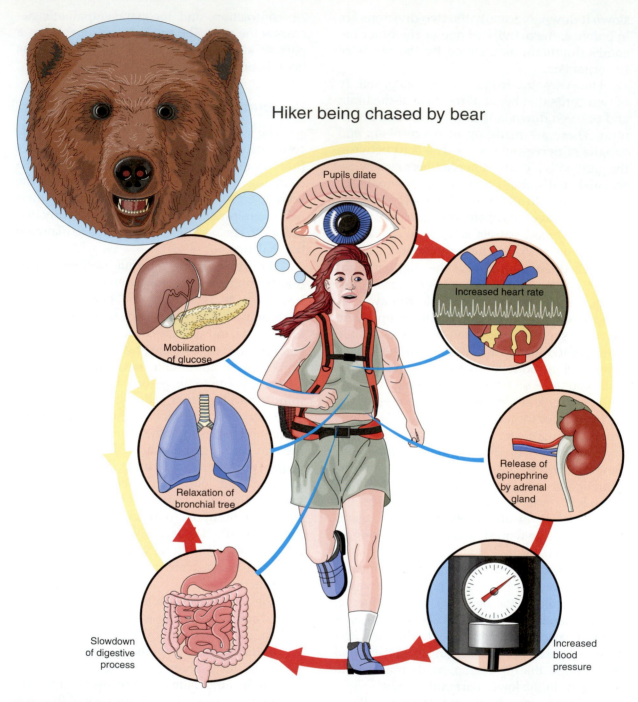

Hiker being chased by bear

Pupils dilate

Increased heart rate

Mobilization of glucose

Release of epinephrine by adrenal gland

Relaxation of bronchial tree

Increased blood pressure

Slowdown of digestive process

● **FIGURE 9–5** *Fight or flight response.*

receptors are further broken down into type 1 and type 2. Each type of receptor, alpha-1, alpha-2, beta-1, and beta-2, causes a target organ to act in a particular way.

For example, alpha-1 receptors cause vaso-constriction of peripheral arterioles, whereas beta-1 receptors cause the kidneys to release a chemical called renin.

Of particular interest to EMS providers are the beta-adrenergic receptors, because they affect the heart and lungs. Stimulation of beta-1 adrenergic receptors causes the heart to increase in rate and strength of contraction, whereas beta-2 adrenergic receptors cause bronchodilation. An easy way to remember these important functions of the adrenergic receptors is the phrase "beta-1, beat faster, beta-2, breathe better."

There is another sympathetic receptor called the dopaminergic receptor. The presence of dopaminergic receptors is debated, but stimulation of the dopaminergic receptors by norepinephrine is thought to increase blood flow to the kidneys.

Like the sympathetic system, the parasympathetic system also has a special set of receptors, called **cholinergic receptors**, which accept the neurotransmitter **acetylcholine**. These cholinergic receptors are also divided into two types. The first type is the **nicotinic receptors**, which cause muscular contraction.

The other type of cholinergic receptor is the **muscarinic receptors**, which affect a large number of organs and are primarily responsible for what is called the "parasympathetic effect." The effect of acetylcholine on muscarinic receptors is to slow the heart rate, dilate arteries, increase gastrointestinal activity, increase mucus production in the lungs, and constrict the pupils.

The importance of understanding each of these neurotransmitters and the effect on the receptors of target organs cannot be overemphasized to EMS providers. Many of the drugs that are used in the field by advanced EMS providers have either a stimulating or blocking effect on these receptors.

Once the neurotransmitter has delivered its message, enzymes present in the organ at the synaptic cleft dissolve the neurotransmitter; for example, the enzyme acetylcholinesterase destroys acetylcholine. Without these enzymes the organ would continue to be stimulated again and again by the neurotransmitter.

Whenever the spinal cord is injured or completely cut as a result of trauma, called a **transection**, such as from a motor vehicle collision (MVC), it disconnects the central nervous system from communication with other portions of the body below the level of the spinal cord injury. This loss of the central nervous system control may result in a loss of motion (efferent nerve injury), called **paralysis**; muscular weakness (**paresis**); or loss of sensation (afferent nerve injury), called **paresthesia**. This loss of feeling, movement, or strength is characteristic of spinal cord injury.

STREET SMART

During an emergency it may be necessary for an EMS provider to place a special breathing tube, called an endotracheal tube, into a patient's lungs so that the patient's airway can be protected and the lungs ventilated. In some cases it may difficult to perform this life-saving technique because the patient is combative. Specially trained EMS providers can use drugs called **neuromuscular blocking agents** to aid intubation. A neuromuscular blocking agent interferes with the neurotransmitters by blocking the nicotinic receptor. Nicotinic receptors are largely responsible for muscle use. The blockade of the nicotinic receptors effectively paralyzes the patient, thereby allowing easier control of the airway for placement of the endotracheal tube.

One popular neuromuscular blocking agent is succinylcholine. Succinylcholine is simply two molecules of acetylcholine that are chemically linked together; the body has natural enzymes that break it down. ∎

If the spinal cord injury is in the cervical area, there may be a loss of feeling and movement in the legs (paraplegia) or a loss of feeling and movement in all four extremities (quadriplegia). Special care must be taken to prevent injury to the spinal cord when caring for patients who could potentially have neck trauma.

If the spinal cord is injured, there is a loss of sympathetic nervous control below the injury. Several other classic symptoms of spinal cord injury may also appear. For example, a male patient may experience a sustained painful erection of the penis (priapism). The patient may also spontaneously empty his or her bladder because of sacral reflexes that are triggered when the bladder is full. These reflexes are usually consciously restrained by the patient; however, spinal cord injury leads to loss of central nervous control and the primitive bladder-emptying sacral reflexes return.

The lack of sympathetic nervous system control because of the spinal cord injury also results in vasodilation of the blood vessels within the body. This has the effect of expanding the size of the blood vessels, that is, the vascular bed, without increasing the amount of blood needed to fill those blood vessels. The result is an insufficient blood volume in relation to the enlarged blood vessels. This state is called a relative hypovolemia, meaning blood is not lost but insufficient amounts of blood exist in the body.

The problem is further compounded because the body also loses its control over the autonomic nervous system, particularly the adrenal medulla. During times of stress the adrenal medulla excretes adrenalin (epinephrine), a hormone that causes the heart rate to accelerate. The increased heart rate helps to supply vital organs with needed blood if there is a loss of blood volume, for example.

The combination of relative hypovolemia and slow heart rate results in inadequate blood flow to the vital organs (hypoperfusion) and can lead to a syndrome called shock. Shock as a result of injury to the spinal cord is called spinal (neurogenic) shock. The patient with spinal shock classically presents with skin that is "cool above and warm below," meaning the skin is warm below the level of spinal cord injury because of vasodilation.

Pain

Pain is the body's early warning system. It tells us when organs or tissues are being injured or inflamed, either internally or externally. In fact, pain is one of the cardinal symptoms of inflammation.

Pain is the result of stimulation of specialized sensory nerves called pain receptors. This sensation, pain, can be described as anything ranging from discomfort to agonizing. Pain is different for every person because to describe a pain that person must have an experience with similar pain in the past. This ability to compare pain is referred to as a pain history.

Many EMS providers ask patients to gauge their pain based on the patients' pain history. The EMS provider asks patients where this pain would fall on a scale of 0 to 10 if 0 means no pain and 10 is the worst pain ever experienced.

Pain is often the result of trauma. An injury to the skin—a cut or laceration, for example—is quickly identified by the patient and can be characterized by an exact descriptor, such as "sharp," and a specific location can be given. This kind of pain is called somatic pain; *soma* means "body."

The kind of pain that a person experiences during a heart attack is harder to pinpoint. For example, a person having a heart attack might say "My whole chest hurts," indicating the entire chest, and may say that it feels something like "an elephant sitting on my chest." This deeper organ pain is called visceral pain.

Visceral pain is usually caused by injury (ischemia) or death (infarction) of organs, or distention or compression of organs within a body cavity. Visceral pain tends to be more disturbing and is frequently continuous, lasting hours.

When visceral pain fibers from one deep organ join with somatic pain fibers from another part of the body in the spinal cord, it is not uncommon for the person to experience somatic pain in that other body part. For example, someone experiencing chest heaviness or discomfort as the result of a heart attack may say that the left arm hurts as well. This type of pain is called **referred pain**.

● DISORDERS OF THE PERIPHERAL NERVOUS SYSTEM

Neuritis is an inflammation of a nerve or a nerve trunk. The symptoms may be severe pain, hypersensitivity, loss of sensation, muscular atrophy, weakness, and paresthesia (tingling, burning, and crawling of the skin). The causes of neuritis may be infectious, chemical, or other conditions such as chronic alcoholism. In the patient who is an alcoholic, neuritis usually occurs because of a lack of vitamin B or an improper diet.

In the treatment of neuritis it is necessary to determine the cause to eliminate the symptoms. The pain of neuritis may be relieved with **analgesics** (painkillers).

Sciatica is a form of neuritis that affects the sciatic nerve. The cause may be a rupture of a lumbar disk or arthritic changes. The most common symptom is pain that radiates through the buttock and behind the knee down to the foot. The person may have difficulty walking. Treatment includes traction, physiotherapy, exercises, and possibly surgery to alleviate the symptoms.

Neuralgia is a sudden severe, sharp, stabbing pain along the pathway of a nerve. The pain is often brief; it may be a symptom of a disease. The various forms of neuralgia are named according to the nerves they affect.

Trigeminal neuralgia is a condition involving the fifth cranial nerve (trigeminal). The cause is unknown, the onset is rapid, and the pain is severe. The spasm of pain can be brought on by a stimulus as slight as a breeze, a piece of food in the mouth, or even a change in temperature. The term "tic douloureux" is sometimes applied to this condition, because the pain lasts only 2 to 5 seconds. The treatment may be analgesics or partial removal of the fifth cranial nerve.

Bell's palsy is a condition that involves the seventh cranial nerve (facial). The patient appears to have had a stroke on one side of the face. Bell's palsy only affects one side of the face. The eye does not close properly, the mouth droops, and there is numbness on the affected side. The cause is unknown. The treatment consists of massage and heat application. The patient must perform exercises such as whistling to prevent atrophy of the cheek muscles. The symptoms usually disappear within a few weeks, with no residual effects.

Shingles, or **herpes zoster**, is an acute viral nerve infection. It is characterized by a unilateral (one-sided) inflammation of a cutaneous nerve. The intercostal nerves are most commonly affected. The course of inflammation can spread to any nerve. Symptoms include extremely painful vesicular eruptions of the skin and mucous membrane along the route of the inflamed nerve. Shingles is frequently seen in the elderly or the debilitated. The causative organism of herpes zoster is the same virus that causes chickenpox. Treatment consists of analgesics for the pain and medications that relieve the **pruritus** (itching).

Carpal tunnel syndrome is a condition affecting the median nerve and the flexor tendons that attach to the carpal bones of the wrist. The syndrome develops because of repetitive movement of the wrist in which the hands are held in an unusual position. Swelling (edema) develops around the carpal tunnel. This is where the median nerve passes. The edema causes pressure on the nerve, which results in pain, muscle weakness, and tingling sensations in the hand. The diagnostic test for carpal tunnel syndrome is an **electromyograph** (EMG). An EMG is a record of muscle electrical activity. Treatment consists of immobilizing the wrist joint. If this treatment is not effective, surgery may be done.

● REVIEW QUESTIONS

Select the letter of choice that best completes the statement.

1. A nerve containing fibers that both send and receive messages is called:
    a. sensory nerve
    b. afferent nerve
    c. efferent nerve
    d. mixed nerve

2. The cranial nerve that is responsible for chewing is the:
    a. trochlear
    b. facial
    c. glossopharyngeal
    d. trigeminal

3. The cranial nerves responsible for eye muscle movement are the oculomotor, trochlear, and:
    a. abducens
    b. acoustic
    c. accessory
    d. hypoglossal

4. A network of spinal nerves is called:
    a. mixed
    b. efferent
    c. plexus
    d. afferent

5. The autonomic nervous system is also called:
    a. voluntary
    b. involuntary
    c. neuralgic
    d. carpal

6. The autonomic nervous system is part of the:
    a. central nervous system
    b. peripheral nervous system
    c. sympathetic nervous system
    d. parasympathetic nervous system

7. The sympathetic nervous system, which acts in the same manner as adrenalin, does the following:
    a. increases the heart rate and dilates the pupils
    b. increases the heart rate and constricts the pupils
    c. slows the heart rate and dilates the pupils
    d. slows the heart rate and constricts the pupils

8. The nerve that activates the diaphragm is the:
    a. sciatic
    b. phrenic
    c. radial
    d. femoral

9. The simplest type of nervous system response is called:
    a. stimulus
    b. effector action
    c. reflex
    d. affector action

10. The acute viral infection that usually affects the intercostal nerves is called:
    a. Bell's palsy
    b. neuralgia
    c. sciatica
    d. shingles

● COMPLETION

Complete the following statements.

1. A nerve is composed of small blood vessels and bundles of fibers called _____.

2. A nerve composed of fibers carrying impulses from sense organs to the brain or spinal cord is called a _____ or _____ nerve.

3. A nerve composed of fibers that carry impulses from the brain or spinal cord to muscles or glands is called a _____ or _____ nerve.

4. A mixed nerve contains both _____ and _____ fibers.

5. The autonomic nervous system is a specialized part of the peripheral system and controls _____.

6. The autonomic nervous system has two parts that counterbalance each other; these are the _____ and _____ systems.

● LABELING

Identify the structures on the following figure. Enter your answers in the spaces provided.

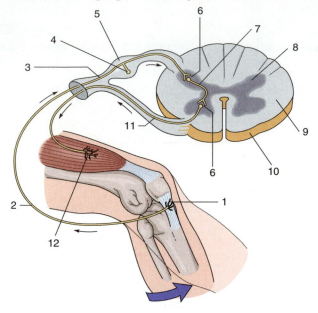

1. _____   7. _____

2. _____   8. _____

3. _____   9. _____

4. _____   10. _____

5. _____   11. _____

6. _____   12. _____

●APPLYING THEORY TO PRACTICE

1. You are passing by a pizzeria and smell the pizza cooking. Describe what happens to your salivary glands. What else are feeling? Relate these reactions to your peripheral nervous system.

2. The knee jerk is the most common reflex we know about in health care. You are born with certain reflexes and you learn some reflexes. Name at least five reflexes with which babies are born and five reflexes that must be learned.

3. A doctor has a patient who is experiencing facial and cheek pain, sometimes called trigeminal neuralgia. Describe this condition and the appropriate treatment.

4. After a lengthy car ride, your elderly uncle gets out of the car and complains, "I can hardly walk. It must be sciatica." Explain what this means.

5. Carpal tunnel syndrome affects many middle-aged Americans. What types of jobs increase the risk of this disease, and what are some of the treatments?

Special Senses

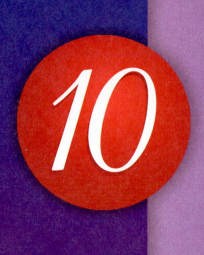

10

Objectives

- Describe the function of the sensory receptors all over our bodies
- Identify the parts of the eye and describe their functions
- Trace the pathway of light from outside to the occipital lobe
- Identify the parts of the ear and describe their functions
- Trace the pathway of sound from pinna to temporal lobe
- Describe the process involved with the sense of smell
- Describe common disorders of the eye, the ear, and the nose
- Define the key words that relate to this chapter

Key Words

amblyopia
American Sign Language
anisocoria
anterior chamber
anvil (incus)
aqueous humor
astigmatism
basilar skull fracture
cataracts
cautery
choroid coat
ciliary body
ciliary gland
cochlea
cochlear duct
cones
conjunctivitis
cornea
cyanotic
detached retina
deviated nasal septum
diplopia
epistaxis
eustachian tube
extrinsic muscle

fovea centralis
glaucoma
hammer (malleus)
hard of hearing (HOH)
hearing aids
hyperopia
   (farsightedness)
interpreter
intrinsic muscle
iris
jaundice
lacrimal gland
lens
macular degeneration
Meniere's disease
miotic
myopia (nearsightedness)
myringotomy
nasal polyp
optic disc (blind spot)
organ of Corti
otitis media
otosclerosis
otorrhea
PEARL

(continues)

Key Words (continued)

pinna	semicircular canals
posterior chamber	six cardinal gazes
presbycusis	stirrup (stapes)
presbyopia	strabismus ("cross eyes")
pupil	sty
raccoon's eyes	suspensory ligament
retina	symbol board
retract	tinnitus
rhinitis	tonometer
rhinorrhea	tympanic membrane
rods	vertigo
sclera	vitreous humor

The special senses are those organs and receptors that are associated with touch (sensory receptors), vision, hearing, smell, and taste. They receive stimuli from the sensory receptors, the eye, the ear, the nose, and the tongue, and transmit these impulses to the brain for interpretation.

● SENSORY RECEPTORS

Sensory receptors are special structures that are stimulated by changes in the environment; these touch, pain, temperature, and pressure receptors are found all over the body, located in the skin or connective tissues. Special sensory receptors include the taste buds of the tongue, special cells in the nose, the retina of the eye, and the special cells in the inner ear that make up the organ of Corti. When a sense organ is stimulated,

the impulse travels along nerve pathways to the brain, where it is registered in a certain area. Sensation actually takes place in the brain, but it is mentally referred back to the sense organ. This is called projection of the sensation.

● THE EYE

The human eye is a tender sphere approximately 1 inch in diameter (about 2.5 centimeters). It is protected by the orbital socket of the skull, a wall of bones surrounding it, and by the eyebrows, eyelids, and eyelashes, Figure 10-1. The eyes are continuously bathed in fluid by tears secreted by lacrimal glands, which are located above the lateral area of each eye. The tears flow across the eye into the lacrimal duct. The lacrimal duct is located in the corner of the eye and empties into the nasal cavity, causing an increase in fluids. This explains why, when we cry, we may also need to blow our noses. Lacrimal secretions have antibiotic properties: Tears cleanse and moisten the eyes on a continuous basis.

Along the border of each eyelid are modified sebaceous glands that secrete an oily substance; that substance lubricates the eye and slows evaporation of water. There are also **ciliary glands**, which have ducts that open into the eyelashes. An infection of the ciliary gland is called a sty.

The conjunctiva is the thin mucous membrane that lines the eyelids and covers part of the eye. It is rich with capillaries and secretes mucus, which helps to lubricate the eye. Many EMS providers pull down, or **retract**, the lower

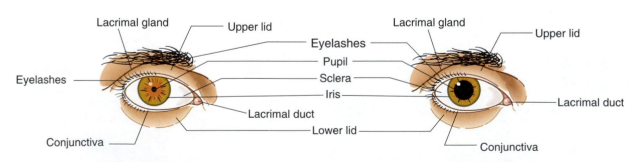

(A) In bright light, circular muscles contract and constrict the pupil.

(B) In dim light, the radial muscles contract and dilate the pupil.

● **FIGURE 10–1**   *External view of the eye.*

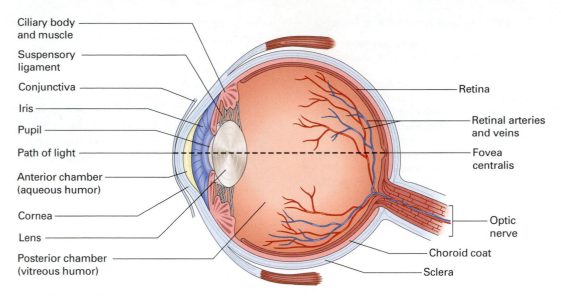

Ciliary body and muscle
Suspensory ligament
Conjunctiva
Iris
Pupil
Path of light
Anterior chamber (aqueous humor)
Cornea
Lens
Posterior chamber (vitreous humor)

Retina
Retinal arteries and veins
Fovea centralis
Optic nerve
Choroid coat
Sclera

● **FIGURE 10–2**   *Internal view of the eye.*

eyelid to observe the capillary bed of the conjunctiva. If the patient's blood is poorly oxygenated, the eyelid may appear bluish, or **cyanotic**. If the patient has lost a significant amount of blood, the conjunctiva may appear pale. If the patient has a liver disease, such as hepatitis, the conjunctiva may be yellowed, or **jaundiced**.

The location of the eyes in the front of the head allows for superimposition of images from each eye. This binocular vision enables us to see stereoscopically in three dimensions (length, width, and depth). The eye's optical system for detecting light is similar to that of a camera.

The wall of the eye is made up of three concentric layers, or coats, each with its specific function. These three layers are the sclera, the choroid, and the retina, Figure 10-2.

Sclera

The outer layer of the eye is called the **sclera**, or white of the eye. It is a tough, unyielding fibrous capsule that maintains the shape of the eye and protects the delicate structures within. Muscles responsible for moving the eye within the orbital socket are attached to the outside of the sclera. These muscles are referred to as the **extrinsic muscles**, Figure 10-3. They include the superior, inferior, lateral, and medial rectus and

the superior and inferior oblique. See Table 10-1 for a listing of the extrinsic and intrinsic eye muscles and their functions.

When an EMS provider suspects an injury to the muscles of an eye, such as when a softball strikes the eye's orbit, an assessment of the eye is performed. A part of that assessment is an evaluation of the **six cardinal gazes**, which involve the use of all the extrinsic muscles.

The patient is asked to look up and then down, from side to side, and from one corner to another. If one eye cannot move in one direction,

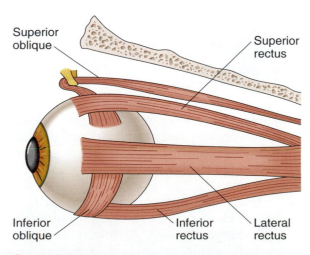

Superior oblique
Superior rectus
Inferior oblique
Inferior rectus
Lateral rectus

● **FIGURE 10–3**   *Extrinsic eye muscles.*

TABLE 10-1 *Extrinsic and Intrinsic Eye Muscles*

EYE MUSCLE	FUNCTION
A. Extrinsic	
1. Superior rectus	Rolls eyeball upward
2. Inferior rectus	Rolls eyeball downward
3. Lateral rectus	Rolls eyeball laterally
4. Medial rectus	Rolls eyeball medially
5. Superior oblique	Rolls eyeball on its axis, moves cornea downward and laterally
6. Inferior oblique	Rolls eyeball on its axis, moves cornea upward and laterally
B. Intrinsic	
1. Sphincter pupillae	Constricts pupil
2. Dilator pupillae	Dilates pupil

it is described as a "loss of gaze" and reported to the physician.

Cornea

In the front center of the sclera coat lies a clear circular area called the **cornea**, sometimes referred to as the "window" of the eye. It is transparent to permit light rays to pass through it. The cornea lacks blood vessels. Corneal cells are fed oxygen and nutrients by the aqueous humor. The cornea is composed of five layers of flat cells arranged much like sheets of plate glass. Possessing pain and touch receptors, it is sensitive to any foreign particles that come in contact with its surface.

An injury to the cornea can cause scarring and impaired vision.

Choroid Coat and the Iris

The middle layer of the eye is the **choroid coat**. It contains blood vessels to nourish the eye and a nonreflective pigment rendering it dark and opaque. The pigment provides the choroid coat with a deep, red-purple color; this darkens the eye chamber, preventing light reflection within the eye. In front the choroid coat has a circular opening called the **pupil**. A circular muscular layer surrounds the pupil; this is the **iris**, the colored part of the eye. The iris may be blue, green, gray, brown, or black. Eye color is related to the number and size of melanin pigment cells in the iris. If there is little melanin present, the eye is blue, because light is scattered to a greater extent. With increasing quantities of melanin, eye color ranges from green to black. The total absence of melanin results in a pink eye color, characteristic of albinism. Such irises are pink because the blood inside the choroid blood vessels shows through the iris.

Within the iris are two sets of antagonistic smooth muscles: the sphincter and the dilator pupillae. These **intrinsic muscles** help the iris to control amounts of light entering the pupil, see Table 10-1. When the eye is focused on a close object or stimulated by bright light, the sphincter pupillae muscle contracts, rendering

STREET SMART

EMS providers regularly check a patient's pupils for a reaction to a bright light. Normal pupils respond to bright light briskly and equally. This response is documented as "pupils equal and reactive to light" (**PEARL**).

Unequal pupils may be a sign of head injury. However, some people naturally have unequal pupils. Naturally occurring unequal pupils, or **anisocoria**, occurs in a very small percentage of the population, Figure 10-4. ■

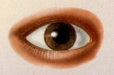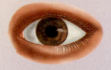

● **FIGURE 10–4** *Unequal pupils (anisocoria).*

the pupil smaller. Conversely, when the eye is focused on a distant object or stimulated by dim light, the dilator pupillae muscle contracts. This causes the pupil to grow larger, permitting as much light as possible to enter the eye. In this way the eye may be compared with a camera; the iris corresponds to the diaphragm.

Lens and Related Structures

The **lens** is a crystalline structure located behind the iris and pupil. It is composed of concentric layers of fibers and crystal-clear proteins in solution. It is an elastic, disk-shaped structure with anterior and posterior convex surfaces, thus forming a biconvex lens. However, the posterior surface is more curved than that of the anterior. The curvature of each surface alters with age. During infancy, the lens is spherical; in adulthood it becomes convex; and it is almost flat in old age. The capsule surrounding the lens also loses its elasticity over time. The lens is held in place behind the pupil by **suspensory ligaments** from the **ciliary body** of the choroid body.

The lens is situated between the **anterior** and **posterior chambers**. The anterior chamber is filled with a watery fluid referred to as the **aqueous humor**, and it is constantly replenished by blood vessels behind the iris, Figure 10-5. **Vitreous humor**, a transparent, jellylike substance, fills the posterior chamber. Vitreous humor

forms in the embryo, is never replaced, and lasts a lifetime. Both these substances help to maintain the eyeball's spherical shape, refracting (bending) light rays as they pass through the eye.

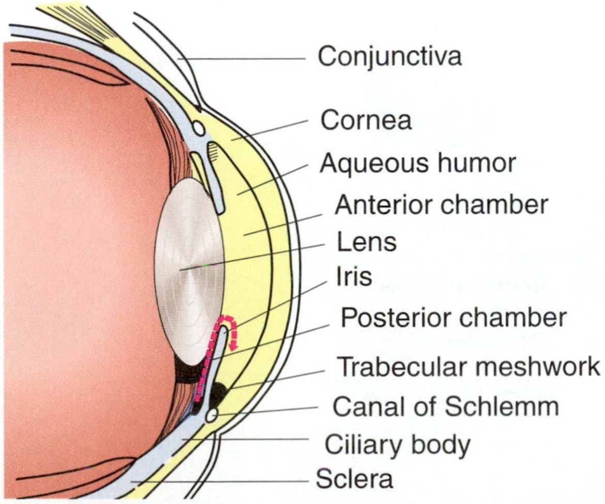

Retina

The **retina** of the eye is the innermost, or third coat of the eye. It is located between the posterior chamber and the choroid coat. The retina does not extend around the front portion of the eye. It is on this light-sensitive layer that light rays from an object form an image. After the image is focused on the retina, it travels via the optic nerve to the visual part of the cerebral cortex (occipital lobe). If light rays do not focus correctly on the retina, the condition may be corrected with properly fitted contact lenses or eyeglasses, which bend the light rays to focus on the retina.

The retina contains pigment and specialized cells known as **rods** and **cones**, Figure 10-6, which are sensitive to light. The rod cells are sensitive to dim light and the cones are sensitive to bright light. The cones are also responsible for color vision. There are three varieties of cone cells. Each type is sensitive to a special color. The part of the retina where the nerve fibers enter the optic nerve to go to the brain does not have these specialized cells.

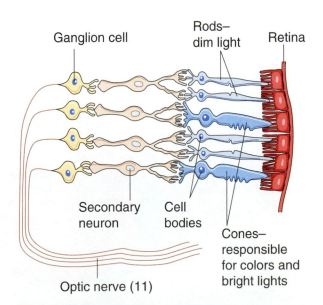

FIGURE 10-6 *Diagram of visual neurons showing rods and cones.*

● **FIGURE 10-5** *Flow of the aqueous humor.*

Conjunctiva

Cornea

Aqueous humor

Anterior chamber

Lens

Iris

Posterior chamber

Trabecular meshwork

Canal of Schlemm

Ciliary body

Sclera

Ganglion cell

Rods—dim light

Retina

Secondary neuron

Cell bodies

Cones—responsible for colors and bright lights

Optic nerve (11)

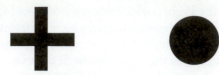

1. Close your left eye and focus your right eye on the cross.
2. Move the page slowly away from your eye and then slowly toward your eye.
3. At a distance of about 6–8 inches the black circle "disappears."

● **FIGURE 10–7** *Testing for the blind spot.*

The Optic Disc and the Fovea. Viewing the retina through an ophthalmoscope, a yellow disc known as the macula lutea can be observed. Within this disc is the **fovea centralis**, which contains the cones for color vision, see Figure 10-2. The area around the fovea centralis is the extrafoveal or peripheral region. This is where the rods for dim and peripheral vision can be found.

Slightly to the side of the fovea lies a pale disc called the **optic disc**, or **blind spot**. Nerve fibers from the retina gather there to form the nerve. The optic disc contains no rods or cones; therefore it is devoid of visual recep-

tion. See Figure 10-7 to help you locate your blind spot.

● **PATHWAY OF VISION**

Light images enter the pupil and pass through the cornea to the lens, where the light rays are bent, or refracted. The inverted image falls on the retina's rods and cones (nerve cells) and the optic nerve picks up the stimulus and transmits the information through the optic chiasma (where the two optic nerves cross) along the optic tracts to the visual cortex in the occipital lobe of the brain for perception and interpretation, Figure 10-8.

● **EYE DISORDERS**

Conjunctivitis is an inflammation of the conjunctival membranes in front of the eye. Redness, pain, swelling, and discharge of mucus occur. Conjunctivitis, or "pink eye," usually begins in one eye and spreads rapidly to the other by contact with contaminated hands. Because it is highly contagious, other family members should not share facial washcloths or hand towels with the infected person. Good

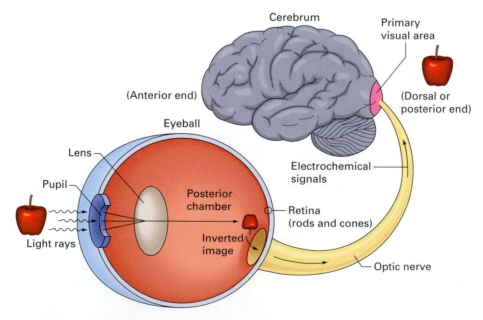

● **FIGURE 10–8** *Pathway of vision.*

hand washing is important to prevent the spread of the infection to others. Treatment includes eye washes or eye irrigations, which will cleanse the conjunctiva and relieve the inflammation and pain. Bacterial conjunctivitis responds to antibiotic and sulfa drug therapy.

Glaucoma is a condition of excessive intraocular pressure leading to the destruction of the retina and atrophy of the optic nerve. The condition results from overproduction of aqueous humor or the obstruction of its outflow through the canal of Schlemm for absorption into the venous circulation. Symptoms are gradual. They include mild aching, a loss of peripheral vision, and a halo around the light.

Glaucoma may occur with aging and has no initial symptoms. It is important for people to be tested for glaucoma annually after age 40. Intraocular eye pressure is measured by a **tonometer**. A puff of air is directed onto the eye or a pressure-sensitive tip is placed gently near the eye to measure the intraocular pressure. The diagnosis is confirmed by viewing characteristic changes in the optic disc through an ophthalmoscope.

Treatment involves **miotic** drugs that constrict the pupil and thus increase the outflow of aqueous humor or drugs that reduce the amount of aqueous fluid produced by the eye. Today laser surgery or incisional surgery help to increase the flow of aqueous humor. All treatments are focused on lowering the intraocular pressure.

Cataracts is a condition in which the lens of the eye gradually becomes cloudy. This frequently occurs in people who are more than 70 years old. The condition causes a painless, gradual blurring and loss of vision. The pupil turns from black to milky white. People with cataracts may complain of seeing halos around lights or being blinded at night by oncoming headlights.

Cataracts are treated by the surgical removal of the cloudy lens and postoperative substitution of contact lenses or eyeglasses. An intraocular lens may also be implanted directly behind the cornea.

Macular degeneration is another eye disorder. The macula, found in the central part of the retina, is responsible for sharp central vision. Symptoms of macular degeneration include a dimming or distortion of vision that is most obvious when reading. In one form of the disease, straight lines look wavy and blind spots may develop in the visual field. There are two types of macular degeneration: dry and wet. In the dry type, the main defect is a gradual thinning of the retina. This is slowly progressive, and there is no known treatment. Central vision is greatly reduced, but usually there is not total blindness.

In the wet type, leakage develops under the retina, causing blister formations that may involve blood vessels. Laser treatment may be used with this type of macular degeneration. The good news about macular degeneration is that the majority of people who develop it are able to maintain their independence of movement with low-vision aids.

A **detached retina** can result from disease or trauma. Symptoms include loss of peripheral vision and then loss of central vision. Early detection is important, because the detachment can be repaired with a laser or freezing technique. NOTE: It is important to have annual eye examinations. Early detection of eye problems can save your vision.

A fracture of the bones that support the eye in the socket, called a blowout fracture, can be the result of a direct blow to the orbit of the eye. If the person leans forward, causing the eye to fall forward out of the eyeball's socket, the retina pulls off the back of the eyeball. The resulting detached retina cannot function and the person is blinded.

A **sty** (hordeolum) is an abscess at the base of an eyelash. It is caused by the inflammation of one of the tiny sebaceous glands of the eyelid. The eye is red, painful, and swollen. Treatment consists of warm, wet compresses to relieve pain and promote drainage.

The second most common cause of blindness is diabetes. Changes to the blood vessels within the eye as a result of the diabetes cause the blood vessels to weaken and rupture. Bleeding into the eyeball's vitreous humor blocks vision; it has been described as "having a curtain fall." Vision remains blocked until the vitreous humor absorbs the blood. Eventually so many

CHANGES OF AGING

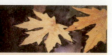

Glaucoma, cataracts, macular degeneration, and detached retina are all common conditions that are caused by aging. As a result, elderly patients are frequently sight impaired. These patients often depend on eyeglasses (especially bifocals).

On occasion, EMS providers are requested to assist a sight-impaired person with walking. The patient will typically grasp the EMS provider by the elbow and walk slightly behind and to the side. The EMS provider should call out obstacles, such as doorways.

In some cases the patient may have a seeing-eye dog. Although many hospitals and ambulances do not permit animals, a seeing-eye dog is considered an exception to the rule. ■

blood vessels break, and other processes occur in the eyes, that permanent blindness results.

Eye Injuries

In most cases of simple eye irritation the natural flow of tears helps to cleanse the eye. In cases in which pieces of glass or other fragments get into the eye, do not attempt to remove the object. Patch both eyes and get medical treatment.

Corneal abrasions and scarring may occur as a result of an accident or irritation. The cornea is avascular; that is, there are no blood vessels present. Therefore corneal transplants can be done readily without fears of tissue rejection.

Eye irritations can be caused by chemicals or fragments that get into the eye. Rinse eyes with water for at least 15 minutes and seek medical treatment.

Night blindness is a condition that makes it difficult to see at night. The rod cells in the retina are affected in this condition.

Color blindness is the inability to distinguish colors. There are three specific types of

STREET SMART

After an injury to the head or face, the patient may develop a bruise around both eyes, called bilateral periorbital ecchymosis, or what is more commonly referred to as **raccoon's eyes**, Figure 10-9. Raccoon's eyes are not the result of an injury to the eye but rather blood collecting in the conjunctiva from a fracture at the base of the skull, called a **basilar skull fracture**. ■

● **FIGURE 10–9**   *Raccoon's eyes. (Courtesy Wayne Triner, DO, Albany Medical Center, Albany, NY.)*

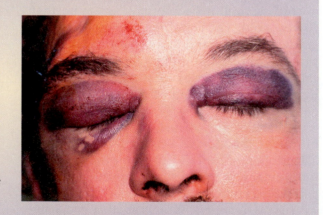

cone cells in the retina related to the primary colors: blue, red, and green. The cone cells are affected in color blindness, which is a genetic disorder carried by the female and transmitted only to male children.

Vision Defects

Presbyopia is a condition in which the lenses of the eye lose their elasticity, resulting in a decrease in the ability to focus on close objects. This usually occurs after age 40.

Hyperopia (hypermetropia; **farsighted-ness**) is a condition in which the focal point is beyond the retina because the eyeball is shorter than normal, Figure 10-10. Objects must be moved farther away from the eye to be seen clearly. Convex lenses help correct this situation.

Myopia (nearsightedness) is a condition in which the focal point is in front of the retina, because the eyeball is elongated, see Figure 10-10. Objects must be brought very close to the eye to be seen clearly. Concave lenses help correct this condition.

Amblyopia is a reduction or dimness of vision.

Astigmatism is a condition in which there is an irregular curvature of the cornea or lens, which causes blurred vision and possible eyestrain. A special prescription eyeglass helps correct this condition.

Diplopia is blurred vision.

Strabismus ("cross-eyes") is a condition in which the muscles of the eyeball do not coordinate their action. This condition is usually seen early in children and can be corrected by eye exercises or surgery.

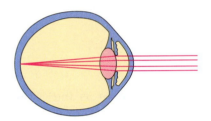

Normal eye
Light rays focus on the retina

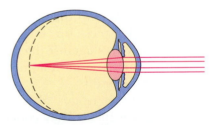

Myopia (nearsightedness)
Light rays focus in front
of the retina

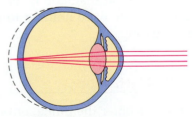

Hyperopia (farsightedness)
Light rays focus beyond
the retina

● **FIGURE 10–10**   *Vision defects.*

● THE EAR

The ear is a special sense organ that is uniquely adapted to pick up sound waves and send these impulses to the auditory center of the brain. The auditory center is located in the temporal area just above the ears. The receptor for hearing is the delicate **organ of Corti**, which is located within the cochlea of the inner ear.

The ear is also involved with equilibrium. The receptors in the inner ear send a message to the cerebellum in the brain about the position of our heads to help us maintain our balance. Other receptors include proprioceptors in our eyes and receptors located around our joints. The information picked up by these receptors is processed by the cerebellum and cerebral cortex to enable the body to cope with changes in our equilibrium. For example, if you become drowsy and feel yourself sliding off a chair, your body becomes alert and makes you sit up straight again.

The ear has three parts: the outer or external ear, the middle ear, and the inner ear, see Figure 10-11.

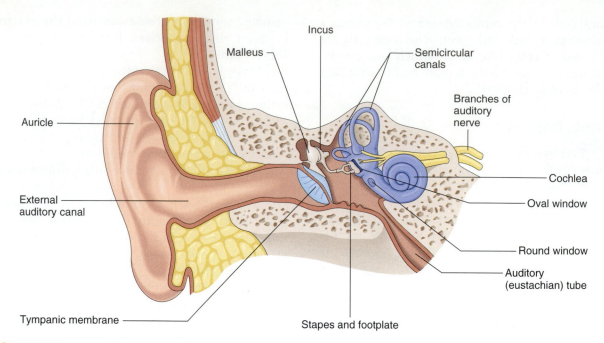

Incus

Malleus

Semicircular canals

Branches of auditory nerve

Auricle

Cochlea

Oval window

External auditory canal

Round window

Auditory (eustachian) tube

Tympanic membrane

Stapes and footplate

● **FIGURE 10–11**   *The ear and its structures.*

The Outer Ear

The **pinna**, or outer ear, also called the auricle, collects sound waves and directs them into the auditory canal. The auditory canal is lined with sebaceous glands, also called ceruminous glands, which secrete a waxlike or oily substance (cerumen). This substance protects the ear. The auditory canal leads to the eardrum, or **tympanic membrane**, which separates the outer and middle ear.

The Middle Ear

The middle ear is really a cavity in the temporal bone. It connects with the pharynx by means of the **eustachian tube**, which serves to equalize the air pressure in the middle ear with that of the outside atmosphere. A chain of three tiny bones is found in the middle ear: the **hammer (malleus)**, the **anvil (incus)**, and the **stirrup (stapes)**; they transmit sound waves from the ear drum to the inner ear.

The Inner Ear

The inner ear consists of several membrane-lined channels that lie deep within the temporal bone. The special organ of hearing is a spiral-shaped passage known as the **cochlea**, which contains a membranous tube called the **cochlear duct**. The duct is filled with fluid that vibrates when the sound waves from the stirrup bone strike against it. Located in the cochlear duct are delicate cells that make up the organ of Corti. These hairlike cells pick up the vibrations caused by sound waves against the fluid, then transmit them through the auditory nerve to the hearing center of the brain.

Three **semicircular canals** also lie within the inner ear, Figure 10-12. They contain a liquid and delicate, hairlike cells that bend when the liquid is set in motion by head and body movements. These impulses are sent to the cerebellum, helping to maintain body balance, or equilibrium. They have nothing to do with the sense of hearing.

● PATHWAY OF HEARING

Sound waves enter the pinna, or outer ear, and traverse the auditory canal to the tympanic membrane; the ear ossicles (hammer, anvil and stirrup) vibrate, stimulating the nerve cell receptors in the cochlea, which transmits the signal through the cochlear nerve

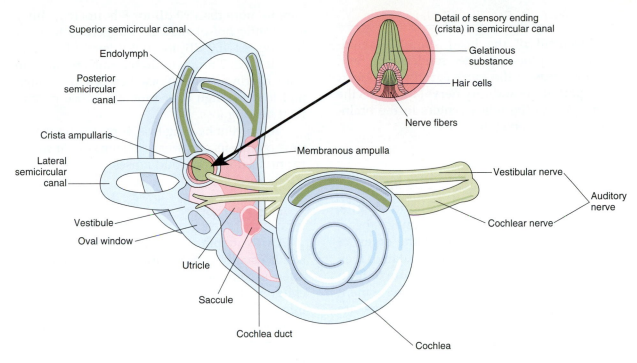

● FIGURE 10–12   *Enlargement of the inner ear showing the three semicircular canals.*

(part of the auditory nerve) to the auditory cortex in the temporal lobe of the brain for perception and interpretation, Figure 10-13.

When the same sound keeps reaching the ears, the auditory receptors adapt to the sound and we do not hear it.

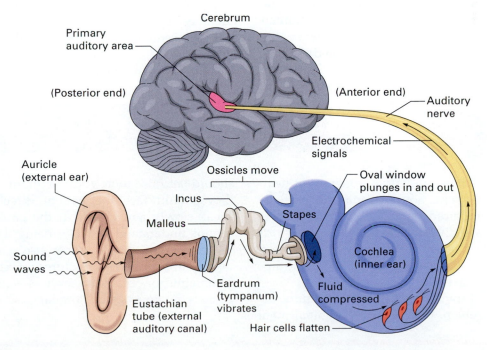

● FIGURE 10–13   *Pathway of hearing.*

PATHWAY OF EQUILIBRIUM

Movement of the head stimulates equilibrium receptors in the semicircular and vestibule areas of the inner ear; the vestibular nerve (part of the auditory nerve) transmits the information to the reflex centers in the brainstem and the cerebellum.

LOUD NOISE AND HEARING LOSS

Hearing is both sensitive and fragile. Loud noise heard for too long damages hearing. If the delicate hair cells in the organ of Corti in the inner ear are overstimulated, they become damaged. Repeated exposure to loud noise causes the loss to become permanent as more cells and their nerve receptors are destroyed.

The alarming increase of hearing loss in young people is most likely caused by loud music. The symptoms of hearing loss may be tinnitus (ringing in the ears) or difficulty in understanding what people are saying (they seem to be mumbling). Words with high-frequency sounds, such as *pill, hill,* and *fill,* may sound alike.

Sound is measured in decibels (dB). The scale runs from the faintest sound the human ear can hear, 0 dB, to the scream of a jet engine or a shotgun blast, at more than 165 dB. Exposure to more than 90 dB for 8 hours (e.g., busy city traffic noise) may be dangerous to your hearing. At 100 dB, the noise level of a chain saw, it takes 2 hours to do the same damage to your hearing. NOTE: Noise heard long enough and loud enough over time can cause permanent hearing loss.

To prevent hearing loss, turn down the volume on music, and wear earplugs or ear muffs for protection from loud noises.

EAR DISORDERS

Otitis media is an infection of the middle ear. It usually causes earache. This disorder is often a complication of the common cold in children. Treatment with antibiotics cures the infection. In some cases there may be a build up of fluid or pus, which can be relieved by a **myringotomy** (an opening made in the tympanic membrane). Tubes may be placed in the ear to allow fluids to drain off, especially in cases of chronic otitis media.

Otosclerosis is an inherited disorder in which the bone stapes of the middle ear first become spongy and then harden. This causes the stirrup, or stapes, to become fixed or immovable. Otosclerosis is a common cause of deafness in young adults. Stapedectomy, a total replacement of the stapes, is the treatment of choice.

STREET SMART

There are varying degrees of hearing impairment. Some people are partially hearing impaired, or **hard of hearing (HOH)**, and use assistive devices called **hearing aids** to hear. Others are totally unable to hear. These patients may have learned to read lips or use **American Sign Language**.

EMS providers trying to communicate with a person with a hearing impairment should *not* raise their voice or shout. Instead they should face the patient directly and speak slowly and clearly. If the patient still cannot understand what is being said, the EMS provider should either use a **symbol board**, a board with pictures of common complaints, or obtain the services of an **interpreter** who knows sign language. ■

CHANGES OF AGING

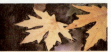

Presbycusis is a condition that causes deafness as a result of the aging process. This can be helped with the use of hearing aids. ■

Tinnitus is a sensation of ringing or buzzing that is perceived in the ear in the absence of an actual sound stimulus. It may be caused by impacted wax, otitis media, otosclerosis, loud noise, blockage of normal blood supply to the cochlea, or the effects of various drugs like the salicylates (e.g., aspirin).

Meniere's disease is a condition that affects the semicircular canals of the inner ear, causing marked **vertigo** (dizziness). Vertigo can occur at any time and without warning, causing the patient to be very frightened. In addition, the vertigo is accompanied by nausea, vomiting, and a ringing sensation, sometimes described as howling, in the ears. Bed rest is sometimes necessary during an acute attack. Medication may be given to relieve vertigo and nausea. The patient should avoid any sudden movement because it may precipitate an attack. The cause is unknown and the symptoms eventually subside; however, attacks occur without any warning.

Types of Hearing Loss

- *Conductive hearing loss* occurs when sounds to the inner ear are blocked by ear wax, there is fluid in the middle ear, or there is abnormal bone growth.

- *Sensorineural damage* to parts of the inner ear of auditory nerve results in a partial or complete deafness. In cases of profound deafness, cochlear implants improve communication ability, which leads to positive psychological and social changes. At the present time, children older than 2 and adults with profound deafness are candidates for cochlear implants.

THE NOSE

The human nose can detect approximately 10,000 different smells. Smell accounts for about 90% of what we think of as taste. Hold your nose and see if you can tell the difference between eating a piece of orange and a piece of pear. Odor molecules inhaled through the nose get warmed and moistened as they pass through the nasal cavity.

In the nasal cavity, Figure 10-14, there is a patch of tissue about the size of a postage stamp called the olfactory epithelium, which has a plentiful supply of nerve cells with specialized receptors. The receptors send signals to the adjoining olfactory bulbs, an extension of the brain. The stimulus is transmitted by the olfactory nerve to the limbic system, thalamus, and frontal cortex. The limbic system generates our basic emotions, such as affection, aggression, and fear. This relationship may explain why odors are tied to feelings. For example, we may associate the smell of something cooking with a good experience.

Scientists are starting to do research on how smells may affect learning, weight loss, aggression levels, and behavior.

DISORDERS OF THE NOSE

Rhinitis is an inflammation of the lining of the nose that may trigger nasal congestion, nasal drainage, sneezing, or itching. The cause may be allergies, infection, or other factors such as fumes, odors, emotional changes, or drugs. Treatment includes eliminating the allergens, if possible, or reducing exposure to them. Some antihistamines are effective for short periods.

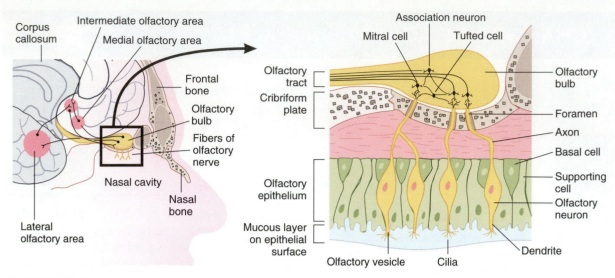

● **FIGURE 10–14**   *The nasal cavity.*

Nasal polyps are growths in the nasal cavity associated with rhinitis. In severe cases, surgery may be necessary to remove the polyps.

Deviated nasal septum is a condition in which there is a bend in the cartilage structure of the septum. Symptoms that result are a blockage in the airflow through one nostril, difficulty sleeping, headaches, loud breathing or snoring, dry nose, and nose bleeds. Treatment traditionally has been surgical correction. In June 1996 a new product was introduced called Breathe Right. This nasal strip is placed across the nose and provides temporary relief of breathing problems associated with a deviated nasal septum. It improves breathing by reducing nasal airflow resistance and can be effective in reducing snoring and in the temporary relief of nasal congestion.

After a trauma, such as a fall or a motor vehicle collision, clear fluid may come from the nose, called rhinorrhea, or from the ears (otorrhea). This clear fluid could be cerebrospinal fluid (CSF) and may be a sign of a more serious condition.

● THE TONGUE

The tongue is a mass of muscle tissue covered with papillae. Located on the papillae are the taste buds, which are stimulated by the flavors of foods. The receptors in the taste buds send stimuli through three cranial nerves to the cerebral cortex for interpretation.

STREET SMART

Bleeding from the nose, or epistaxis, is a common medical complaint that can result from trauma, such as a fall, or from dry mucous membranes, as occurs during the winter months from being indoors where furnaces pull humidity from the air. Epistaxis can also be a sign of dangerously high blood pressure. Frequent nose bleeds can be a medical emergency. A person with frequent nose bleeds should be evaluated by a physician. ■

MEDICAL HIGHLIGHTS

Laser, short for **l**ight **a**mplification by **s**timulated **e**mission of **r**adiations, is based on the principle that certain atoms, molecules, or ions can be excited by absorption of thermal, electrical, or light energy. After such energy absorptions, the atoms, molecules, or ions give off a beam of synchronized light waves. The laser beam is a narrow, intense, and monochromatic (single-color) light beam that can be used for a variety of purposes. For example, it can stop bleeding, make incisions, or remove tissue.

Lasers are often used to burn bleeding blood vessels within the eye, called cautery. Some patients, especially diabetics, have a large number of bleeding vessels. All these offending vessels can be cauterized using computers and lasers to map the posterior chamber.

Blood vessels within the eyes are primarily at the periphery. Such cauterization thus preserves the central vision, but at a loss of peripheral vision. Night vision, via the rod cells found in the periphery, is also lost. ■

● REVIEW QUESTIONS

Select the letter of the choice that best completes the statement.

1. The outer tough coat of the eye is the:
   a. retina
   b. sclera
   c. choroid
   d. lens

2. The clear anterior portion of the sclera is the:
   a. cornea
   b. lens
   c. pupil
   d. iris

3. The muscle that regulates how much light enters the eye is the:
   a. conjunction
   b. iris
   c. cornea
   c. lens

4. The posterior chamber of the eye is filled with fluid called:
   a. tears
   b. ciliary body
   c. vitreous humor
   d. aqueous humor

5. The area of the eye that contains the rods and cones is the:
   a. retina
   b. choroid
   c. sclera
   d. cornea

6. The tube that connects the throat to the ear is the:
   a. pinna
   b. eustachian
   c. cochlear
   d. auditory

7. Hardening of the bones of the middle ear is called:
   a. otitis media
   b. presbycusis
   c. otosclerosis
   d. presbyopia

8. Nearsightedness is also known as:
   a. myopia
   b. hyperopia
   c. presbyopia
   d. strabismus

9. A clouding of the lens is called:
   a. myopia
   b. glaucoma
   c. hyperopia
   d. cataract

10. An infectious disease known as "pink eye" is also called:
    a. kernicterus
    b. otitis
    c. conjunctivitis
    d. strabismus

● LABELING

Identify the structures on the following figure and write and your answers in the spaces provided.

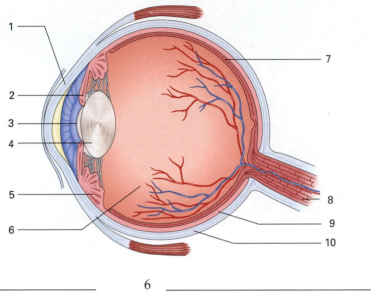

1 _____	6 _____
2 _____	7 _____
3 _____	8 _____
4 _____	9 _____
5 _____	10 _____

●APPLYING THEORY TO PRACTICE

1. You have heard that your eye works like a camera. Explain how you see and track the pathway of light from the cornea to the occipital lobe of the brain.

2. Explain to a friend how your outer ear catches a sound and where in the brain it is interpreted.

3. One of the most serious side effects of aging is sensory loss. Explain how the aging process affects vision and hearing in the elderly.

4. A patient comes to the doctor's office for treatment of glaucoma. She states, "I am so tired of taking these eyedrops. I don't want to use them anymore." How would you respond and what instructions would you give her?

5. The phrase "stop and smell the roses" means slow down and enjoy life. What conditions may interfere with your ability to smell the roses?

11 Endocrine System

Objectives

- List the glands that make up the endocrine system
- Describe negative feedback hormonal control
- Name the hormones of the endocrine system and their function
- Describe the role of prostaglandins
- List the causative factors for endocrine gland disorders
- Describe some disorders of the endocrine system
- Define key words that relate to this chapter

Key Words

acromegaly
Addison's disease
adrenal crisis
adrenal gland
Adrenalin (epinephrine)
adrenocorticotropic
   hormone (ACTH)
androgen
anterior pituitary lobe
calcitonin
cretinism
Cushing's syndrome
diabetes insipidus
diabetes mellitus
dwarfism
endocrine gland
estrogen
exocrine gland
exophthalmos
follicle-stimulating
   hormone (FSH)
gigantism
glucagon
glucocorticoids (G-Cs)
goiter
gonads
growth hormone (GH)
hyperglycemia
hyperthyroidism
hypoglycemia
hyponatremia
hypothyroidism
insulin
interstitial
   cell–stimulating
   hormone (ICSH)
islets of Langerhans
luteinizing hormone
   (LH)
melatonin
mineralocorticoids
   (M-Cs)
myxedema
negative feedback
norepinephrine
oxytocin
pancreas
parathormone
parathyroid gland
pheochromocytoma
(continues)

Key Words (continued)

pineal gland	antidiuretic hormone
pituitary gland	(SIADH)
polydipsia	testosterone
polyphagia	tetany
polyuria	thymus
posterior pituitary lobe	thyroid gland
progesterone	thyroid-stimulating
prolactin hormone	hormone (TSH)
(PRL)	thyroxin (T_4)
prostaglandin	triiodothyronine (T_3)
somatotropin	vasopressin
syndrome of	
inappropriate	

A gland is any organ that produces a secretion. **Endocrine glands**, Figure 11-1, are organized groups of tissues that use materials from the blood or lymph to make new compounds called hormones. Endocrine glands are also called ductless glands and glands of internal secretion; the hormones are secreted directly into the bloodstream as the blood circulates through the gland. The secretions are often transported to all areas of the body, where they have a special influence on cells, tissues, and organs. There is another type of gland called an **exocrine gland**, in which the secretions from the gland must go through a duct. This duct then carries the secretion to a body surface or organ. Exocrine glands include sweat, salivary,

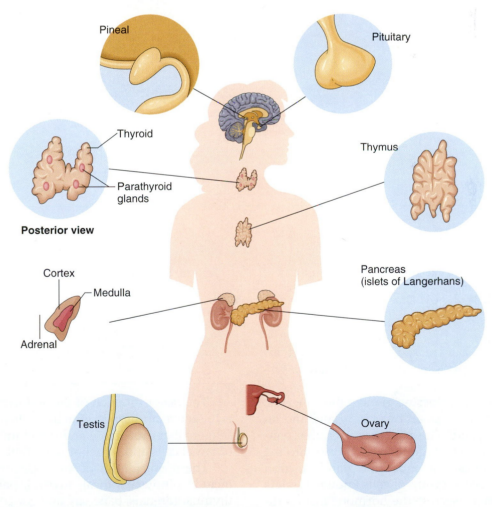

Pineal

Pituitary

Thyroid

Thymus

Parathyroid glands

Posterior view

Cortex

Medulla

Adrenal

Pancreas (islets of Langerhans)

Testis

Ovary

● **FIGURE 11–1**   *Locations of the endocrine glands.*

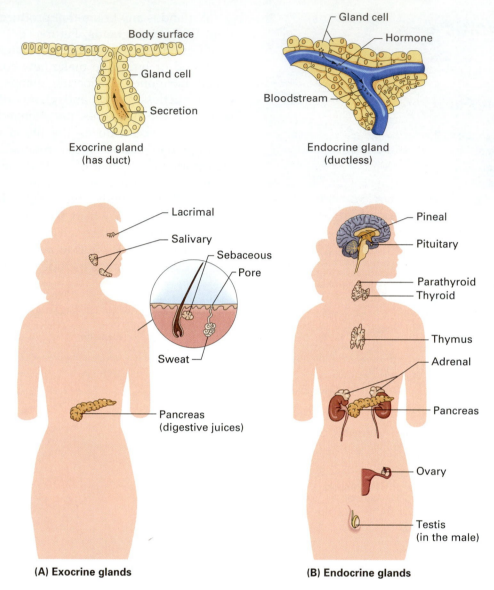

● **FIGURE 11–2**   *(A) Exocrine glands. (B) Endocrine glands.*

lacrimal, and pancreas. Their functions are included in chapters on the relevant body systems, Figure 11-2.

One of the endocrine glands, the pancreas, can perform both as an exocrine gland and an endocrine gland. The pancreas produces pancreatic juices, which go through a duct into the small intestines. The endocrine gland function is when a special group of cells known as **islets of Langerhans** secrete the hormone insulin directly into the bloodstream.

● FUNCTION OF THE ENDOCRINE SYSTEM

The major function of the endocrine system is to secrete hormones, which are chemical messengers that coordinate and direct the activities of target cells and target organs, Table 11-1.

The major glands of the endocrine system include pituitary, pineal, thyroid, parathyroid, thymus, adrenals, pancreas, and gonads (ovaries in the female and testes in the male).

TABLE 11-1 *Endocrine Glands*

GLAND	LOCATION	HORMONE	PRINCIPAL EFFECTS
PITUITARY Anterior lobe	Undersurface of the brain in the sella turcica of the skull	Growth hormone (GH) Thyroid stimulating hormone (thyrotropin; TSH) Adrenocorticotropic hormone (ACTH) Melanocyte-stimulating hormone (MSH) Follicle-stimulating hormone (FSH) Luteinizing hormone (LH) Interstitial cell–stimulating hormone (ICSH)	Normal growth of body tissues. Stimulates growth and activity of thyroid cells to produce thyroid hormone. Stimulates the cortex of the adrenal gland. Increases skin pigmentation. Stimulates the maturity of the graafian follicle to rupture and to produce estrogen in the female. In the male it stimulates the development of the testes and the production of sperm. Causes the development of the corpus luteum, which then secretes progesterone in the female. ICSH in the male stimulates the interstitial cells of the testes to produce testosterone.
Posterior lobe		Prolactin (PRL) Oxytocin Vasopressin (antidiuretic hormone; ADH)	Develops breast tissue and stimulates secretion of milk from mammary glands Stimulates contraction of uterus, especially during childbirth; causes ejection of milk from mammary glands. Acts on cells of kidney tubules to concentrate urine and conserve fluid in the body. Also acts to constrict blood vessels.
THYROID	Lower portion of anterior neck	Thyroxine (T_4) and triiodothyronine (T_3) Thyrocalcitonin	Increases metabolism; influences both physical and mental activity; promotes normal growth and development. Causes calcium to be stored in bones; reduces blood level of calcium.
PARATHYROID	Posterior surface of thyroid gland	Parahormone	Regulates exchange of calcium between the bones and blood.
ADRENAL Medulla	Superior surface of each kidney	Epinephrine (adrenaline) Aldosterone (mineralocorticoid)	Increases heart rate, blood pressure, and flow of blood; decreases intestinal activity. Controls electrolyte balances by regulating the reabsorption of sodium and the excretion of potassium.
Cortex		Glucocorticoids Sex hormones (androgens)	Affect the metabolism of protein, fat, and glucose, thereby increasing blood sugar. Govern sex characteristics, especially those that are masculine.
PANCREAS	Behind the stomach	Insulin Glucagon	Essential to the metabolism of carbohydrates; reduces the blood sugar level. Stimulates the liver to release glycogen and converts it to glucose to increase blood sugar levels.
THYMUS	Under the sternum	Thymosin	Induces lymphoid tissue to produce T-lymphocyte cells to develop immunity to certain diseases.
PINEAL BODY	Third ventricle in the brain	Melatonin	Controls onset of puberty.
OVARIES	Female pelvis	Estrogen Progesterone	Promotes growth of primary and secondary sexual characteristics. Develops excretory portion of mammary glands; aids in maintaining pregnancy.
TESTES	Male scrotum	Testosterone	Develops primary and secondary sexual characteristics; stimulates maturation of sperm.

Figure 11-1 shows the locations of the endocrine glands in the body. Each has specific functions to perform. Any disturbance in the functioning of these glands may cause changes in the appearance or functioning of the body.

HORMONAL CONTROL

The secretion of the hormones operates on a negative feedback system or under the control of the nervous system.

Negative Feedback

In **negative feedback** there is a drop in the level of the hormone, which triggers a chain reaction of responses to increase the amount of hormone in the blood. A description follows of how the negative feedback system functions as it relates to the thyroid gland:

1. The blood level of thyroxine (thyroid hormone) falls.

2. The hypothalamus in the brain gets the message.

3. The hypothalamus responds by sending a hormone to the anterior pituitary gland in-

structing it to release thyroid-stimulating hormone (TSH).

5. TSH stimulates the thyroid gland to produce thyroxine.

6. Thyroxine blood level rises, which in turn shuts off the releasing hormone for TSH.

Nervous Control

The nervous system controls the glands by stimulation, as in the adrenal medulla, where the gland is stimulated by the sympathetic nervous system. For example, when we become afraid, the adrenal medulla secretes epinephrine (adrenaline).

PITUITARY GLAND

The **pituitary gland** is a tiny structure having a diameter of about 10 millimeters and a weight of approximately 0.5 grams, about the size of a grape. It is located at the base of the brain within the sella turcica, a small bony depression in the sphenoid bone of the skull, Figure 11-3. The pituitary gland is connected to the hypothalamus by a stalk called the infundibu-

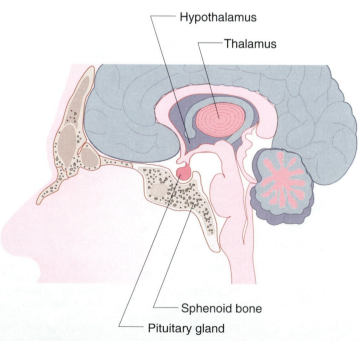

Hypothalamus

Thalamus

Sphenoid bone

Pituitary gland

FIGURE 11–3   *The pituitary gland in relation to the brain.*

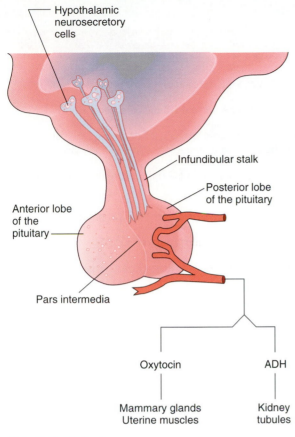

Hypothalamic
neurosecretory
cells

Infundibular stalk

Posterior lobe
of the pituitary

Anterior lobe
of the
pituitary

Pars intermedia

Oxytocin   ADH

Mammary glands   Kidney
Uterine muscles   tubules

● **FIGURE 11–4**   *Pituitary gland.*

lum, Latin for funnel. The pituitary gland is divided into an anterior lobe and a posterior lobe, Figure 11-4.

Pituitary-Hypothalamus Interaction

The hormones of the anterior pituitary are controlled by the releasing chemicals or factors produced by the hypothalamus in the brain. As the pituitary hormones are needed by the body, the hypothalamus emits a specific releasing factor for each hormone, see Figure 11-4. For example, the thyroid-stimulating hormone has a TSH releasing factor. In addition, when a sufficient amount of the hormone is produced, a different releasing factor inhibits the anterior pituitary from secreting TSH.

The hypothalamus is considered part of the nervous system. However, it produces two hormones: vasopressin, which converts to antidiuretic hormone (ADH), and oxytocin.

These hormones are stored in the posterior lobe of the pituitary and are released into the bloodstream in response to nerve impulses from the hypothalamus.

● HORMONES OF THE PITUITARY GLAND

The pituitary gland is known as the "master gland" because of its major influence on the body's activities, Table 11-2. It is even more amazing when you consider the size of this incredible gland.

Anterior Pituitary Lobe

The **anterior pituitary lobe** secretes the following hormones:

1. **Growth hormone (GH)** or **somatotropin** is responsible for growth and development. This hormone also helps use fat for energy, store glucose, and maintain blood sugar levels.

2. **Prolactin hormone (PRL)** develops breast tissue and stimulates the production of milk after childbirth. The function in males is unknown.

3. **Thyroid-stimulating hormone** stimulates the growth and secretion of the thyroid gland.

4. **Adrenocorticotropic hormone (ACTH)** stimulates the growth and secretion of the adrenal cortex.

5. **Follicle-stimulating hormone (FSH)** stimulates the growth of the graafian follicle and the production of estrogen in females and stimulates the production of sperm in males.

6. **Luteinizing hormone (LH)** stimulates ovulation and the formation of the corpus luteum, which produces progesterone in females.

7. **Interstitial cell–stimulating hormone (ICSH)** is necessary for the production of testosterone by the interstitial cells of the testes in men.

TABLE 11-2 *Pituitary Hormones and Their Known Functions*

PITUITARY HORMONE	KNOWN FUNCTION
Anterior Lobe	
TSH—Thyroid-stimulating hormone (thyrotropin)	Stimulates the growth and the secretion of the thyroid gland.
ACTH—Adrenocorticotropic hormone	Stimulates the growth and the secretion of the adrenal cortex.
FSH—Follicle-stimulating hormone	Stimulates growth of new graafian (ovarian) follicle and secretion of estrogen by follicle cells in the female and production of sperm in the male.
LH—Luteinizing hormone (female)	Stimulates ovulation and formation of the corpus luteum. Corpus luteum secretes progesterone.
ICSH—Interstitial cell–stimulating hormone (male)	Stimulates testosterone secretion by the interstitial cells of the testes.
PRL—Prolactin	Stimulates secretion of milk in females. Function in males is unknown.
GH—Growth hormone (somatotropin; STH)	Accelerates body growth and causes fat to be used for energy; this helps to maintain blood sugar.
Posterior Lobe	
VASOPRESSIN—Antidiuretic hormone (ADH)	Maintains water balance by reducing urinary output. Acts on kidney tubules to reabsorb water into the blood more quickly. In large amounts it causes constriction of arteries.
OXYTOCIN	Promotes milk ejection and causes contraction of the smooth muscles of the uterus.

Posterior Pituitary Lobe

The hormones produced by the hypothalamus are stored in the **posterior pituitary lobe**.

1. **Vasopressin** converts to antidiuretic hormone in the bloodstream. The principal function of vasopressin is to regulate extracellular fluids. ADH maintains water balance by increasing the absorption of water in the kidney tubules. Sometimes drugs called diuretics are used to inhibit the action of ADH. The result is an increase in urinary output and a decrease in blood volume, thus decreasing blood pressure.

2. **Oxytocin** is released during childbirth, causing strong contractions of the uterus. It also causes strong contractions when a mother is breastfeeding. Pitocin, a synthetic form of oxytocin, is given to help start labor or make uterine contractions stronger.

STREET SMART

Recently vasopressin (arginine vasopressin) has been used during the resuscitation of persons experiencing cardiac arrest. It is believed that vasopressin constricts arterial blood vessels, increasing blood pressure and increasing blood flow to the coronary arteries. ■

THYROID AND PARATHYROID GLANDS

The thyroid and parathyroid glands are located in the neck, inferior to the laryngeal prominence formed by the thyroid cartilage, which houses the voice box. The thyroid cartilage is more prominent in males and is referred to as the "Adam's apple." The thyroid regulates body metabolism. The parathyroid maintains the calcium-phosphorus balance.

THYROID GLAND

The thyroid gland is a butterfly-shaped mass of tissue located in the anterior part of the neck, Figure 11-5. It lies on either side of the larynx, over the trachea. Its general shape is that of the letter H. It is about 2 inches long, with two lobes joined by strands of thyroid tissue called the isthmus. Coming from the isthmus is a fingerlike lobe of tissue known as the intermediate lobe. This intermediate lobe projects upward toward the floor of the mouth, as far up as the hyoid bone. The thyroid gland has a rich blood supply. In fact, it has been estimated that approximately 4 to 5 liters (8½ to 10½ pints) of blood pass through this gland every hour.

The thyroid gland secretes three hormones: thyroxine, triiodothyronine, and calcitonin. The first two are iodine-bearing derivatives of the amino acid tyrosine. Triiodothyronine is 5 to 10 times more active than thyroxine, but its activity is less prolonged. However, the two have the same effect. Both hormones are produced in the follicle cells of the thyroid gland. These cells are stimulated to secretory activity by a hormone from the anterior lobe of the pituitary gland. This thyroid-stimulating hormone (TSH) controls the production and secretion of the thyroid hormone from the thyroid gland. The thyroid hormones contain iodine. Most of the iodine needed for their synthesis comes from the diet. Iodides are circulated to the thyroid gland, where they are "trapped." There the iodides combine with the amino acid tyrosine to form triiodothyronine (T3) and thyroxine (T4).

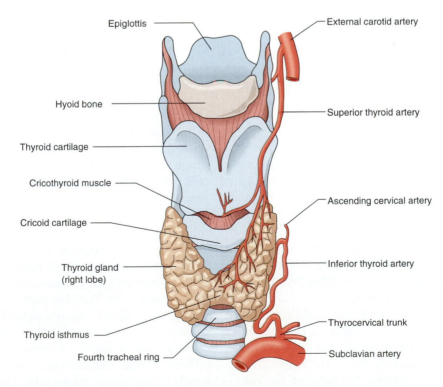

Epiglottis

External carotid artery

Hyoid bone

Superior thyroid artery

Thyroid cartilage

Cricothyroid muscle

Ascending cervical artery

Cricoid cartilage

Thyroid gland
(right lobe)

Inferior thyroid artery

Thyroid isthmus

Thyrocervical trunk

Fourth tracheal ring

Subclavian artery

● **FIGURE 11–5** *Thyroid gland.*

Under normal circumstances, the presence of these two hormones (T_3 and T_4) in the bloodstream serves to regulate the system. On the other hand, an excess of these hormones suppresses TSH secretion. When the concentration of thyroid hormones is lowered in the bloodstream, the pituitary gland secretes more TSH. This in turn stimulates thyroid gland activity. (The consequences of hyposecretion and hypersecretion of the thyroid hormones are discussed later in this chapter.)

Thyroxine controls the rate of metabolism, heat production, and oxidation of all cells, with the possible exception of the brain and spleen cells. It can speed up or slow down the activities of the body as needed. In the liver the two thyroid hormones affect the conversion of glycogen from sources other than sugar. It also helps to change glycogen into glucose, raising the glucose level of the blood.

To summarize, the functions of thyroxin are as follows:

1. Controls the rate of metabolism in the body; controls how cells use glucose and oxygen to produce heat and energy.

2. Stimulates protein synthesis and thus helps in tissue growth.

3. Stimulates the breakdown of liver glycogen.

Calcitonin

Calcitonin is another hormone produced and secreted by the thyroid gland. It controls the calcium ion concentration in the body by maintaining a proper calcium level in the bloodstream.

Calcium is an essential body mineral. Approximately 99% of the calcium in the body is stored in the bones. The rest is located in the blood and tissue fluids. Calcium is necessary for blood clotting, holding cells together, and neuromuscular functions. The constant level of calcium in the blood and tissues is maintained by the actions of calcitonin and parathormone (produced by the parathyroid gland).

When blood calcium levels are higher than normal, calcitonin secretion is increased. Calcitonin lowers the calcium concentration in the blood and body fluids by decreasing the rate of the bone resorption, or osteoclastic activity, and by increasing the calcium absorption by bones, or osteoblastic activity. Proper secretion of calcitonin into the bloodstream prevents hypercalcemia, a harmful rise in the blood calcium level.

● PARATHYROID GLANDS

The parathyroid glands, usually four in number, are tiny glands the size of grains of rice. These are attached to the posterior surface of the thyroid gland and secrete the hormone parathormone. Parathormone, like calcitonin, also controls the concentration of calcium in the bloodstream. When the blood calcium level is lower than normal, parathormone secretion is increased.

Parathormone stimulates an increase in the number and size of specialized bone cells referred to as osteoclasts. Osteoclasts quickly invade hard bone tissue, digesting large amounts of the bony material containing calcium. As this process continues, calcium leaves the bone and is released into the bloodstream, increasing the blood calcium level.

Bone calcium is bonded to phosphorus in a compound called calcium phosphate ($CaPO_4$). When calcium is released into the bloodstream, phosphorus is released along with it. Parathormone stimulates the kidneys to excrete any excess phosphorus from the blood; at the same time, it inhibits calcium excretion from the kidneys. Consequently the concentration of blood calcium rises.

Thus parathormone and calcitonin of the thyroid have opposite, or antagonistic, effects to one another (see Figure 11-6 for a summary of their actions). Parathormone, however, acts much more slowly than calcitonin. It may be hours before the effects of parathormone become apparent. In this manner the secretion of parathormone and calcitonin serve as complementary processes controlling the level of calcium in the bloodstream.

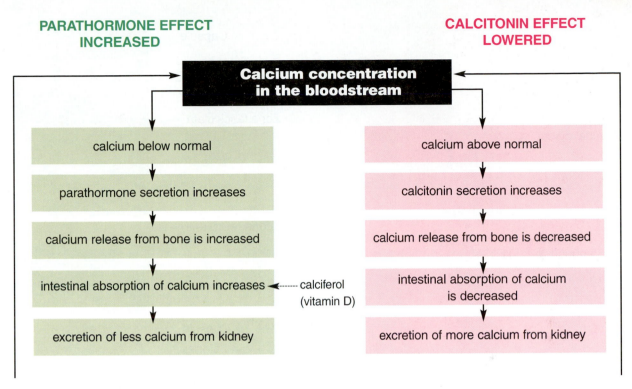

**PARATHORMONE EFFECT
INCREASED**

**CALCITONIN EFFECT
LOWERED**

Calcium concentration
in the bloodstream

calcium below normal	calcium above normal
parathormone secretion increases	calcitonin secretion increases
calcium release from bone is increased	calcium release from bone is decreased
intestinal absorption of calcium increases ◄----- calciferol (vitamin D)	intestinal absorption of calcium is decreased
excretion of less calcium from kidney	excretion of more calcium from kidney

● **FIGURE 11–6**   *Effects of parathormone and calcitonin on the level of calcium in the blood.*

● THYMUS GLAND

The **thymus** gland is both an endocrine gland and a lymphatic organ. It is located under the sternum, anterior and superior to the heart. Fairly large during childhood, it begins to disappear at puberty. Recent research has discovered that the thymus gland secretes a large number of hormones. The major hormone is thymosin, which helps to stimulate the lymphoid cells that are responsible for the production of T cells, which fight certain diseases.

● ADRENAL GLANDS

One of the two **adrenal glands** is located on top of each kidney, Figure 11-7. Each gland has two parts: the cortex and the medulla. Adrenocorticotropic hormone (ACTH) from the pituitary glands stimulates the activity of the cortex of the adrenal gland. The hormones secreted by the adrenal cortex are known as corticoids. The corticoids are very effective as antiinflammatory drugs.

The cortex secretes three groups of corticoids, each of which is of great importance:

1. **Mineralocorticoids (M-Cs)**, mainly aldosterone, affect the kidney tubules by speeding up the reabsorption of sodium into the blood circulation and increasing the excretion of potassium from the blood. They also speed up the reabsorption of water by the kidneys. Aldosterone (M-C) is used in the treatment of Addison's disease to replace deficient secretion of mineralocorticoids.

2. **Glucocorticoids (G-Cs)**, namely cortisone and cortisol, increase the amount of glucose in the blood. This is presumably done by (1) conversion of the protein brought to the liver into glycogen, followed by (2) breakdown of the glycogen into glucose. These glucocorticoids also help the body resist the aggravations caused by various everyday stresses. In addition, these hormones seem to decrease edema in inflammation and reduce pain by inhibiting pain-causing **prostaglandin**.

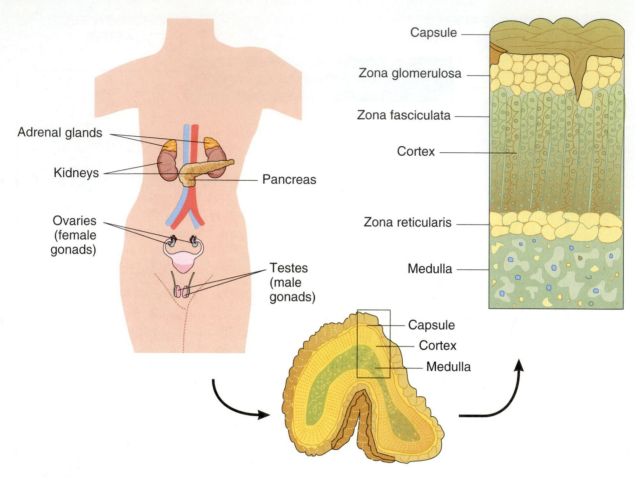

Capsule

Zona glomerulosa

Zona fasciculata

Cortex

Zona reticularis

Medulla

Adrenal glands

Kidneys

Pancreas

Ovaries
(female
gonads)

Testes
(male
gonads)

Capsule
Cortex
Medulla

● **FIGURE 11–7**   *Locations of adrenal glands and gonads.*

3. Sex hormones are present in both males and females. **Androgens** are male sex hormones that, together with similar hormones from the gonads, bring about masculine characteristics. Some estrogens are also present.

Medulla of the Adrenal Gland

The medulla of the adrenal gland secretes **epinephrine** and **norepinephrine**. Epinephrine (**Adrenaline**) is a powerful cardiac stimulant. Epinephrine stimulates the liver to release more glucose from its glycogen stores for use by the muscles and increases the force and rate of the heartbeat. The adrenal medulla is a major organ in the sympathetic nervous system. The hormones produced are referred to as the "fight or flight" hormones, because they prepare the body for an emergency situation. Table 11-3 highlights the effects of epinephrine.

GONADS

The **gonads**, or sex glands, include the ovaries in the female and the testes in the male.

TABLE 11-3 *Physiological Effects of Epinephrine*

EPINEPHRINE
1. Bronchial relaxation
2. Dilation of iris
3. Excitation of central nervous system
4. Increased conversion of stored glycogen to glucose
5. Increased heart rate
6. Increased cardiac output and venous return
7. Increased blood flow to muscles
8. Increased myocardial strength
9. Increased basal metabolic rate (BMR)
10. Increased systolic blood pressure
11. Increased lipolytic effects; frees fatty acids from fat deposits
12. Relaxation of uterine myometrial muscles

The ovary is responsible for producing the ova, or egg, and the hormones **estrogen** and **progesterone**. The testes are responsible for producing sperm and the hormone **testosterone**.

Female Hormones: Estrogen and Progesterone

Estrogen is produced by the graafian follicle cells of the ovary. It stimulates the development of the reproductive organs, including the breasts, and secondary sex characteristics such as pubic and axillary hair.

Progesterone is produced by the cells of the corpus luteum of the ovary. Progesterone works with estrogen to build up the lining of the uterus for the fertilized egg. If no fertilization occurs, menstruation takes place. This cycle depends on the secretion of the progesterone from the corpus luteum. (See Chapter 20.)

Male Hormone: Testosterone

Testosterone is produced by the interstitial cells of the testes and is responsible for the development of the male reproductive organs and secondary sex characteristics. Testosterone influences beard growth and the growth of other body hair, the deepening of the voice, the increase in musculature, and the production of sperm. The secretion of the hormone depends on the pituitary gland. (See Chapter 20.)

PANCREAS

The **pancreas** is located behind the stomach and functions as both an exocrine and endocrine gland. The exocrine portion secretes pancreatic juices, which are excreted through a duct into the small intestines. There they become part of the digestive juices. The endocrine portion is involved in the production of insulin by the beta (B) cells of the islets of Langerhans on the pancreas.

The islet cells are distributed throughout the pancreas. These cells were named the **islets of Langerhans**, after the doctor who discovered them. B cells produce **insulin**, which (1) promotes the utilization of glucose in the cells, necessary for maintenance of normal levels of blood glucose, Figure 11-8; (2) promotes fatty acid

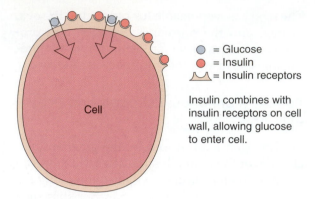

= Glucose
= Insulin
= Insulin receptors

Insulin combines with insulin receptors on cell wall, allowing glucose to enter cell.

● **FIGURE 11–8**   *Insulin carries sugar from the blood into the cells.*

transport and fat deposition into cells; (3) promotes amino acid transport into cells; and (4) facilitates protein synthesis. Lack of insulin secretion by the islet cells causes diabetes mellitus.

The alpha (A) cells contained in the islets of Langerhans secrete the hormone **glucagon**. The action of glucagon is antagonistic, or the opposite of insulin. Glucagon's function is to increase the level of glucose in the blood-

stream. This is done by stimulating the conversion of glycogen in the liver to glucose. The control of glucagon secretion is achieved by negative feedback (refer to Negative Feedback, page 184.) Low glucose levels in the bloodstream stimulate the A cells to secrete glucagon, which quickly increases the glucose level in the bloodstream.

● PINEAL GLAND

The **pineal gland** or body is a small, pine cone–shaped organ attached by a slim stalk to the roof of the third ventricle in the brain. The hormone produced by the pineal gland is called **melatonin**. The pineal gland is stimulated by a group of nerve cells called the suprachiasmatic nucleus (SCN), which are located in the brain over the pathway of fibers of the optic nerve. The amount of light entering the eye stimulates the SCN, which then stimulates the pineal gland to release its hormone. The amount of light affects the amount of melatonin secreted. The less light there is, the more

STREET SMART -

The brain is very sensitive to the level of blood glucose. During periods of low blood glucose (hypoglycemia), such as what might occur during a diabetic emergency, the patient may become unconscious. If the patient is unconscious, then he or she is unable to swallow foods containing sugar, which are needed to reverse the hypoglycemia.

During a diabetic emergency, or any time a patient has a decreased level of blood glucose, EMS providers should establish intravenous (IV) access and quickly administer glucose directly into the bloodstream of the patient.

In those cases when IV access cannot be obtained by EMS providers, an intramuscular (IM) injection of glucagon can be administered. Glucagon is another hormone that

breaks glycogen (a complex form of glucose found in the liver) into simple glucose to be excreted into the bloodstream from the liver.

This treatment assumes that the patient has glycogen stores in the liver. A patient who has poor nutrition, such as an alcoholic, may not have sufficient reserves of glycogen in the liver.

Intramuscular injection of glucagon can raise blood sugar levels, often within 20 minutes, and the patient may regain consciousness. NOTE: family members of patients with diabetes are frequently trained to administer glucagon IM when the patient becomes unconscious. It is important for EMS providers to ascertain what treatments family members may have initiated before they administer any other medications to the patient. ■

MEDICAL HIGHLIGHTS

It is called "cabin fever" or "winter blues." It is the depression or anxiety many people feel during the dark days of winter. To feel better many people look for a winter vacation in the sunshine. Scientists call this phenomena seasonal affective disorder, or SAD. Scientist Norman Rosenthal and his colleagues at the National Institute of Mental Health described SAD and documented the preliminary findings regarding a form of treatment with light.

They conducted a study to observe how a group of people reacted to differing amounts of daylight. As daylight began decreasing during the fall, people started to develop symptoms of lethargy, anxiety, mood changes, appetite increases (especially a craving for carbohydrates), and a decrease in physical activity. As winter progressed and the days shortened, the symptoms increased. When spring arrived, the symptoms diminished; by the end of May almost everyone in the study group exhibited no symptoms at all.

During this study, the scientists found that they could reverse the symptoms by supplying light. They used two different kinds of light: dimmer yellow light had no effect, but brighter light (with a frequency spectrum approximately simulating the frequencies in sunlight) produced a marked change in mood in most of the patients who received this treatment.

Our bodies have evolved to respond to a "biological clock," being alert during daylight and becoming sleepy as the sun fades into the night. A small cluster of brain cells called the suprachiasmatic nucleus (SCN) has been identified as the probable site for the biological clock in our bodies. One type of information has to do with the amount of light coming in through the eyes. *Supra* means "over"; *chiasmatic* refers to the optic chiasma, which is the site where the fibers (nerve endings) from the retinas of the right and left eyes cross. The SCN nerve cluster is located directly above a part of our vision system.

The SCN sends its message about the amount of light through the sympathetic nervous system to the pineal gland. The pineal gland secretes melatonin—the more light, the less secretion of melatonin; the less light, the more melatonin is secreted. Light suppresses the secretion of melatonin.

For people affected by SAD, the suggested treatment is bright light exposure for 30 minutes to 3 hours, usually in the morning. In addition, prepare for the change in daylight hours by planning special activities during the shorter days of winter. Expose yourself to as much bright light as possible. On sunny days, go outside; on dark days, use bright lights. Proper diagnosis is essential for proper treatment. If these symptoms develop, seek professional advice. ■

melatonin is produced; the more light there is, the less melatonin is produced. There are no clear answers to the function of melatonin; however melatonin may help regulate our circadian rhythm (biological clock). It is also thought that melatonin combines with a hypothalamic substance to prevent the early onset of puberty.

● OTHER HORMONES PRODUCED IN THE BODY

A host of hormones are produced throughout the body. They can originate from many different glands or other organs. A complete description of all the hormones of the body is beyond the intent of this anatomy text.

Prostaglandins

In various tissues throughout the body, hormones called prostaglandins are secreted. Their activity depends on which tissue secretes them. Some prostaglandins can cause constriction of the blood vessels; others may cause dilation. Prostaglandins can be used to induce labor and cause severe muscular contractions of the uterus. The exact nature and function of the prostaglandins are being extensively studied by scientists.

● DISORDERS OF THE ENDOCRINE SYSTEM

Endocrine gland disturbances may be caused by several factors, such as disease of the gland itself, infections in other parts of the body, autoimmune causes, and dietary deficiencies. Most disturbances result from (1) hyperactivity of the glands, causing oversecretion of hormones; or (2) hypoactivity of the gland, resulting in undersecretion of hormones.

● PITUITARY DISORDERS

Disturbances of the pituitary gland may produce a number of body changes. This gland is chiefly involved in the growth function. However, as the master gland, the pituitary indirectly influences other activities.

Hyperfunction of Pituitary

Hyperfunctioning of the pituitary gland (often caused by a pituitary tumor) causes hypersecretion of the pituitary growth hormone. When this occurs during preadolescence, it causes **gigantism**, an overgrowth of the long bones leading to excessive tallness. If hypersecretion of the growth hormone occurs during adulthood, **acromegaly** results. This is an overdevelopment of the bones of the face, hands, and feet. In adults whose long bones have already matured, the growth hormone attacks the cartilaginous regions and the bony joints. Thus the chin protrudes, and the lips, nose, and extremities enlarge disproportion-

ately. Lethargy and severe headaches frequently set in as well. Treatment of acromegaly and gigantism is drug therapy (which inhibits growth hormone) and radiation therapy.

Hypofunction of Pituitary

Hypofunctioning of the pituitary gland during childhood leads to pituitary **dwarfism**. Growth of the long bones is abnormally decreased by an inadequate production of growth hormone. Despite the small size, however, the body of a dwarf is normally proportioned and intelligence is normal. Unfortunately, the physique remains juvenile and sexually immature. Treatment involves early diagnosis and injections of human growth hormone. The treatment period is 5 years or more.

Diabetes Insipidus

Another disorder caused by posterior lobe dysfunction is **diabetes insipidus**. In this condition, there is a drop in the amount of ADH, which causes an excessive loss of water and electrolytes. The affected person complains of excessive thirst (**polydipsia**).

With diabetes insipidus, the patient's urine output increases (**polyuria**) from 2 to 6 liters a day to as much as 18 liters a day. The urine is diluted, unlike urine in diabetes mellitus, which is laden with sugar.

Diabetes insipidus can be caused by head trauma, brain tumors, and brain surgery. Untreated, a patient suffering from diabetes insipidus can lapse into a coma and die.

Drinking alcohol (ethyl alcohol, often abbreviated as EtOH; *Et* stands for "ethyl" and *OH* is the chemical symbol of alcohol) is thought to inhibit vasopressin (ADH) secretion, resulting in excessive urination after a bout of drinking.

The opposite can occur as well. When an individual drinks too much fluid, more vasopressin than the body needs is excreted and the person suffers water intoxication. Excessive consumption of beer (beer potomania) can cause this condition.

Syndrome of Inappropriate Antidiuretic Hormone

The **syndrome of inappropriate antidiuretic hormone (SIADH)** occurs when the posterior lobe of the pituitary excretes excessive amounts of ADH, which results in excessive water retention.

The kidneys, in an effort to rid the body of the excess water, start to eliminate salt (sodium) from the body, hoping that the water will follow the salt out of the body. The resulting low sodium levels (**hyponatremia**) can cause hypertension, confusion, convulsions, and coma.

Causes of SIADH include certain medications, including psychotic medications, lung diseases, and tumors, as well as intracranial bleeding that may create increased intracranial pressure (ICP).

● THYROID DISORDERS

Because the thyroid gland controls metabolic activity, any disorder involving this gland also affects other structures. Persons at risk include those with other immune system problems, such as arthritis. Common signs and symptoms of the disorders are discussed in this unit.

● DIAGNOSTIC TESTS FOR THYROID

To diagnose thyroid function, a blood test is done; blood levels of TSH, T_3, and T_4 are checked to see if they are within normal limits.

A thyroid scan is another diagnostic tool used to determine the activity of the thyroid gland. The patient takes radioactive iodine; after the dye is taken, a scan is done to measure how the radioactive iodine is taken up by the thyroid gland. A large uptake indicates hyperthyroidism.

The radioactive iodine uptake test measures the activity of the thyroid gland. Diluted radioactive iodine is given orally. The amount that accumulates in the thyroid gland is calculated by use of a scan.

Hyperthyroidism

Hyperthyroidism is a condition caused by overactivity of the thyroid gland. Too much thyroxin is secreted (hypersecretion), leading to enlargement of the gland. People with hyperthyroidism consume large quantities of food but nevertheless suffer a loss of body fat and weight. Symptoms include feeling too hot, fast-growing and rougher fingernails, and weakened muscles. They may suffer from increased blood pressure and heartbeat, hand tremors, perspiration, and irritability. In addition, the liver releases excess glucose into the bloodstream, increasing the blood sugar level and causing a mild case of glycosuria. The most pronounced symptoms of hyperthyroidism include enlargement of the thyroid gland (**goiter**), bulging of the eyeballs (**exophthalmos**), dilation of the pupils, and wide-open eyelids. In the United States, 70% to 80% of people who have hyperthyroidism have the type also known as Graves' disease.

The immediate cause of exophthalmos is not completely known. It is not directly caused by the hyperthyroidism, because removal of the thyroid does not always cause the eyeballs to return to their normal state. Treatment of hyperthyroidism includes total or partial removal of the thyroid and administration of drugs like propylthiouracil and methylthiouracil to reduce the thyroxin secretion. The use of radioactive iodine to suppress the activity of the thyroid gland is another treatment for hyperthyroidism.

Hypothyroidism

Hypothyroidism is a condition in which the thyroid gland does not secrete sufficient thyroxin (hyposecretion). This is manifested by low T_3 or T_4 levels or increased TSH blood levels.

Adult hypothyroidism may occur because of iodine deficiency. A simple goiter may indicate this condition. Because iodized salt is commonly used in the United States, that is not the usual cause of a hypothyroid condition. The major cause is an inflammation of the thyroid that destroys the ability of the gland to make thyroxine. This inflammation is an autoimmune disease that attacks the body's own thyroid gland. Symptoms include dry and itchy skin, dry and brittle hair, constipation, and muscle cramps at night.

Depending on when hypothyroidism strikes, two different sets of disorders may occur: myxedema or cretinism.

Myxedema. The face becomes swollen, weight increases, and initiative and memory fails when a person experiences **myxedema**. Treatment is daily medication of thyroid hormone. It is important for the health care worker to be sure the patient understands the necessity of taking the medication. Follow-up tests to measure TSH blood levels are also important.

Cretinism. **Cretinism** develops in early infancy or childhood. It is characterized by a short and disproportionate body, and mental retardation. Hypothyroidism in children causes cretinism. The sexual development and physical growth of cretins does not proceed beyond that of a 7- or 8-year-old child.

In treating cretinism, thyroid hormones or thyroid extract may restore a degree of normal development if administered in time. In most cases, however, normal development cannot be completely restored once the affliction has set in.

PARATHYROID DISORDERS

The parathyroid glands regulate the use of calcium and phosphorus. Both these minerals are involved in many of the body systems.

Hyperfunctioning of the parathyroid glands may cause an increase in the amount of blood calcium, thereby increasing the tendency for the calcium to crystallize in the kidneys as kidney stones. Excess amounts of calcium and phosphorus are withdrawn from the bones; this may lead to eventual deformity. So much calcium can be removed from the bones that they become honeycombed with cavities. Afflicted bones become so fragile that even walking can cause fractures.

Hypofunctioning of the parathyroid glands leads to a condition known as **tetany**. In this case, severely diminished calcium levels affect the normal function of nerves. Convulsive twitching develops, and the afflicted person dies of spasms in the respiratory muscles. Treatment consists of administering vitamin D, calcium, and parathormone to restore a normal calcium balance.

ADRENAL DISORDERS

The adrenal glands produce glucocorticoid hormones. Therefore disorders of the adrenal glands result in either an abundance or a deficiency of these hormones. Changes in glucocorticoid hormone levels always affect blood glucose levels.

Hyperfunction of Adrenal

Cushing's syndrome results from the hypersecretion of the glucocorticoid hormones from the adrenal cortex, Figure 11-9. This hypersecretion may be caused by an adrenal cortical tumor or the prolonged use of prednisone. (More women than men tend to develop this endocrine disorder.) Symptoms include high blood pressure, muscular weakness, obesity, poor healing of skin lesions, a tendency to bruise easily, hirsutism (excessive hair growth), menstrual disorders in women, and hyperglycemia. The most noticeable characteristics are a rounded "moon" face and a "buffalo hump" that develops from the redistribution of body fat. Therapy consists of surgical removal of the adrenal cortical tumor.

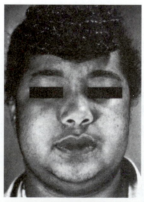 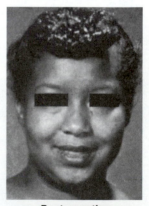

Preoperative   **Postoperative (6 months later)**

● **FIGURE 11–9**   *Cushing's syndrome.*

Hypofunction of Adrenal

Hypofunctioning of the adrenal cortex can also lead to **Addison's disease**. Persons with Addison's disease exhibit the following symptoms: excessive pigmentation, prompting the characteristic "bronzing" of the skin; decreased levels of blood glucose (hypoglycemia); low blood pressure that falls further when standing; pronounced muscular weakness and fatigue; diarrhea, weight loss, and vomiting; and a severe drop of sodium in the blood and tissue fluids, causing a serious imbalance of electrolytes.

The medical treatment of Addison's disease is focused on the replacement of the deficient hormones.

● STEROID ABUSE IN SPORTS

Athletes of today have turned to the use of androgenic anabolic steroids to build bigger, stronger muscles, hoping to achieve status in the world of sports. The risks of taking steroids far outweigh any temporary improvement that an athlete may hope to gain. Effects on males who abuse steroids include liver changes, decrease in spleen production, atrophy of the testicles, breast enlargement, and increased risk of cardiovascular disease. Effects on females include amenorrhea (loss of menstrual cycle), abnormal placement of body hair, baldness, and voice changes. In addition, both sexes complain of headaches, dizziness, hypertension, mood swings, and aggressiveness.

● GONAD DISORDERS

Disturbances in the ovaries may consist of cysts and tumors, abnormal menstruation, and menopausal changes. Turner's syndrome may occur in either the male or female; this is a chromosomal disorder. (See Chapter 20.)

PANCREATIC DISORDERS

Diabetes mellitus is a condition caused by decreased secretion of insulin from the islet cells of the pancreas or by the ineffective use of insulin. Insulin is necessary for the cells to use glucose. Carbohydrate metabolism is disturbed in persons with diabetes mellitus, which has an adverse effect on protein and fat metabolism.

Diabetes is divided into two types: insulin dependent (type I) and non–insulin dependent (type II). The insulin-dependent type is also known as juvenile diabetes, because the onset usually occurs during childhood or young adulthood. The cause of type I is thought to be an autoimmune reaction involving genetic and viral factors that destroy the islets of Langerhans cells. Individuals with type I diabetes must take insulin and monitor daily blood glucose levels.

Symptoms of type I, or insulin-dependent, diabetes mellitus (IDDM) include the following:

- polyuria—excessive urination
- polydipsia—excessive thirst
- polyphagia—excessive hunger
- weight loss
- blurred vision
- possible diabetic coma

Insulin deficiency causes glucose to accumulate in the bloodstream, rather than be transported to the cells and converted into energy. Eventually the excess becomes too much for the kidneys to reabsorb, and the excess glucose is excreted in the urine. Excretion of excess glucose requires an accompanying excretion of large amounts of water. This ensures that the sugar concentration does not rise too high. Diabetics are constantly thirsty because the lost water must be replaced.

Because sufficient glucose is not available for cellular oxidation in diabetes mellitus, the body starts to burn up protein and fats. The diabetic is constantly hungry and usually eats voraciously but loses weight nonetheless.

When fats are utilized as a fuel source, they are rapidly but incompletely oxidized. One product of this abnormal rate of fat oxidation is ketone bodies. Ketone bodies are highly toxic; the type most commonly formed is acetoacetic acid. These ketone acids accumulate in the blood, promoting the development of acidosis and giving the breath and urine an odor of "sweet" acetone. If acidosis is severe, diabetic coma and death may result. Prolonged diabetes leads to atherosclerosis, heart disease, and kidney damage. Therapy consists of daily insulin injections and a controlled diet.

Patient education is critical in the treatment of diabetes. The person with insulin-dependent diabetes must be educated in the signs of **hypoglycemia** (low blood sugar; insulin shock) and **hyperglycemia** (high blood sugar; diabetic coma), as illustrated in Table 11-4.

Characteristics and symptoms of type II, or non–insulin-dependent, diabetes (NIDDM) include the following:

- gradual onset
- most common in adults over age 55
- feelings of tiredness or illness
- frequent urination, especially at night
- unusual thirst
- frequent infections and slow healing of sores

Non–insulin-dependent (type II) diabetes makes up 90% to 95% of cases of diabetes. It is usually a familial disease that occurs later in life. In this condition, insulin is secreted but in lowered amounts. The treatment focus is on diet, weight reduction, and medication.

Because insulin is a protein, as well as a hormone, the digestive juices in the stomach digest any insulin that is swallowed. Thus persons with diabetes need insulin to carry carbohydrates (sugar) into the body's cells.

However, for every hormone, there is an enzyme that breaks down the hormone in the blood after it has been used. Insulinase is the enzyme that breaks down insulin. Special oral medications can decrease the creation of insulinase, resulting in more circulating insulin left in the blood. Many persons with non–insulin-dependent diabetes mellitus take these oral hypoglycemic agents (drugs). Other oral

TABLE 11-4 *Signs of Hypoglycemia (Insulin Shock) and Hyperglycemia (Diabetic Coma)*

	HYPERGLYCEMIA (LOW BLOOD SUGAR)	HYPOGLYCEMIA (HIGH BLOOD SUGAR)
Onset	Sudden	Slow
Reason	Too much insulin Too much exercise Not enough food	Not enough insulin Not enough exercise Too much food
Skin	Pale, moist to wet Sweating	Flushed, dry, hot No sweating
Symptoms	Nervous, trembling, confused, irritable	Drowsy, lethargic, weak, lapses into unconsciousness
Breath	Normal odor	Fruity odor
Respiration	Normal to rapid	Kussmaul's breathing (air hunger)
Glycosuria	Little to none	High amount
Ketonuria	None	Present
Blood sugar	Low—below 80	High—above 150
Treatment	Rapid response; give sugar in form of soft drink or orange juice Glucagon (IM); glucose 50% IV	Slow response IV fluids Regular insulin

STREET SMART

Low blood sugar (hypoglycemia) is a medical emergency. The patient with low blood sugar becomes confused, perhaps combative, and then lapses into unconsciousness. Convulsions can occur when the blood sugar is dangerously low.

Hypoglycemia can occur for a number of reasons, including too much insulin, too much exercise, or not eating. Whatever the reason, the blood sugar falls.

If the patient is conscious, he or she should be encouraged to eat. When the patient becomes unconscious, EMS is needed. Advanced EMTs who are capable of starting an IV can administer glucose (50% dextrose in water) directly into the bloodstream and reverse this potentially lethal condition, Figure 11-10. ∎

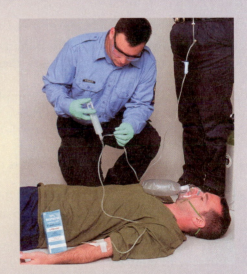

● **FIGURE 11–10** *Advanced life support personnel can rapidly reverse hypoglycemia with sugar (dextrose) via an intravenous infusion.*

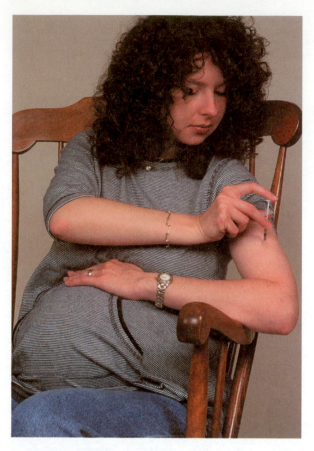

● **FIGURE 11–11**   *A pregnant woman can develop diabetes during her pregnancy.*

hypoglycemic drugs encourage the pancreas to produce more insulin. In both cases these agents can help treat diabetes.

Some women develop diabetes as a complication of pregnancy, and they often take insulin for the duration of the pregnancy, Figure 11-11. After the baby is born, the mother's body returns to normal and supplemental insulin is no longer needed.

Babies born to women with gestational diabetes are usually large and may have an increased risk for hypoglycemia and an inability to maintain body temperature, which can cause complications with delivery.

Treatment of Diabetes Mellitus

Patients with diabetes can lead normal, productive lives if they follow their treatment.

Diabetics need instruction on how to use the glucose monitoring system, how to inject insulin, exercise and its effects on the blood sugar, and how to use their calculated diet and the food exchange listings.

Diabetes is widely recognized as one of the leading causes of death and disability in the United States. It is associated with long-term complications that affect almost every part of the body, including blindness, heart disease, stroke, kidney failure, amputations, and nerve damage.

Persons with diabetes should wear a Medic Alert bracelet and carry an identification card stating that they are diabetic. EMS providers should look for a Medic Alert bracelet or necklace during the rapid trauma assessment or rapid physical examination, Figure 11-12.

Tests for Diabetes Mellitus

The diagnostic tests to determine the presence of glucose are done on urine and blood samples. The most common test is a finger prick to obtain a blood sample that is then mea-

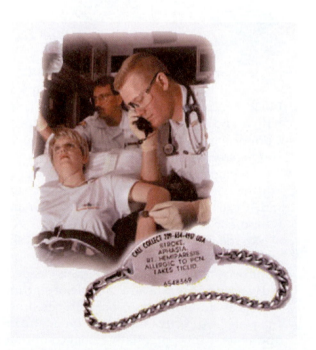

● **FIGURE 11–12**   *Always check for a Medic Alert bracelet. (Courtesy The Medic Alert Foundation, Turlock, Calif.)*

sured in a glucometer (glucose monitor). This test may be done by the patient at home. The normal blood sugar is 80 to 120 milligrams of glucose per 100 milliliters of blood.

Another blood test for diabetes is glycosylated hemoglobin (HbA$_{1c}$). The glucose exposed to hemoglobin attaches itself to the protein in a way that reflects the average blood glucose concentration for the preceding 2 to 3 months. The test is done every 3 months.

Urine also may be tested by using a specifically coded dipstick. A urine sample is obtained, then the tape is dipped into the urine and compared with the special coding bar that is found on the outside of the dipstick container.

MEDICAL HIGHLIGHTS

Approximately 14 million persons in the United States have diabetes mellitus, a serious, lifelong disorder that is as yet incurable. Half these people do not know they have the disease and are not under medical care. Researchers in the past 15 years have made advances in managing diabetes and treating its complications. Major advances include:

- New forms of purified insulin, such as human insulin produced through genetic engineering

- Development of better ways for patients to monitor blood glucose levels at home

- Development of external and implantable insulin pumps that deliver appropriate amounts of insulin and replace daily injections

- The use of laser treatment for diabetic eye disease, reducing the risk of blindness

- Successful transplantation of kidneys in diabetics with kidney failure

- Better ways of managing diabetic pregnancies and improving chances of a successful outcome

- Development of new drugs to treat NIDDM and better ways to manage this type through weight control

- Proof that intensive management of blood glucose levels reduces and may prevent development of microvascular complications of diabetes, such as peripheral vascular disease

- Firm evidence that antihypertensive drugs called ACE inhibitors prevent or delay kidney failure in people with diabetes

- Ongoing research to develop insulin that may be administered through nasal sprays or taken in the form of a pill

- Ongoing research to develop devices that read blood glucose levels without having to prick a finger to get the blood sample

Researchers continue to look for the exact cause of diabetes and methods to prevent and cure it. Some genetic markers for IDDM have been identified, and it is now possible to screen relatives of people with IDDM to see if they are at risk for diabetes. Studies are now under way using drugs that stop the immune system from attacking the beta cells, to try to prevent IDDM from developing in people who are at high risk for IDDM. ■

● REVIEW QUESTIONS

Select the letter of the choice that best completes the statement.

1. The master gland is known as:
   a. pituitary
   b. thyroid
   c. adrenal
   d. ovary

2. The hormone that governs metabolism is:
   a. FSH
   b. MSH
   c. TSH
   d. ACTH

3. The hormones that affect neuromuscular functioning, blood clotting, and holding the cells together are:
   a. thyroxine and calcitonin
   b. thyroxine and parathormone
   c. calcitonin and thymosin
   d. calcitonin and parathormone

4. The gland that governs the production of antibodies is the:
   a. thymus
   b. thyroid
   c. parathyroid
   d. pituitary

5. The hormone that is responsible for stimulating ovulation is:
   a. TSH
   b. ICSH
   c. FSH
   d. LTH

6. The hormone that prepares us to fight or flee is:
   a. aldosterone
   b. epinephrine
   c. cortisol
   d. corticoid

7. The secretions of the ovaries are:
   a. estrogen and LTH
   b. estrogen and LH
   c. progesterone and LTH
   d. progesterone and estrogen

8. A decrease in the production of insulin causes:
   a. diabetes mellitus
   b. diabetes insipidus
   c. cretinism
   d. exophthalmos

9. A hypofunction of the thyroid gland causes:
    a. exophthalmos
    b. glycosuria
    c. cretinism
    d. Graves' disease

10. An oversecretion of the adrenal cortex is known as:
    a. myxedema
    b. Cushing's syndrome
    c. Addison's disease
    d. dwarfism

● COMPLETION

Complete the following chart.

GLAND	HORMONE	NORMAL FUNCTION	DISORDERS
Pituitary			
Pineal			
Thyroid			
Parathyroid			
Thymus			
Adrenal			
Gonads			
Pancreas			

● MATCHING

Match each term in Column A with its correct description in Column B.

Column A	Column B
_____ 1. ACTH	a. master gland of the endocrine system
_____ 2. adrenals	b. any gland of internal secretion
_____ 3. cortisone	c. a hormone secreted by the adrenals
_____ 4. gonad	d. regulates use of calcium
_____ 5. endocrine	e. the secretion of any endocrine gland
_____ 6. hormone	f. helps body meet emergencies
_____ 7. insulin	g. sex gland
_____ 8. parathyroid	h. regulates body metabolism
_____ 9. pituitary	i. one of the hormones secreted by the pituitary gland
_____ 10. thyroid	j. a hormone that regulates carbohydrates and metabolism
	k. hypofunction of the endocrine glands

● APPLYING THEORY TO PRACTICE

1. You have a thermostat in your house that regulates the heat or the air conditioner. When a certain temperature is reached, it automatically shuts off. This principle applies also to negative feedback in hormonal control. Explain how this functions in relation to the thyroid gland.

2. A patient comes to the doctor's office and tells the doctor she is experiencing leg cramping, which she has heard has to do with calcium. Explain to the patient how calcium is affected by the action of the thyroid gland and parathyroid.

3. Upon arrival at the scene, a patient calls out to you. He is near hysteria; he tells you he is experiencing heart palpitations and feels he is "jumping out of his skin." The patient's history reveals that he has been on thyroid medication. Explain to the patient what you think may be the cause of his symptoms and what action should be taken.

4. Your brother wants to be a football player. He is 5' 7"; he heard "steroids" could help him. Explain the action of steroids and why they should not be used.

5. Remember a time when you were frightened; think about it. How did your body react?

6. Diabetes mellitus affects 1 in 10 persons in the United States. You have to do a presentation to the class. Explain diabetes: its causes, treatments, signs of insulin shock (hypoglycemia), diabetic coma (hyperglycemia), diet, and research currently being conducted.

Blood

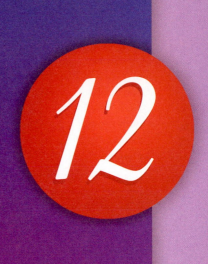

12

Objectives

- List the important components of blood
- Describe the function of each component
- Recognize the significance of the various blood types
- Describe venipuncture
- Describe some disorders of the blood
- Define the key words that relate to this chapter

Key Words

abscess
agranulocyte (agranular
    leukocyte)
albumin
anemia
antibody
anticoagulant
antigen
antiprothrombin
    (heparin)
antithromboplastin
aplastic anemia
B-lymphocyte
basophil
clotting time
coagulation
coagulation cascade
Cooley's anemia
diapedesis
disseminated
    intravascular
    coagulation (DIC)
embolism
eosinophil
erythroblastosis fetalis

erythrocyte
erythropoiesis
fibrin
fibrinogen
fibrinolytic
gamma globulin
globin
globulin
granulocyte (granular
    leukocyte)
hematocrit
hematoma
heme
hemoglobin
hemolysis
hemolytic reaction
hemophilia
inflammation
iron deficiency anemia
leukemia
leukocyte
leukocytosis
leukopenia
lymphocyte
lysis

(continues)

Key Words (continued)

macrophage	Rh factor
monocyte	RhoGAM
myeloblast	sedimentation rate
myocardial infarction	septicemia
neutrophil	sickle cell anemia
oxyhemoglobin	stroke
pathogenic	thrombin
pernicious anemia	thrombocyte
phagocytosis	thrombocytopenia
physiological jaundice	thrombolytic
plasma	thromboplastin
polycythemia	thrombosis
polymorphonuclear	thrombus
leukocyte	T-lymphocyte
prothrombin	type and crossmatch
pus	universal donor
pyrexia	universal recipient

From the time of antiquity to the present day, blood's fundamental role in life has been recognized. An unrelenting loss of blood, whether internal or external, will surely lead to death. That is in part due to blood's purpose in the body. Blood is, literally and figuratively, a connective tissue. Blood connects all the cells inside the body with the world outside the body. Blood transports life-giving oxygen and nutrients, in the form of blood sugar, to all the cells in the body.

The average body has approximately 70 milliliters of blood for every kilogram of weight, less if there is a great deal of fat. Therefore the average 154-pound (70-kilogram) male has about 5 liters of circulating blood volume.

FUNCTION OF BLOOD

Blood is the transporting fluid of the body. It carries nutrients from the digestive tract to the cells, oxygen from the lungs to the cells, waste products from the cells to the various organs of excretion, and hormones from secreting cells to other parts of the body. It aids in the distribution of heat formed in the more active tissues (such as the skeletal muscles) to all parts of the body. Blood also helps to regulate the acid-base balance and to protect against infection. Consequently, it is vital to our life and health, Table 12-1.

BLOOD COMPOSITION

Blood is made up of these major components:

- **Plasma**, the liquid portion of blood without its cellular elements. *Serum* is the name given to plasma after a blood clot is formed. Serum = plasma − (fibrinogen + prothrombin).

- Cellular (formed) elements, which include erythrocytes, or red blood cells (RBCs), leukocytes, or white blood cells (WBCs), and thrombocytes (platelets), Figure 12-1.

TABLE 12-1 *Summary of the Various Functions of Blood*

FUNCTION	EFFECT ON BODY
Nutritive	Transports nutrient molecules (glucose, amino acids, fatty acids, and glycerol) from the small intestine or storage sites to the tissues.
Respiratory	Transports oxygen from the lungs to the tissues and carbon dioxide from the tissue to the lungs.
Excretory	Transports waste products (lactic acid, urea, and creatinine) from the cells to the excretory organs.
Regulatory	Transports hormones and other chemical substances that control the proper functioning of many organs.
	Circulates excess heat to the body surfaces and to the lungs, through which it is lost (controls body temperature).
	Maintains water balance and a constant environment for tissue cells.
Protective	Circulates antibodies and defensive cells throughout the body to combat infection and disease.

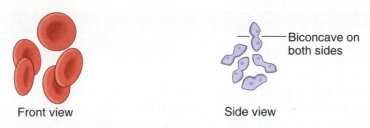

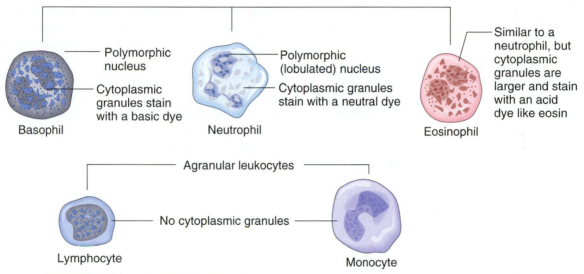

● FIGURE 12–1   *Cellular elements of the blood.*

● BLOOD PLASMA

Plasma is a straw-colored, complex liquid, composing about 55% of the blood volume and containing the following seven substances in solution:

1. *Water*—Water makes up about 92% of the total volume of plasma. This percentage is maintained by the kidneys and by water intake and output.

2. *Blood proteins*—There is a protein found in red blood cells known as hemoglobin, which composes about two thirds of the blood proteins.

3. *Plasma proteins*—These three proteins are the most abundant of those found in plasma: fibrinogen, serum albumin, and serum globulin.

a. **Fibrinogen** is necessary for blood clotting. Without fibrinogen, the slightest cut or wound would bleed profusely. It is synthesized in the liver.

b. **Albumin** is the most abundant of all the plasma proteins. Another product of the liver, albumin helps to maintain the blood's osmotic pressure and volume. It provides the "pressure" needed to hold and pull water from the tissue fluid back into the blood vessels. Normally plasma proteins do not pass through the capillary walls, because their molecules are relatively large. They are colloidal substances; they can give up or take up water-soluble substances, thus regulating the osmotic pressure within the blood vessels.

c. **Globulin** is formed not only in the liver but also in the lymphatic system (discussed in Chapter 15). **Gamma globulin** has been fractionated (separated) from globulin. This portion helps in the synthesis of antibodies, which destroy or render harmless various disease-causing organisms. **Prothrombin** is yet another globulin, formed continually in the liver, which helps blood to coagulate. Vitamin K is necessary in aiding the process of prothrombin synthesis.

4. *Nutrients*—Nutrient molecules are absorbed from the digestive tract. Glucose, fatty acids, cholesterol, and amino acids are dissolved in the blood plasma.

5. *Electrolytes*—The most abundant electrolytes are sodium chloride and potassium. These come from foods and chemical processes occurring in the body.

6. *Hormones, vitamins, and enzymes*—These three substances are found in very small amounts in the blood plasma. They generally help the body to control its chemical reactions.

7. *Metabolic waste products*—All the body's cells are actively engaged in chemical reactions to maintain homeostasis. As a result of this, waste products are formed and subsequently carried by the plasma to the various excretory organs.

RED BLOOD CELLS

Red blood cells, or **erythrocytes**, are biconcave, disk-shaped cells. They are caved in on both sides, with a thin center and thicker mar-

gins. When viewed from above, they appear to have a doughnut shape, see Figure 12-1.

Physicians are often interested in the amount of red blood cells in a volume of blood. This amount, measured by percentage, is called the **hematocrit**. A hematocrit is determined after a tube of blood is rapidly spun in a centrifuge to separate the formed blood, including red blood cells, from the plasma.

A typical hematocrit for a man is about 40% to 55% and 35% to 45% percent for a woman. If a patient's hematocrit is decreasing, a physician looks for signs of internal or external bleeding.

Hemoglobin

Erythrocytes contain a red pigment (coloring agent) called **hemoglobin**, which provides blood's characteristic color. Hemoglobin is composed of a protein molecule called **globin** and an iron compound called **heme**. A single blood cell contains several million molecules of hemoglobin. Hemoglobin is vital to the function of the red blood cell, helping it to transport oxygen to the tissues and some carbon dioxide away from the tissues. Normal hemoglobin count for men is 14 to 18 grams per 100 milliliters; for women it is 12 to 16 grams per 100 milliliters.

Function

In the capillaries of the lung, erythrocytes pick up oxygen from the inspired air. The oxygen chemically combines with the hemoglobin, forming the compound **oxyhemoglobin**. The oxyhemoglobin-laden erythrocytes circulate to the capillaries of tissues, where oxygen is released to the tissues. The carbon dioxide that is formed in the body's tissues during metabolism chemically combines with the hemoglobin, forming the compound carbaminohemoglobin. The red blood cells then circulate back to the lungs to release the carbon dioxide and absorb more oxygen. Blood cells that travel in the arteries (except for pulmonary arteries) carry oxyhemoglobin, which gives blood its bright red color. Blood cells in the veins (except for pulmonary veins) carry carbaminohemoglobin, which is responsible for the dark, crimson-blue color characteristic of venous blood.

Erythropoiesis

Erythropoiesis, the manufacturing of red blood cells, occurs in the red bone marrow of essentially all bones until adolescence. (In the fetus, red blood cells are also produced by the spleen and liver.) As persons grow older, the red marrow of the long bones is replaced by fat marrow; erythrocytes are thereafter formed only in the short and flat bones.

Erythrocytes come from stem cells in the red bone marrow called hemocytoblasts, Figure 12-1. As the hemocytoblast matures into an erythrocyte, it loses its nucleus and cytoplasmic organelles. The hemocytoblast also becomes smaller, gains hemoglobin, develops a biconcave shape, and enters into the bloodstream. To aid in erythropoiesis, vitamin B_{12},

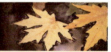

CHANGES OF AGING

When red blood cells are broken down by the spleen and liver after cell death, two molecules result: heme and globin. In some cases the heme, the iron-containing molecule, is recycled. However, some heme is converted into an orange pigment called bilirubin and excreted with the bile in stool.

The liver of a newborn is immature and cannot excrete the bilirubin into the bile. The result can be that the orange-pigmented bilirubin builds up in the body and the infant's skin and eyes appear yellow. Approximately one third of all infants develop this mild disorder, called **physiological jaundice**.

Physiologic jaundice can be treated by simply using fluorescent lights called bili-lights during the infant's stay in the nursery. The condition usually resolves without treatment. ■

folic acid, copper, cobalt, iron, and proteins are needed.

Red blood cells (erythrocytes) lack a cell nucleus (enucleated) necessary to permit the cell to fabricate new cell components and repair itself. Because erythrocytes are enucleated and unable to repair themselves, they only live approximately 120 days. As the cells age they become more vulnerable to rupture and fragmentation. The fragments that remain in the bloodstream are further broken down by the spleen and liver. Hemoglobin breaks down into globin and heme; the iron content of heme is used to make new red blood cells. The normal count of red blood cells ranges from 4.5 to 6.2 million per microliter of venous blood for men and 4.2 to 5.4 million per microliter of venous blood for women.

Hemolysis

A rupture or bursting of the red blood cell (erythrocyte) is called **hemolysis**. This sometimes occurs as a result of a blood transfusion reaction or other disease processes.

● WHITE BLOOD CELLS

White blood cells are known as **leukocytes**. They are larger than erythrocytes, ranging from 1.25 to 2 times their diameter. They are granular or agranular, translucent, and ameboid in shape. Leukocytes are manufactured both in red bone marrow and in lymphatic tissue.

Types of Leukocytes

Leukocytes are classified into two major groups of cells: the **granulocytes (granular leukocytes)** and the **agranulocytes (agranular leukocytes)**. This classification is due to the presence of cytoplasmic granules, nuclear structure, and reactions to stains like Wright's stain. Granulocytes are synthesized in red bone marrow from cells called **myeloblasts**. Granulocytes are destroyed as they age and as a result of participating in bacterial destruction. The life span of white blood cells is variable, but most granulocytes live only a few days.

There are three types of granulocytes: neutrophils, eosinophils, and basophils.

Neutrophils, also called **polymorphonuclear leukocytes**, phagocytize bacteria with lysosomal enzymes. (**Phagocytosis** is a process that surrounds, engulfs, and digests harmful bacteria.) **Eosinophils** phagocytize the remains of antibody-antigen reactions. They also increase in great numbers when a person experiences allergic conditions, malaria, or worm infestations. **Basophils** perform phagocytosis, and their count increases during chronic inflammation and during healing from an infection. Basophils produce histamine, a vasodilator, and heparin, an anticoagulant.

Agranulocytes are divided into lymphocytes and monocytes. **Lymphocytes** are further subdivided into **B-lymphocytes**, which are synthesized in the bone marrow, and **T-lymphocytes** from the thymus gland. Still others are formed by the lymph nodes and spleen. Their life span ranges from a few days to several years. They basically help the body by synthesizing and releasing antibody molecules and by protecting against the formation of cancer cells.

Monocytes are formed in bone marrow and the spleen. They assist in phagocytosis and are able to leave the bloodstream to attach themselves to tissues; here they become tissue **macrophages**, or histiocytes. During an inflammation, histiocytes help to wall off and isolate the infected area.

The aforementioned types of leukocytes (basophils, neutrophils, eosinophils, and monocytes), which can perform phagocytosis, are called phagocytes. Unlike erythrocytes, they can move through the intercellular spaces of the capillary wall into neighboring tissue. This process is known as **diapedesis**.

A normal leukocyte count averages from 3200 to 9800 per cubic millimeter of blood per microliter.

To summarize, leukocytes help protect the body against infection and injury. This is achieved through (1) phagocytosis and destruction of bacteria, (2) synthesis of antibody molecules, (3) "cleaning up" of cellular remnants at the site of inflammation, and (4) walling off of the infected area, Tables 12-2 and 12-3.

TABLE 12-2 *The Different Types of Leukocytes and Their Sizes*

MAJOR TYPES OF LEUKOCYTES	SPECIFIC KINDS OF LEUKOCYTES	SIZE
Granulocytes 60%–70%	Neutrophils Eosinophils Basophils	9–12 mu 10–14 mu 8–10 mu
Agranulocytes Lymphocytes 20%–30%	Small Large	7–10 mu up to 20 mu
Monocytes 5%–8%	Mononuclear Transitional	9–12 mu 9–12 mu

mu, *Micron.*

TABLE 12-3 *Characteristics and Functions of the Leukocytes*

LEUKOCYTE	WHERE FORMED	TYPE OF NUCLEUS	CYTOPLASM	FUNCTION
Agranular leukocytes 1. Lymphocyte	Lymph glands and nodes, bone marrow, spleen	One large, spherical nucleus; may be indented; sharply defined and stains dark blue.	Cytoplasm stains a pale blue and contains scattered violet granules.	Helps to form antibodies at a site of inflammation; protects against cancer.
2. Monocyte (macrophage)	Lymph glands and nodes, bone marrow, spleen	One lobulated or horse-shoe-shaped nucleus that stains blue.	Abundant cytoplasm that stains a gray-blue.	Phagocytosis of cellular debris and foreign particles.
Granular leukocytes 1. Neutrophil	Formed in bone marrow from neutrophilic myelocytes	Lobulated; contains 1–5 or more lobes; stains deep blue.	Cytoplasm has a pink tinge with very fine granules.	Displays marked phagocytosis toward bacteria during infections and inflammations. Contributes to pus formation.
2. Eosinophil	Formed in bone marrow from eosinophilic myelocytes	Irregularly shaped with 2 lobes; stains blue, but less deeply than neutrophils.	Cytoplasm has a sky-blue tinge with many coarse, uniform, round or oval bright red granules.	Marked increase during parasitic and worm infections and allergic attacks.
3. Basophil (mast cell)	Formed in bone marrow from basophilic myelocytes	Centrally located, slightly lobulated nucleus; stains a light purple; hidden by granules.	Cytoplasm has a mauve color with many large deep purple granules.	Phagocytosis; releases heparin and histamine and promotes the inflammatory response.

● INFLAMMATION

If living tissue is damaged in any way, the body usually responds to the damage by either neutralizing or eliminating the cause of the damage. When this happens, the damaged body part goes through an inflammation process. **Inflammation** occurs when tissues are subjected to chemical or physical trauma (cut or heat). Invasion by **pathogenic** (disease-causing) microorganisms such as bacteria, fungi, protozoa, and viruses also can cause inflammation.

The characteristic symptoms of inflammation are redness, localized heat, swelling, and pain. This is due to irritation by bacterial toxins, increased blood flow, congestion of blood vessels, and collection of blood plasma in the surrounding tissues (edema). Histamine released from the basophil and other chemical substances increase blood flow to the injured area, as well as increasing capillary permeability. Thus large amounts of blood plasma and fibrinogen enter the damaged area, which is walled off as a result of the clotting action of fibrinogen on the damaged tissue and macrophage action.

Neutrophils move very quickly through the capillary walls, by diapedesis, to the damaged area. There they begin phagocytosis of the pathogenic microorganisms. Macrophages also participate in phagocytosis.

In most inflammations, a cream-colored liquid called **pus** forms. Pus is a combination of dead tissue, dead and living bacteria, dead leukocytes, and blood plasma. If the damaged area is below the epidermis, an **abscess** (pus-filled cavity) forms. If it is on the skin or a mucosal surface, it is called an ulcer. In many inflammations, chemical substances called pyrogens are formed, which are circulated to the hypothalamus. In the hypothalamus the pyrogens affect the temperature control center, which raises the body's temperature, causing fever (**pyrexia**).

When inflammation is present there is an increased production of neutrophils by bone marrow. If the white blood cell count exceeds 10,000 cells per cubic millimeter of blood, a condition called **leukocytosis** exists. After healing, the leukocyte count returns to normal. Sometimes a decrease in the number of white blood cells occurs. This is called **leukopenia**. Leukopenia can be caused by taking marrow-depressant drugs, by pathological conditions, or by radiation.

● THROMBOCYTES (BLOOD PLATELETS)

Thrombocytes are the smallest of the solid components of blood. They are ovoid-shaped structures, synthesized from the larger megakaryocytes in red bone marrow. Thrombocytes

are not cells but fragments of the megakaryocytes' cytoplasm, see Figure 12-1.

The normal blood platelet count ranges from 250,000 to 450,000 per cubic millimeter of blood. Platelets function in the initiation of the blood clotting process. When a blood vessel is damaged, as in a cut or wound, the vessel's collagen fibers come into contact with the platelets. The platelets are then stimulated to produce sticky projecting structures, allowing them to adhere to the collagen fibers. This reaction occurs countless times, creating a "platelet plug" to stop the bleeding. The platelets secrete a chemical called serotonin, which causes the blood vessel to spasm and narrow and decreases blood loss until the clot forms. Subsequently, the blood clotting process follows to "harden" the platelet plug.

Coagulation

Blood clotting, or **coagulation**, is a complicated and essential process that depends in large part on thrombocytes. When a cut or other injury ruptures a blood vessel, clotting must occur to stop the bleeding.

Although the exact details of this process are not clear, there is a general agreement that the following reaction occurs:

Whenever a blood vessel or tissue is injured, platelets and injured tissue release **thromboplastin**. An injury to a blood vessel makes the lining rough; as blood platelets flow over the roughened area, they disintegrate, releasing thromboplastin.

Thromboplastin is a complex substance that can only cause coagulation if calcium ions and prothrombin are present. Prothrombin is a plasma protein synthesized in the liver.

The thromboplastin and calcium ions act as enzymes in a reaction that converts prothrombin into **thrombin**. This reaction occurs only in the presence of bleeding, because normally there is no thrombin in the blood plasma.

In the next stage of coagulation, the thrombin just formed acts as an enzyme, changing fibrinogen (a plasma protein) into **fibrin**. These gel-like fibrin threads layer themselves over the cut, creating a fine, meshlike network. This fibrin network traps the red blood cells, platelets,

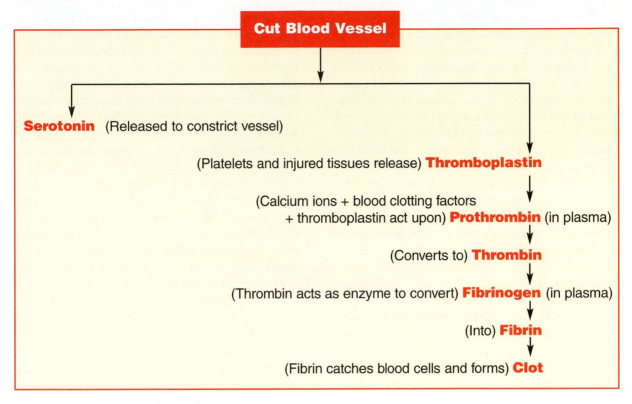

Cut Blood Vessel

Serotonin (Released to constrict vessel)

(Platelets and injured tissues release) **Thromboplastin**

(Calcium ions + blood clotting factors
+ thromboplastin act upon) **Prothrombin** (in plasma)

(Converts to) **Thrombin**

(Thrombin acts as enzyme to convert) **Fibrinogen** (in plasma)

(Into) **Fibrin**

(Fibrin catches blood cells and forms) **Clot**

● **FIGURE 12–2**   *Blood clotting process.*

and plasma, creating a blood clot. At first, serum (a pale yellow fluid) oozes out of the cut. As the serum slowly dries, a crust (scab) forms over the fibrin threads, completing the common clotting process.

For coagulation to occur successfully, two **anticoagulants** (substances preventing coagulation) must be neutralized. These are called **antithromboplastin** and **antiprothrombin (heparin)**; they are neutralized by thromboplastin.

STREET SMART -

Approximately 70% of heart attacks (**myocardial infarctions**) and the majority of brain attacks (**strokes**) are caused by a blood clot (**thrombus**) blocking (occluding) a blood vessel. The resulting blockage dooms the tissues distal to the blockage to oxygen starvation and death. Fortunately, new drugs can break up (**lysis**) these clots before permanent damage can occur.

These new clot-busting drugs, called **thrombolytics**, act to reverse the clotting process (**coagulation cascade**) in the fibrin-

ogen phase. More properly termed **fibrinolytics**, these drugs activate special enzymes, such as plasminogen, to start the process of dismantling a clot.

In some cases it is easier to prevent clot formation. Using chemicals naturally found in the body, such as heparin, or drugs such as aspirin, clots may be prevented. Self-administration of aspirin may prevent clot formation and decrease the incidence of heart attack by approximately 25%. ■

Prothrombin depends on vitamin K. Vitamin K is manufactured in the body by a type of bacteria found in the intestines. See Figure 12-2 for a summary of the coagulation process. It is important to note that prothrombin and fibrinogen are plasma proteins, which are manufactured in the liver; therefore serious liver disease may interfere with the blood clotting process.

Clotting Time. The time it takes for blood to clot is known as its **clotting time**. The clotting time for humans is from 5 to 15 minutes. This information is useful when trying to estimate the time of injury. If a bruise (coagulated blood) has formed, the injury occurred at least 5 minutes prior to examination.

● BLOOD TYPES

There are four major groups, or types, of blood: A, B, AB, and O. Blood type is inherited from one's parents. It is determined by the presence—or absence—of the blood protein called agglutinogen, or **antigen**, on the surface of the red blood cell. People with type A blood have the A antigen on their red blood cells; type B blood has the type B antigen; type AB has both A and B antigen; and type O has neither of the antigens.

There is a protein present in the plasma known as agglutinin, or **antibody**. An individual with type A blood has b antibodies in the blood plasma. Type B blood possesses a antibodies; type O contains both a and b antibodies; and type AB contains no antibodies.

Knowledge of a person's correct blood type is important in cases of blood transfusions and surgery. A test known as **type and crossmatch** is done before receiving a blood transfusion. This determines the blood type of both recipient and donor. Antibodies react with the antigens of the same type, causing the red blood cells to clump together. The clumping of blood, a process known as agglutination, clogs up the blood vessels, impeding circulation and causing death.

For example, if a person with type A blood needs a transfusion, he or she must receive only type A blood. Should the person receive type B, the B antigens of the type B blood would clump with the b antibodies of the person's type A blood. This would prove fatal. In an emergency, persons with type A blood can receive both types A and O blood. How is this possible? Because the red blood cells of type O contain no A or B antigens. Therefore they will not clump with the b antibodies of type A or the a antibodies of type B. Thus blood type O can be donated to all four blood types, for which reason it is known as the **universal donor**. This is only done in an emergency situation.

Conversely, type AB, having no antibodies in its plasma, can receive all four blood types. The reason is that, lacking antibodies, AB cannot agglutinate the red blood cells of any donor. It is thus called the **universal recipient**. This is only done in emergency situations. Blood of the same type should always be given to the recipient to avoid serious reactions. Table 12-4 provides a summary of pertinent facts about blood types.

TABLE 12-4 *Blood Types*

BLOOD TYPE	PERCENT OF U.S. POPULATION	ANTIGEN ON RED BLOOD CELLS	ANTIBODY IN PLASMA	CAN RECEIVE	CAN DONATE TO
A	41%	A	b	A or O only	A or AB only
B	12%	B	a	B or O only	B or AB only
AB	3%	A and B	none	A, B, AB, O (universal recipient)	AB only
O	44%	None	a and b	O only	A, B, AB, O (universal donor)

STREET SMART

Reactions to blood transfusions are infrequent. This is due to the work of blood banks that accurately compare the person's blood with the blood from a potential donor (typing and crossmatching).

In rare cases a breakdown of red blood cells because of incompatibility, called a **hemolytic reaction**, can occur. The body's immune system, sensing a foreign protein from the donor blood, attacks and hemolyzes the donor's blood.

Symptoms of a hemolytic reaction are similar to the symptoms of an anaphylactic reaction, including flushed skin, wheezing, and hives. The patient may also experience chills, fever, flank pain, and hyperventilation. Without prompt treatment, the patient may experience permanent kidney damage. ■

● Rh FACTOR

Human red blood cells, in addition to containing antigens A and B, also contain the Rh antigen. We know it as the **Rh factor** because it was found in the Rhesus monkey. The Rh factor is found on the surface of red blood cells. People possessing the Rh factor are said to be Rh positive (Rh+). Those without the Rh factor are Rh negative (Rh−).

About 85% of U.S. residents are Rh positive and 15% are Rh negative. Neither Rh negative nor Rh positive blood contains antibodies, or agglutinins, in its plasma. However, if an Rh negative individual receives a transfusion of Rh positive blood, he or she will develop antibodies to it. The antibodies take 2 weeks to develop. Generally there is no problem with the first transfusion. But if a second transfusion of Rh positive blood is given, the accumulated Rh antibodies clump with the Rh antigen (agglutinogen) of the blood being received. Therefore both blood type and Rh factor must be taken into account for safe and successful transfusions.

STREET SMART

Problems arise when an Rh negative mother is pregnant with an Rh positive fetus. The mother's blood can develop anti-Rh antibodies to the fetus's Rh antigens. The firstborn child normally suffers no harmful effects. However, subsequent pregnancies are affected because the mother's accumulated anti-Rh antibodies clump the baby's red blood cells. If the condition is left untreated, the baby is usually born with the condition known as **erythroblastosis fetalis** (hemolytic disease of the newborn). This condition is rare today because of the use of the drug **RhoGAM**, which is a special preparation of immune globulin. RhoGAM is given to the Rh negative mother within 72 hours after delivery. (Some doctors also give this drug during the last trimester of pregnancy.) The antibodies in the RhoGAM destroy any Rh positive cells of the baby's that may have entered the mother's bloodstream; therefore the mother's immune system is not stimulated to produce antibodies. ■

BLOOD NORMS

Tests have been devised to use physiological blood norms in diagnosing and following the course of certain diseases. Some of these norms are listed in Table 12-5.

TABLE 12-5 *Selection of Routine Blood Tests*

TEST	RANGE	TUBE
Venous Blood		
Electrolytes		Red-topped tube
Sodium	135–145 mEq/L	
Potassium	3.5–4.5 mEq/L	
Magnesium	1.5–2.5 mEq/L	
Chloride	100–106 mEq/L	
Calcium	8.5–10.5 mg/100 ml	
Glucose	70–100 mg/100 ml	
Kidney Study		Red-topped tube
Creatinine	0.7–1.5 mg/ml	
BUN	8–25 mg/ml	
Toxicology		Special tube
Ethanol	Less than 0.3%	
Lead	Less than 5 μg/100 ml	
Salicylate	Less than 30 mg/100 ml	
Cardiac Panel		Red-topped tube
CPK	5–25 mu/ml	
LDH	60–120 u/ml	
Lipid Study		Red-topped tube
Cholesterol	150–280 mg/100 ml	
Fatty acids	190–420 mg/100 ml	
Complete Blood Count		Purple-topped tube
Hematocrit	42%–50% (male)	
	40%–48% (female)	
Hemoglobin	12–16 g/100 ml	
WBC count	4800–10,800/mm^3	
RBC count	4.2–5.9 million/mm^3	
Coagulation Study		Blue-topped tube
Prothrombin	Less than 2 seconds from control	
Partial thromboplastin time	22–37 seconds	
Arterial Blood Gases		Heparinized syringe
PH	7.35–7.45	
PO_2	75–100 mmHg	
PCO_2	35–45 mmHg	

BUN, *Blood urea nitrogen;* CPK, *creatine phosphokinase;* g, *gram;* LDH, *lactate dehydrogenase;* mEq/L, *milliequivalents per liter;* μg/ml, *micrograms per milliliter;* mg/ml, *milligrams per milliliter;* mm^3, *cubic millimeter;* mu, *micron;* PCO_2, *carbon dioxide pressure;* PO_2, *oxygen pressure;* u, *units.*
Laboratories often group blood samples according to a group, called a panel. For example, blood electrolytes and cardiac panels are often part of an emergency profile (EP).
NOTE: *Always refer to the laboratory for standards and for the exact ranges of blood test results, as well as blood tubes preferred for sample.*

MEDICAL HIGHLIGHTS

The blood found in the umbilical cord contains the same immunity-producing stem cells found in the bone marrow and is far easier to transplant. Although bone marrow transplants require an almost exact match, cord blood stem cells are too young and the brand-new donor has not yet developed antibodies that turn against the recipient. At this time these transplants are highly experimental and have been used mainly in children. Proponents of this treatment say it will give a new chance for life to people with some forms of leukemia, anemia, Hodgkin's disease, and other conditions. ■

Patients who are taking anticoagulant medications to prolong the clotting time of their blood must have prothrombin time (PT) and partial thromboplastin time (PTT) tests done frequently. The dosage of their medication is based on their clotting times.

Sedimentation rate is the time required for erythrocytes to settle to the bottom of an upright tube at room temperature. It indicates whether disease is present and is valuable in observing the progression of inflammatory conditions.

● DISORDERS OF THE BLOOD

Anemia is a deficiency in the number or percentage of red blood cells and the amount of hemoglobin in the blood. Anemia results from a large or chronic loss of blood (hemorrhage), which decreases the number of erythrocytes. Extreme erythrocyte destruction and malformation of the hemoglobin of red blood cells also cause this condition. Because some hemoglobin deficiency always exists, there is never enough oxygen transported to the cells of cellular oxidation. Consequently, not enough energy is released. Anemia is characterized by varying degrees of dyspnea, pallor, palpitation, and fatigue.

Iron deficiency anemia is a common condition in women, children, and adolescents. It is caused by a deficiency of iron in the diet. This leads to insufficient hemoglobin synthesis in the red blood cells. The condition is easily alleviated by ingestion of iron supplements and green, leafy vegetables that contain the mineral iron.

Pernicious anemia is a form of anemia caused by a deficiency of vitamin B_{12} or lack of the intrinsic factor. The intrinsic factor, produced by the stomach mucosa, is necessary for the absorption and utilization of vitamin B_{12}. Vitamin B_{12} and folic acid are necessary for the development of mature red blood cells. Symptoms such as dyspnea, pallor, and fatigue are present, as well as specific neurological changes. Foods that contain vitamin B_{12} are animal proteins such as liver and organ meats. Treatment for pernicious anemia involves injections of vitamin B_{12}.

Aplastic anemia is a disease caused by the suppression of the bone marrow chemical agents, certain drugs, or radiation therapy. In this condition, bone marrow does not produce enough red blood cells and white blood cells. Treatment consists of removing the toxic substances or discontinuing the drugs and radiation. In severe conditions a bone marrow transplant may be performed.

Sickle cell anemia is a chronic blood disease inherited from both parents. The disease causes red blood cells to form in the abnormal crescent shape. These cells carry less oxygen and break easily, causing anemia. The sickling trait, a less serious disease, occurs with inheritance from only one parent. Sickle cell anemia occurs almost exclusively among African-Americans. Treatment of sickle cell anemia consists of the affected person's receiving blood transfusions when necessary. Drug therapy and bone marrow transplants are being considered as treatment.

Cooley's anemia, also known as *thalassemia major*, is a blood disease caused by a defect in hemoglobin formation. It affects people of Mediterranean descent.

Polycythemia is a condition in which too many red blood cells are formed. This may be a temporary condition that occurs at high altitudes where there is less oxygen pressure, encouraging the production of red blood cells.

Primary polycythemia (polycythemia vera) is due to a cancer of the bone marrow, where red blood cells are produced.

Polycythemia can also be due to chronic hypoxia (secondary polycythemia) subsequent to chronic pulmonary conditions, such as emphysema or morbid obesity.

The increase in the number of red blood cells causes a thickening of the blood, which slows or blocks the flow of blood. Treatment for this condition includes phlebotomy (removal of blood) or dilution of the blood with IV fluid.

Disseminated intravascular coagulation (DIC) is a disorder in which the blood clots inappropriately in some places while failing to clot correctly in others. DIC is an outcome seen in several diseases, including severe trauma, massive infection, and certain complications of pregnancy. Mucosal bleeding is usually seen early in the disorder. Kidney failure is a common complication. Extensive hemorrhage can occur and may lead to life-threatening exsanguination.

Embolism is a condition in which an embolus is carried by the bloodstream until it reaches an artery too small for passage. An embolus is a substance foreign to the bloodstream. It may be air, a blood clot, cancer cells, fat, bacterial clumps, a needle, or even a bullet that was lodged in tissue and breaks free.

Thrombosis is the formation of a blood clot in a blood vessel. The blood clot formed is called a **thrombus**. It is caused by unusually slow blood circulation, changes in the blood or blood vessel walls, immobility, or a decrease in mobility.

Hematoma is a localized clotted mass of blood found in an organ, tissue, or space. It is caused by an injury, such as a blow, that can cause a blood vessel to rupture.

Hemophilia is a hereditary disease in which the blood clots slowly or abnormally. This causes prolonged bleeding from even minor cuts and bumps. Although sex-linked hemophilia occurs mostly in males, it is transmitted genetically by females to their sons. The person with hemophilia may be treated with the missing clotting factor and is taught to avoid trauma, if possible, and report promptly any bleeding, no matter how slight.

Thrombocytopenia is a blood disease in which there is a decrease in the number of platelets (thrombocytes). In this condition, blood does not clot properly.

Leukemia is a cancerous or malignant condition in which there is a great increase in the number of white blood cells. The overabundant immature leukocytes replace the erythrocytes, thus interfering with the transport of oxygen to

MEDICAL HIGHLIGHTS

One of the most severe problems related to sickle cell anemia is that the rigid sickle red blood cells clog the blood vessels, causing vaso-occlusion and painful episodes. Daily administration of the drug hydroxyurea reduces the painful episodes by about 50%. However, this drug may not be appropriate for some patients with sickle cell anemia. It is a cytotoxic agent and has the potential to cause life-threatening cytopenia (a decrease in the number of cells). Hydroxyurea is a treatment, not a cure, and positive results only occur as long as the patient takes the prescribed dose. The Food and Drug Administration (FDA) has not given its full approval for the drug at this time; however, the results were so promising after the initial trials that doctors were permitted to prescribe hydroxyurea for patients with sickle cell anemia. ■

the tissues. They can also hinder the synthesis of new red blood cells from bone marrow. The acute form of the disease, which develops quickly and runs its course rapidly, occurs most often in children and young adults. Treatment today consists of drug therapy, bone marrow transplants, and radiation therapy, which has given people with leukemia remissions that may last for several years.

Septicemia describes the presence of pathogenic (disease-producing) organisms or toxins in the blood.

● REVIEW QUESTIONS

Select the letter of the choice that best completes the statement.

1. Blood of the universal donor is:
   a. type B
   b. type A
   c. type AB
   d. type O

2. Blood of the universal recipient is:
   a. type B
   b. type A
   c. type AB
   d. type O

3. Negative Rh blood is found in:
   a. 5% of the population
   b. 10% of the population
   c. 15% of the population
   d. 20% of the population

4. The blood type found in the largest percent of the population is:
   a. type O
   b. type A
   c. type AB
   d. type B

5. The prothrombin in the blood clotting process depends on:
   a. vitamin A
   b. vitamin K
   c. vitamin P
   d. vitamin D

6. Which of the following is not a blood cell?
   a. erythrocyte
   b. leukocyte
   c. osteocyte
   d. monocyte

7. Erythrocytes contain all but one of the following elements:
   a. Rh factor
   b. leukocytes
   c. hemoglobin
   d. globin and heme

8. What characteristic is not true of normal thrombocytes?
    a. They average 4500 for each cubic millimeter of blood.
    b. They are also called platelets.
    c. They are plate-shaped cells.
    d. They initiate the blood-clotting process.

9. The normal leukocyte cell:
    a. can only be produced in the lymphatic tissue
    b. goes to the infection site to engulf and destroy microorganisms
    c. is too large to move through the intracellular spaces of the capillary wall
    d. exists in numbers that amount to an average of 12,000 cells per cubic millimeter of blood

10. The blood clotting process:
    a. requires a normal platelet count, which is 5000 to 9000 per cubic millimeter of blood
    b. is delayed by the rupture of platelets, which produces thromboplastin
    c. occurs in less time with persons having type O blood
    d. requires vitamin K of the synthesis of prothrombin

● COMPLETION

Briefly answer the following questions.

1. Name the three major types of blood cells.

2. What name is given to the straw-colored liquid portion of the blood?

3. What five proteins are contained in the blood and what are their functions?

4. Describe the process of blood clot formation.

●APPLYING THEORY TO PRACTICE

1. You hear that your friend has been in a car accident and needs a blood transfusion; you want to donate blood. You friend has type O+ blood and you have A+ blood. Can your blood be given to your friend? Explain the reason for your answer.

2. Why is blood considered the "gift of life"?

3. A patient comes to the doctor's office. She is pregnant and states she is Rh negative and her husband is Rh positive. She has heard that there may be a problem with the baby. Explain to her about the Rh factor and how this situation is dealt with today.

4. You are caring for a 6-year-old girl with leukemia. The mother asks what she did that caused the disease. What will your response be?

Heart

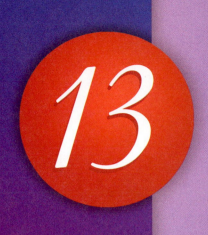

Objectives

- Describe the functions of the circulatory system
- List the components of the circulatory system
- Describe the structure of the heart
- Describe the functions of the various structures of the heart
- Describe the control of heart contractions
- Describe the method of taking an ECG
- Discuss the diseases of the heart
- Define the key words that relate to this chapter

Key Words

acute coronary syndrome (ACS)
acute myocardial ischemia (AMI)
anastomose
angina pectoris
angioplasty (balloon surgery)
anterior wall
aorta
aortic semilunar valve
apex
arrhythmia
ascites
atrial kick
atrial-septal defect
atrioventricular bundle (bundle of His)
atrioventricular (AV) node
atrium
AV blocks
bicuspid (mitral) valve
bradycardia
bundle
cardiac arrest
cardiac output (CO)
cardiopulmonary resuscitation (CPR)
cardiotonics
conduction defect
congestive heart failure
coronary artery bypass graft (CABG)
coronary bypass
coronary sinus
defibrillation
defibrillator
deoxygenated
diastole
diuretics
dyspnea
dysrhythmia
edema
ejection fraction
electrocardiogram (ECG)
endocarditis
endocardium
fibrillation
functional syncytium

(continues)

Key Words (continued)

heart block	public access
heart failure	defibrillation
infarction	pulmonary artery
inferior wall	pulmonary circulation
intra-aortic balloon	pulmonary semilunar
pump (ABP)	valve
ischemia	pulmonary veins
lateral wall	Purkinje fibers
leaflet	rheumatic heart disease
left coronary artery	right coronary artery
(LCA)	(RCA)
left ventricle	right ventricle
left ventricular assist	S_3
device	septal wall
lubb dupp	septum
mitral valve prolapse	sinoatrial (SA) node
murmur	(pacemaker)
myocardial infarction	sinus of Valsalva
myocarditis	Starling's law
myocardium	stethoscope
oxygenated	stroke volume
palpitations	systemic circulation
penumbra	systole
pericarditis	tachycardia
pericardium	tricuspid valve
point of maximum	vena cava
intensity (PMI)	ventricular bundle
posterior wall	ventricular fibrillation
progressive	ventricular gallop
atherosclerosis	whorl

The circulatory system is the longest system of the body. If one were to lay all the blood vessels in a single human body end to end, they would stretch one fourth of the way from earth to the moon, a distance of some 60,000 miles*.

● FUNCTIONS OF THE CIRCULATORY SYSTEM

1. The heart is the pump necessary to circulate blood to all parts of the body.

---

*I. Sherman and V. Sherman, *Biology: A Human Approach* (New York: Oxford University Press, 1979).

2. Arteries, veins, and capillaries are the structures that take blood from the heart to the cells and return blood from the cells back to the heart.

3. Blood carries oxygen and nutrients to the cells and carries the waste products away.

4. The lymph system (see Chapter 15) returns excess fluid from the tissues to the general circulation. The lymph nodes produce lymphocytes and filter out pathogenic bacteria.

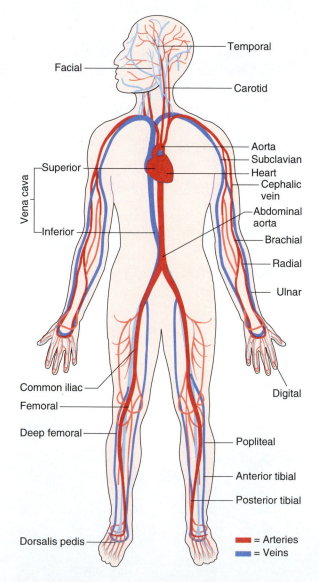

Temporal
Facial
Carotid
Aorta
Subclavian
Superior
Heart
Vena cava
Cephalic vein
Abdominal aorta
Inferior
Brachial
Radial
Ulnar
Common iliac
Digital
Femoral
Deep femoral
Popliteal
Anterior tibial
Posterior tibial
Dorsalis pedis

■ = Arteries
■ = Veins

● **FIGURE 13–1** *General or systemic circulation.*

COMPONENTS OF THE CIRCULATORY SYSTEM

The organs of the circulatory system include the heart, arteries, veins, and capillaries. The blood and lymphatic system are part of the circulatory system.

The heart is the muscular pump responsible for circulating the blood throughout the body.

MAJOR BLOOD CIRCUITS

Blood leaves the heart through arteries and returns by veins. The blood uses two circulation routes:

1. The systemic (general) circulation carries blood throughout the body, Figure 13-1.

2. The pulmonary circulation carries blood from the heart to the lungs and back, Figure 13-2.

CHANGES IN THE COMPOSITION OF CIRCULATING BLOOD

The major substances added to and removed from the blood as it circulates through organs along the various sites of the circulatory system are outlined in Table 13-1. (This table includes only the major changes in the blood as it passes through certain specialized organs or structures.)

THE HEART

The blood's circulatory system is extremely efficient. The main organ responsible for this efficiency is the heart, a tough, simply constructed muscle about the size of a closed fist.

The adult human heart is about 5 inches long and 3.5 inches wide, weighing less than 1 pound (12 to 13 ounces). The importance of a healthy, well-functioning heart is obvious: It circulates life-sustaining blood throughout the body. When the heart stops beating, life stops as well. If blood

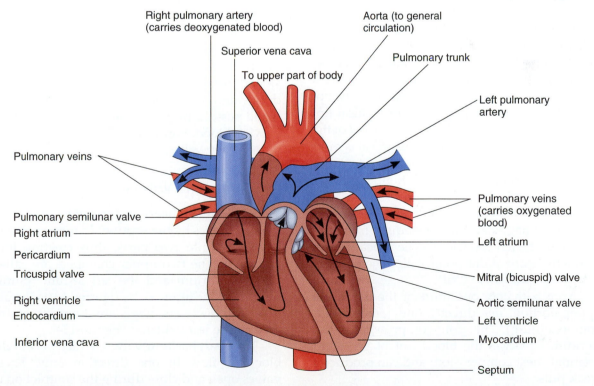

● **FIGURE 13–2** *Schematic of heart pulmonary circulation.*

TABLE 13-1 *Changes in the Composition of the Blood*

ORGANS	BLOOD LOSSES	BLOOD GAINS
Digestive glands	Raw materials needed to make digestive juices and enzymes	Carbon dioxide
Kidneys	Water, urea, and mineral salts	Carbon dioxide
Liver	Excess glucose, amino acids, and worn-out red blood cells	Released glucose, urea, and plasma proteins
Lungs	Carbon dioxide and water	Oxygen
Muscles	Glucose and oxygen	Lactic acid and carbon dioxide
Small intestinal villi	Oxygen	End products of digestion (glucose and amino acids)

flow to the brain ceases for 15 seconds or more, the subject starts to lose consciousness. After 4 to 6 minutes without blood flow, some brain cells are irreversibly damaged.

The heart is located in the thoracic cavity. This places the heart between the lungs, behind the sternum, in front of the thoracic vertebrae, and above the diaphragm. Although the heart is centrally located, its axis of symmetry is not along the midline. The heart's **apex** (conical tip) lies on the diaphragm and points to the left of the body. It is at the apex where the heartbeat is most easily felt and heard through a **stethoscope**.

Try this simple demonstration: Place the bell of a stethoscope over the heart's apex. This is the area between the fifth and sixth ribs, along an imaginary line extending from the middle of the left clavicle. The heartbeat can be distinctly heard at this point, called the **point of maximum intensity (PMI)**.

Approximately one third of the heart, the upper portion, lies directly under the breastbone (sternum). Therefore compression of the sternum squeezes the blood out of the heart (manual chest compression) and can produce a weak pulse.

Knowledge of the correct position of the heart can make all the difference in the treatment of **cardiac arrest**. During such a medical emergency, the combination of manual heart compression and artificial respiration can save a life. This life-saving technique is known as **cardiopulmonary resuscitation (CPR)** and should be performed only by those specifically trained in CPR.

● STRUCTURE OF THE HEART

The heart is a hollow, muscular double pump that circulates the blood through the blood vessel to all parts of the body. At rest, the heart pumps 2 ounces of blood with each beat, 5 quarts per minute, 75 gallons per hour. The heart contracts about 72 times per minute, or about 100,000 times each day.

Layers of Heart Wall

Surrounding the heart is a double layer of fibrous tissue called the **pericardium**. Between these two pericardial layers is a space filled with lubricating pericardial fluid, which prevents the two layers from rubbing against each other and creating friction. The thin inner layer covering the heart is the visceral or serous pericardium. The tough outer membrane is the parietal, or fibrous, pericardium.

The inner lining of the heart consists of a smooth tissue called the **endocardium**. The endocardium covers the heart valves and lines the blood vessels, providing smooth transit for the flowing blood. Figure 13-3 illustrates the layers of the heart wall.

Chambers and Valves

The human heart is separated into right and left halves by the **septum**. In turn, each half is divided into two parts, thus creating four chambers. The two upper chambers are called the right atrium and the left atrium (plural, atria). The **atrium** may be referred to as the auricle. The lower chambers are the **right ventricle** and the **left ventricle**, Figure 13-4.

The heart has four valves, which permit the blood to flow in one direction only. These valves open and close during the contraction of the heart, preventing the blood from flowing backward, Figure 13-5.

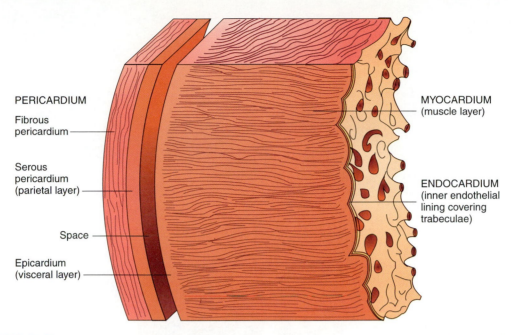

● **FIGURE 13–3** *The layers of the pericardial sac (left) and the layers of the walls of the heart (right).*

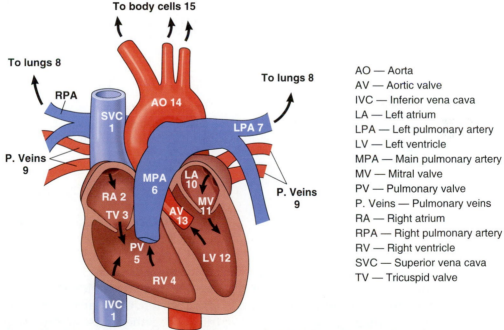

AO — Aorta
AV — Aortic valve
IVC — Inferior vena cava
LA — Left atrium
LPA — Left pulmonary artery
LV — Left ventricle
MPA — Main pulmonary artery
MV — Mitral valve
PV — Pulmonary valve
P. Veins — Pulmonary veins
RA — Right atrium
RPA — Right pulmonary artery
RV — Right ventricle
SVC — Superior vena cava
TV — Tricuspid valve

1. Blood reaches heart through superior vena cava and inferior vena cava
2. To right atruim
3. To tricuspid valve
4. To right ventricle
5. To pulmonary valve (semilunar)
6. To main pulmonary artery
7. To left pulmonary artery and right pulmonary artery
8. To lungs—blood receives O_2
9. From lungs to pulmonary veins
10. To left atrium
11. To mitral (bicuspid) valve
12. To left ventricle
13. To aortic valve (semilunar valve)
14. To aorta (largest artery in the body)
15. Blood with oxygen then goes to all cells of the body

● **FIGURE 13–4** *Normal heart.*

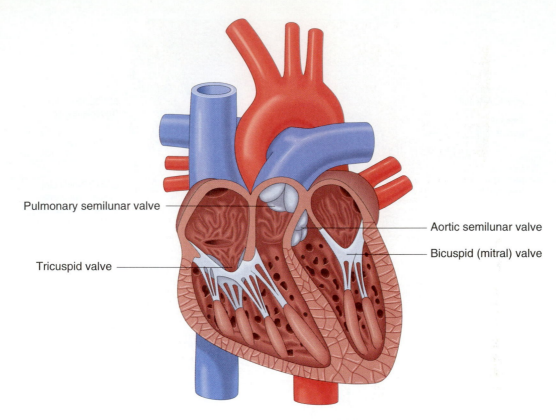

Pulmonary semilunar valve

Aortic semilunar valve

Bicuspid (mitral) valve

Tricuspid valve

● **FIGURE 13–5**   *The heart and its valves.*

Atrioventricular valves are located between the atria and the ventricles.

- The **tricuspid valve** is positioned between the right atrium and the right ventricle. Its name comes from the fact that there are three points, or cusps, of attachment. It allows blood to flow from the right atrium into the right ventricle, but not in the opposite direction.

- The **bicuspid**, or **mitral**, **valve** is located between the left atrium and the left ventricle. Blood flows from the left atrium into the left ventricle; backflow from the left ventricle to the left atrium is prevented.

Semilunar valves are located where blood leaves the heart:

- The **pulmonary semilunar valve** is found at the orifice (opening) of the pulmonary artery. It lets blood travel from the right ventricle into the pulmonary artery and then into the lungs.

- The **aortic semilunar valve** is at the orifice of the aorta. This valve permits the blood to pass from the left ventricle into the aorta, but not backward into the left ventricle, see Figure 13-5.

Cardiac Skeleton and Muscle

Fibrous rings create the base of the valves and perform several functions. First, these fibrous rings create a firm point of attachment for the muscles of the heart. These fibrous rings also functionally divide the cardiac muscle, or **myocardium**, of the atria from those of the ventricles. Together these fibrous rings create the cardiac skeleton.

Cardiac muscle fibers within each portion of the heart, the atrium and the ventricle, interconnect, creating a collection of muscles called a **functional syncytium**. As a result, when one muscle fiber contracts, the entire group of muscle fibers, or the **bundle**, contracts as one unit.

STREET SMART ------------------------------

The source of sudden cardiac death, and where the majority of cell death occurs during a heart attack, is the left ventricle. The left ventricle logically becomes the center for discussion among all health care providers. For this reason, when physicians and EMS providers are speaking of the anterior heart, they are discussing the anterior portion of the left ventricle.

The ventricles, shaped like an inverted pyramid lying on its side, has four walls. The front portion of the left ventricle is referred to as the **anterior wall**. The portion of the left ventricle that lies on top of the diaphragm at the bottom of the heart is called the **inferior wall**. The wall that is shared between the right and left ventricles, proximal to the sternum, is called the **septal wall**, and the wall that lies next to the lateral chest is called the **lateral wall**. There is a fifth side, the base of the pyramid, where the valves are located. This wall, the **posterior wall**, has very little muscle mass and is not frequently discussed. ■

It is because of separate syncytium that the atrial syncytium can contract a moment (0.12 second) earlier than the ventricular syncytium. This phenomena is described in more detail during the discussion of cardiac cycles.

Cardiac muscle tissue, or myocardium, makes up the major portion of the heart. The muscle fibers in the lower half of the heart, the **ventricular bundles**, form the greatest portion of the mass of the heart.

The origin of these ventricular bundles is at the fibrous rings of the valves, part of the cardiac skeleton; the terminus, or insertion, of these bundles is also at the valves.

With the same origin as insertion, these muscular bundles form a double-looped, spiral-like configuration called a **whorl**. Because of this unique muscle fiber arrangement, when a whorl contracts, in a twisting motion, it squeezes the blood out of the heart's ventricles, like wringing out a hand towel.

Arteries and Veins

The following are structures leading to and from the heart:

- Superior **vena cava** and inferior vena cava—the large venous blood vessels that bring **deoxygenated** blood (which has lesser amounts of oxygen) to the right atrium from all parts of the body.

- **Coronary sinus**—transports blood from the heart muscle to the right atrium.

- **Pulmonary artery**—takes blood away from the right ventricle to the lungs for oxygen.

- **Pulmonary veins**—bring **oxygenated** blood from the lungs to the left atrium.

- **Aorta**—takes blood away from the left ventricle to the rest of the body.

Physiology of the Heart

The structure of the heart allows it to function as a double pump. (Think of the heart as having a right side and a left side.) Two major functions occur each time the heart beats:

- *Right side of the heart*—Blood (deoxygenated) flows into the heart from the superior and inferior vena cava to the right atrium, to the tricuspid valve, to the right ventricle, through the pulmonary semilunar valves, to the pulmonary artery, which takes blood to the lungs for oxygen.

- *Left side of the heart*—Blood (oxygenated) flows into the heart from the lungs by the pulmonary veins to the left atrium, through the bicuspid valve (mitral), to the left ventricle, to the aorta, and then to general circulation.

It is sometimes hard to imagine this idea of two pumping actions occurring at the same time. Each time the ventricles contract, blood leaves the right ventricle to go to the lungs and blood leaves the left ventricle to go to the aorta.

Cardiac Cycle

Normally the two halves of the heart contract (beat) together. This synchronous beat propels blood to either the pulmonary circuit (right side of the heart) or the systemic circuit (left side of the heart).

The contraction of the heart, and the subsequent ejection of the blood in the ventricles, is called **systole**. Immediately after systole, the heart rests in **diastole**. Diastole starts when the last blood leaves the ventricles and as new blood pours into the atriums from the vena cava (right) or pulmonary vein (left).

Once the atrium and ventricles fill, the atrium contracts once more and pushes blood into the ventricles. This additional volume of blood in the ventricles helps to distend the ventricles further. When the walls of the ventricles are maximally distended, they contract with greater force, like a rubber band that is stretched to its maximum. This principle is called **Starling's law**.

The contraction of the atriums therefore helps to improve systole, according to Starling's law, and is thus called the **atrial kick**. Atrial kick increases a single contraction's effectiveness by approximately 30%.

The entire volume of blood ejected from the ventricle in a single heartbeat is called the **stroke volume**. The average ventricle can hold a total volume of 110 to 120 milliliters of blood, and the average stroke volume is about 70 to 80 milliliters. Therefore the amount of blood pumped out can also be called the **ejection fraction**—the fraction of blood pumped out. The ejection fraction can be estimated using special medical imaging equipment or invasive monitors, and the health of the patient's heart can thus be evaluated.

The amount of blood that the heart can pump is a function of two factors. The first factor is the health of the heart, which can be assessed by estimating the stroke volume. The second factor is the speed of contraction, which is measured in beats per minute (BPM). These two factors, stroke volume (milliliters, or ml) and heart rate (bpm) create the patient's **cardiac output (CO)**. The average person's cardiac output is approximately 5 liters per minute.

$$CO = SV \times HR \ \ (5 \text{ L/min} = 70 \text{ ml} \times 72 \text{ bpm})$$

Diseases, drugs, and treatments can affect either one of these variables and therefore affect cardiac output. Blood pressure, discussed in the next chapter, is one way for EMS providers to estimate cardiac output and heart health.

Coronary Circulation

The heart receives its blood supply from the coronary artery, which branches into right and left coronary arteries.

The openings for these two coronary arteries are found immediately past the aortic valve and behind the aortic valve's flaps, or **leaflets**, in a hollow called the **sinus of Valsalva**.

The coronary arteries are the first arteries in the systemic circulation. However, because of their position behind the leaflets of the aortic valve, the coronary arteries are obstructed by the aortic valve's leaflets during ventricle contraction, or systole. The coronary arteries thus depend on backflow from the aorta during diastole for filling. The coronary arteries are the only arteries in the body that fill during diastole.

Both ventricles receive their blood from these two main coronary arteries. The larger share of blood goes to the left ventricle, where the majority of the oxygen in the blood is utilized by the left ventricle.

The **left coronary artery (LCA)** supplies blood to the left ventricle. It almost immediately divides into its major branches: the left anterior descending (LAD) coronary artery and the circumflex artery (Cx).

The LCA and its tributaries, the LAD and the Cx, provide blood to anterior portions of the left ventricle, as well as lower portions of the conduction system.

Occlusion of the left coronary artery is common and may result in loss of blood flow (hypoperfusion) of the left ventricle and **acute myocardial ischemia (AMI)**.

The **right coronary artery (RCA)** supplies blood to the right ventricle and an upper portion of the conduction system. The right coronary artery divides late, into the posterior descending coronary artery and the marginal artery.

In about 90% of the population, the right coronary artery, found along the inferior wall of the ventricle, supplies blood to a vital portion of the conduction system called the **atrioventricular (AV) node**. The upper portion of heart, the atria, communicates with the lower portion of the heart, the ventricles, through the AV node. Loss of circulation and subsequent AV node ischemia can lead to disturbances in conduction, called **AV blocks**, discussed later in the chapter.

The two coronary arteries are interconnected by smaller arteries. This connection is called an **anastomose**. The combination of the major arteries, their tributaries, and their anastomoses encircles the heart and has the appearance of a thorny crown (hence the name coronary). Table 13-2 highlights the coronary arteries.

Heart Sounds

The physician listens at specific locations on the chest wall to hear how the heart is functioning. During the cardiac cycle, the valves make a sound when they close. These are referred to as the **lubb dupp** sounds. The lubb sound is heard first and is made by the valves (tricuspid and bi-

TABLE 13-2 *Coronary Arteries*

RIGHT CORONARY ARTERY	LEFT CORONARY ARTERY

1. Posterior descending coronary artery
   a. Branches to both ventricles
	1. Left anterior descending coronary artery
	   a. Branches to both ventricles

2. Marginal artery
   a. Branch to the AV node
   b. Branch to the right ventricle
	2. Circumflex artery
	   a. Branch to left ventricle
	   b. Branch to left atrium

NOTE: *There is a high degree of variability in branch locations among normal people.*

cuspid) closing between the atria and ventricles. The physician refers to it as the S_1 sound. It is best heard at the apex of the heart.

The dupp sound is heard second and is shorter and higher pitched. It is caused by the semilunar valves in the aorta and the pulmonary artery closing. The physician refers to it as the S_2 sound. Certain conditions can cause changes in the action of the heart valves.

When a heart valve fails, blood can flow back into the chamber. The resultant turbulent blood flow results in a sound called a **murmur**. Some murmurs have no effect on the patient and are called functional murmurs.

Other murmurs, especially those that occur during a heart attack, can indicate valve damage. These pathological murmurs are often the first indication of valvular damage. Open-heart surgery

STREET SMART

During moments of excitement or distress, the left side of the heart beats a little more forcefully than the right side. This increased force of contraction tends to cause the right and left ventricles to beat at slightly different times, or asynchronously.

This asynchronous beating, resulting in different times of closure for the aortic and pulmonic valves (the dupp sound) causes the

heart sound (S_2) to split. The result is a new sound called S_3.

Because S_3 sounds like a three-legged horse in a race, it is also called a **ventricular gallop**. The presence of a ventricular gallop can indicate a serious abnormality, especially if the patient is at rest. S_3 may be heard in patients with congestive heart failure. ■

can replace these valves with artificial valves, restoring the heart back to its original condition.

In some instances an infant is born with a hole between the right and left portions of the heart, a condition called an **atrial-septal defect**. The result is that blood flows from one side of the heart to the other, without circulating throughout the body, and a loud machinery-like murmur is heard. The infant becomes cyanotic. These "blue babies" eventually undergo an operation in which a patch is placed over the hole to correct the condition.

● CONTROL OF HEART CONTRACTIONS

A heart removed from the body continues to beat rhythmically, which demonstrates that heartbeat generates in the heart muscle itself. The heart rate is also affected by the endocrine and nervous systems. The myocardium contracts rhythmically to perform its duty as a forceful pump.

Control of heart muscle contractions is found within a group of conducting cells located at the opening of the superior vena cava in the right atrium. These cells are known as the **sinoatrial (SA) node**, or **pacemaker**. The SA node sends out an electrical impulse that starts and regulates the heart. The impulse spreads out over the atria, making them contract or depolarize. This causes blood to flow downward from the upper atrial chamber to the atrioventricular openings. The electrical impulse eventually reaches the AV node, which is another conducting cell group located between the atria and ventricle.

From the AV node, the electrical impulse is carried to conducting fibers in the septum. These conducting fibers are known as the **atrioventricular bundle**, or the bundle of His. It divides into a right and left branch; each branch then subdivides into a fine network of branches spreading throughout the ventricles, called the Purkinje network. The electrical impulse shoots along the **Purkinje fibers** to the ventricles, causing them to contract. The heart then rests briefly (repolarizes), Figure 13-6.

The combined action of the SA and AV nodes is instrumental in the cardiac cycle. The cardiac cycle comprises one complete heartbeat, with both atrial and ventricular contractions.

1. The SA node stimulates the contraction of both atria. Blood flows from the atria into the ventricles through the open tricuspid and mitral valves. At the same time, the ventricles are relaxed, allowing them to fill with blood. At this point, because the semilunar valves are closed, the blood cannot enter the pulmonary artery or aorta.

2. The AV node stimulates the contraction of both ventricles so that the blood in the ventricles is pumped into the pulmonary artery and the aorta through the semilunar valves, which are now open. At this point the atria are relaxed and the tricuspid and mitral valves closed.

3. The ventricles relax; the semilunar valves are closed to prevent the blood flowing back into the ventricles. The heart rests briefly (repolarization). The cycle begins again with the signal from the SA node.

This action of the heart is known as the cardiac cycle and represents one heartbeat. Each cardiac cycle takes 0.8 second. The average person's heart rate is between 72 to 75 bpm.

Electrocardiogram

The **electrocardiogram (ECG)** is a device used to record the electrical activity of the heart that causes the contraction (systole) and the relaxation (diastole) of the atria and ventricles during the cardiac cycle, see Figure 13-6.

The baseline, or isoelectric line, of the ECG is the flat line that separates the various waves. It is present when there is no current flowing in the heart. The waves are either deflecting upward, known as positive deflection, or deflecting downward, known as negative deflection. The P, QRS, and T waves recorded during the ECG represent the depolarization (contraction) and repolarization (relaxation) of the myocardial cells. The P wave represents atrial depolarization; QRS represents ventricular depolarization; and the T wave represents ventricular repolarization.

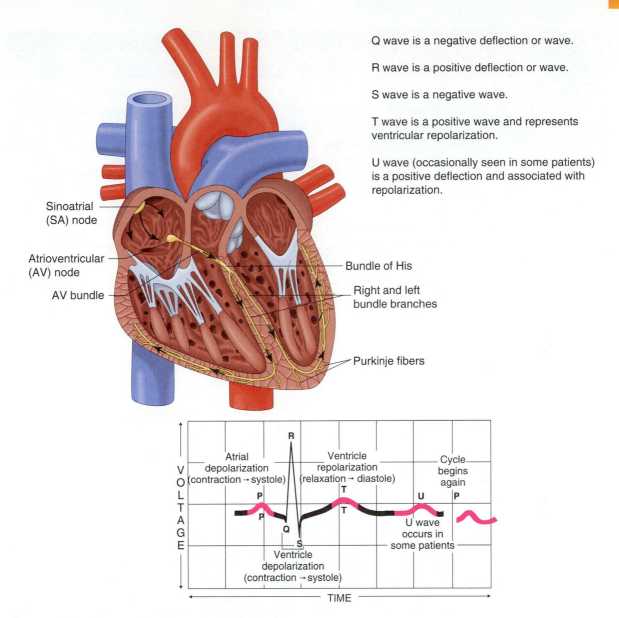

Q wave is a negative deflection or wave.

R wave is a positive deflection or wave.

S wave is a negative wave.

T wave is a positive wave and represents ventricular repolarization.

U wave (occasionally seen in some patients) is a positive deflection and associated with repolarization.

Sinoatrial (SA) node

Atrioventricular (AV) node

AV bundle

Bundle of His

Right and left bundle branches

Purkinje fibers

VOLTAGE

Atrial depolarization (contraction → systole)

R

Ventricle repolarization (relaxation → diastole)

Cycle begins again

P

P

T

T

U

P

Q

S

Ventricle depolarization (contraction → systole)

U wave occurs in some patients

TIME

● **FIGURE 13–6** *Cardiac cycle and ECG reading.*

By observing the size, shape, and location of each wave, the physician can analyze and interpret the conduction of electricity through the cardiac cells, the heart's rate, the heart's rhythm, and the general health of the heart.

● DISEASES OF THE HEART

One of the leading causes of death is cardiovascular disease. Some of the common symptoms of heart disease are the following:

- **Arrhythmia** or dysrhythmia—the terms used to discuss any change or deviation from the normal rate or rhythm of the heart.

- **Bradycardia**—the term used for slow heart rate (less than 60 bpm).

- **Tachycardia**—the term used for rapid heart rate (more than 100 bpm).

- **Murmurs**—indicate some defects in the valves of the heart. When valves fail to close properly, a gurgling or hissing sound occurs.

STREET SMART

EMS providers often monitor the heart with an ECG to detect and treat any irregularity in the heart's normal rhythm, called a dysrhythmia, that would result in sudden cardiac death. Typical monitoring leads for the EMS provider are leads II and MCL[1], demonstrated in Figure 13-7.

Advanced EMS providers in some localities have also been trained and equipped to provide 12-lead ECGs, demonstrated in Figure 13-8. These 12-lead ECGs provide a more comprehensive view of the heart and can be used to diagnosis a heart attack (myocardial ischemia or infarction).

The prehospital use of 12-lead ECGs improves the speed at which care can be delivered to the patient. This practice has been encouraged by such groups as the American Heart Association in its Advanced Cardiac Life Support (ACLS) standards. ■

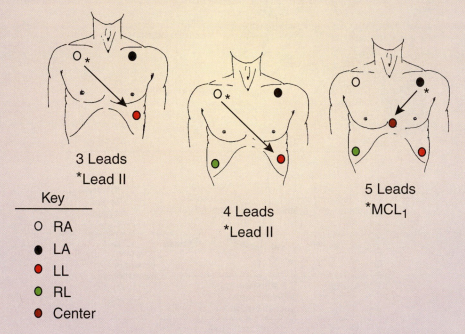

3 Leads
*Lead II

Key
○   RA
●   LA
●   LL
●   RL
●   Center

4 Leads
*Lead II

5 Leads
*MCL₁

● **FIGURE 13–7**   *Proper placement of cardiac electrodes for three-, four-, and five-lead systems.*

(continues)

CHANGES OF AGING

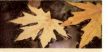

Heart valves tend to thicken and become more rigid as persons age, as a result of calcification. These changes in the valves are coupled with changes in the conduction system as well, and the heart becomes a little less effective each year. In fact, cardiac output typically decreases about 1% per year after a person reaches age 20. By age 65 a person's muscles may be receiving 40% less blood flow than a 30-year-old. ■

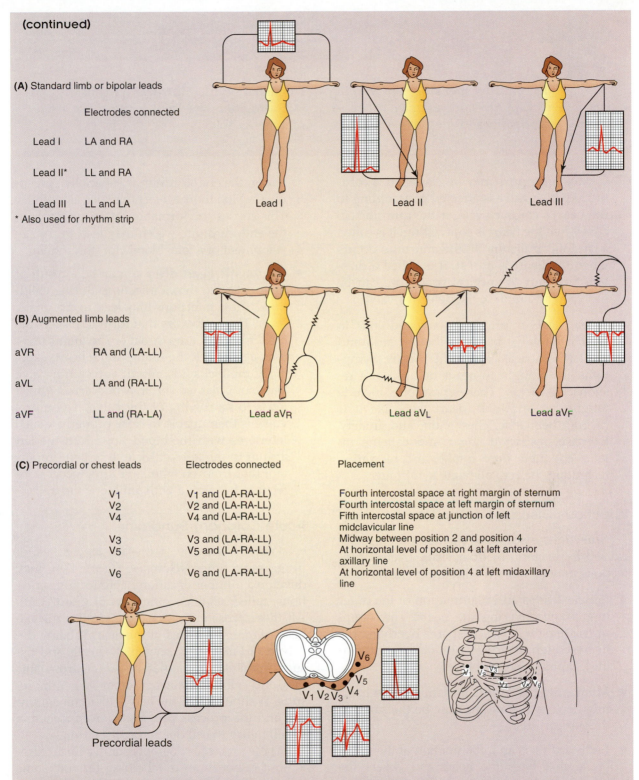

(continued)

(A) Standard limb or bipolar leads

	Electrodes connected
Lead I	LA and RA
Lead II*	LL and RA
Lead III	LL and LA

* Also used for rhythm strip

Lead I   Lead II   Lead III

(B) Augmented limb leads

aVR	RA and (LA-LL)
aVL	LA and (RA-LL)
aVF	LL and (RA-LA)

Lead aV$_R$ Lead aV$_L$ Lead aV$_F$

(C) Precordial or chest leads

	Electrodes connected	Placement
V$_1$	V$_1$ and (LA-RA-LL)	Fourth intercostal space at right margin of sternum
V$_2$	V$_2$ and (LA-RA-LL)	Fourth intercostal space at left margin of sternum
V$_4$	V$_4$ and (LA-RA-LL)	Fifth intercostal space at junction of left midclavicular line
V$_3$	V$_3$ and (LA-RA-LL)	Midway between position 2 and position 4
V$_5$	V$_5$ and (LA-RA-LL)	At horizontal level of position 4 at left anterior axillary line
V$_6$	V$_6$ and (LA-RA-LL)	At horizontal level of position 4 at left midaxillary line

Precordial leads

V$_1$ V$_2$ V$_3$ V$_4$ V$_5$ V$_6$

● **FIGURE 13–8**   *Lead types, connections, and placement:* **(A)** *Standard limb or bipolar leads.* **(B)** *Augmented limb leads.* **(C)** *Precordial or chest leads.*

STREET SMART

Technically speaking, an *arrhythmia* is a lack of rhythm, as may occur in cardiac standstill, and *dysrhythmia* is an irregular rhythm. However, physicians and EMS providers frequently use these terms interchangeably. ∎

Cardiac murmurs may be classified according to which valve is affected or according to the heart's cardiac cycle. If the murmur occurs when the heart is contracting, it is called a systolic murmur. If the murmur occurs when the heart is at rest, it is called a diastolic murmur. A surgical procedure can be performed to replace the defective valve.

- **Mitral valve prolapse**—a condition in which the valve between the left atria and the left ventricle closes imperfectly. Symptoms are thought to occur because of a response to stress. These symptoms include fatigue, **palpitations** (heart feels like it is racing), headache, chest pain, and anxiety. Exercise, restricted sugar and caffeine intake, adequate fluid intake, and relaxation techniques help to alleviate symptoms.

Infectious Diseases of the Heart

Infectious diseases of the heart are usually caused by bacteria or by a virus. Bacterial infections may be treated with antibiotic therapy.

- **Pericarditis** is an inflammation of the outer membrane covering the heart. The symptoms are pain in the chest area overlying the heart, cough, **dyspnea** (difficulty in breathing), rapid pulse, and fever.

- **Myocarditis** is an inflammation of the heart muscle. The symptoms may be the same as the pericarditis.

- **Endocarditis** is an inflammation of the membrane that lines the heart and covers the valves. Unlike the rest of the heart, the lining of the heart, the endocardium, receives its oxygen and nourishment directly from the systemic blood within the chambers. For this reason the endocardium is especially susceptible to bloodborne infections such as syphilis. This causes the formation of rough spots in the endocardium, which may lead to the development of a fatal blood clot (thrombus).

- **Rheumatic heart disease** may be a result of frequent strep throat infections during childhood; these infections may lead to rheumatic fever. The antibodies that form to protect the child from the strep throat or rheumatic fever may also attack the lining of the heart, especially the bicuspid (mitral) valve. The valve becomes inflamed and may be scarred, which leads to narrowing of the valve. The mitral valve is then unable to close properly, which interferes with the blood flow from the left atrium to the left ventricle. It is very important that children who have streptococcal infections be treated with antibiotic therapy.

Acute Coronary Syndrome

Patients with heart disease as a result of **progressive atherosclerosis**, Figure 13-9, may develop a number of different clinical presentations, called **acute coronary syndrome (ACD)**. All these presentations have a similar mechanism of injury. An area of the heart is being deprived of life-giving oxygen. The cells and tissues involved immediately suffer from this loss, and cellular malfunction, or **ischemia**, results. Without relief, the cell's dilemma continues and the process progresses from ischemia to cell injury to cell death, or **infarction**.

These processes do not occur in a linear fashion but rather in an overlapping fashion; some cells die (infarct), while new cells suffer from ischemia. This is a concept called **penumbra**.

In about 70% of the cases of myocardial infarction the cause is a blood clot. As dis-

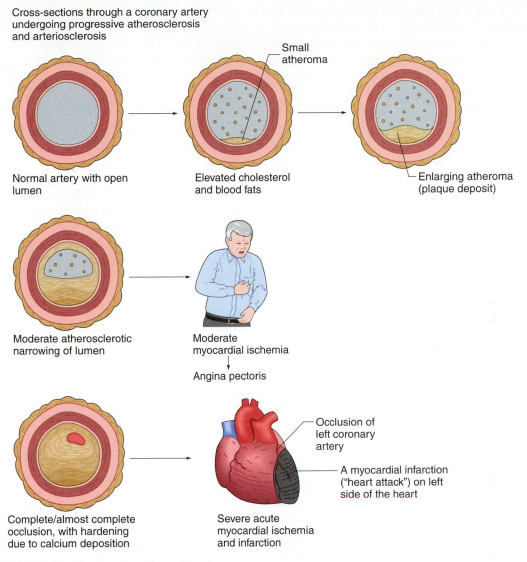

Cross-sections through a coronary artery
undergoing progressive atherosclerosis
and arteriosclerosis

Small
atheroma

Normal artery with open
lumen

Elevated cholesterol
and blood fats

Enlarging atheroma
(plaque deposit)

Moderate atherosclerotic
narrowing of lumen

Moderate
myocardial ischemia

Angina pectoris

Occlusion of
left coronary
artery

A myocardial infarction
("heart attack") on left
side of the heart

Complete/almost complete
occlusion, with hardening
due to calcium deposition

Severe acute
myocardial ischemia
and infarction

● **FIGURE 13–9**   *Progressive atherosclerosis.*

cussed previously, timely treatment with special fibrinolytic drugs (clot busters) can mean cell recovery.

Unfortunately, in as many as 25% of cases the presenting symptom for the patient is sudden cardiac death resulting from a lethal dysrhythmia called **ventricular fibrillation**. More than 50% of all cardiac-related mortality can be directly related to ventricular fibrillation that occurs within the first hour of symptoms, such as chest pain.

The only definitive treatment for ventricular fibrillation is **defibrillation**. A defibrillator applies an electrical charge across the heart,

hoping to return it to normal rhythm. For every minute that a patient remains in ventricular fibrillation, mortality increases by 10%.

Special programs such as **public access defibrillation (PAD)** and rapid-response EMS systems are hopeful steps toward improving the prehospital survival of many patients.

The following is a review of the spectrum of illnesses that result from acute coronary syndrome.

● **Angina pectoris** is the severe chest pain that arises when the heart does not receive enough oxygen. It is not a disease in itself, but a symptom of an underlying problem with the coronary circulation. The chest pain radiates from the precordial area to the left shoulder, down the arm along the ulnar nerve. Victims often experience a feeling of impending death. Angina pectoris occurs quite suddenly; it may be brought on by stress or physical exhaustion. It may be treated with the drug nitroglycerin, which helps to dilate the coronary arteries to permit blood flow to the heart.

• **Myocardial infarction**, commonly known as an "MI" or "heart attack," is caused by a lack of blood supply to the heart muscle, the myocardium. This may be due to blocking of the coronary artery by a blood clot, narrowing of the coronary artery as a result of arteriosclerosis (a loss of elasticity and thickening of the wall), or atherosclerosis (caused by plaque build up in the arterial walls), Figure 13-9. The heart muscle becomes damaged because of lack of blood supply. The amount of tissue affected depends on how much of the heart area is deprived of blood. Symptoms are crushing, severe chest pain radiating to the left shoulder, arm, neck, and jaw. Patients may also complain of nausea, increased perspiration, fatigue, and dyspnea. Mortality is highest when treatment is delayed; therefore immediate medical care is critical. Treatment consists of bed rest, oxygen, and medications. Morphine or meperidine (Demerol) is given to alleviate the pain, drugs such as tPA are used to dissolve the blood clot, and **cardiotonic** drugs such as digitalis are used to slow and strengthen the heartbeat. Anticoagulant therapy is used to prevent further clots from forming. Angioplasty and bypass surgery may also be necessary.

Prevention of Heart Disease

The National Institutes of Health has stated that the following lifestyle changes reduce the risk of heart attacks: smoking cessation, regular exercise, maintenance of ideal weight, estrogen replacement therapy for postmenopausal women, reduction of blood cholesterol levels, and maintenance of normal blood pressure. There are two types of blood cholesterol: high-density lipoprotein (HDL) and low-density lipoprotein (LDL). HDL helps to remove a portion of the cholesterol plaque deposited by a related LDL. The benefits of increasing the HDL to LDL ratio are significant; medication and diet help to increase HDL.

Heart Failure

Heart failure occurs when the ventricles of the heart are unable to contract effectively and blood pools in the heart. Different symptoms can arise depending on which ventricle fails to beat properly. If the left ventricle fails, dyspnea occurs. If the right ventricle fails, engorgement of organs with venous blood occurs, as well as **edema** (excessive fluid in tissues) and **ascites** (abnormal accumulation of serous fluid in the abdominal cavity). Other symptoms may include lung congestion and coughing.

Congestive Heart Failure

Congestive heart failure is similar to heart failure, but in addition there is edema of the lower extremities. Blood backs up into the lung vessels, and fluid extends into the air passages. Treatment consists of cardiotonics (drugs used to slow and strengthen the heartbeat, such as digoxin) and **diuretics** (drugs that reduce the amount of fluid in the body).

Rhythm/Conduction Defects

A **conduction defect**, or rhythm defect, is said to occur when the conduction system of the heart is affected.

• **Heart block** is the interruption of the AV node message from the SA node.

• The interruption can occur in varying degrees. The abnormal patterns are seen on an electrocardiograph. First-degree block is characterized by a momentary delay at the AV node before the impulse is transmitted to the ventricles. Second-degree block can be of two forms: Wenckebach, or second degree type I, block occurs in cycles of increasingly delayed impulses through the AV node until the AV node fails to conduct the impulse to the ventricles and the beat is dropped. Immediately afterward the heart's conduction system recovers, returns to near normal, and the cycle resumes. Classic, or second-degree type II, block is characterized by a pattern in which every second, third, or fourth impulse is blocked to the ventricles. These dropped beats cause a decrease in cardiac output and a loss of blood pressure. Third-degree block is known as "complete heart block." In the case of complete heart block there is no impulse carried through the AV node to the ventricles. Because the heart is essential to life, there is a built-in safety mechanism. The atria continue to beat normally while the ventricles contract independently at about less than the atrial rate, fast enough to sustain life, but resulting in a severe decrease in cardiac output and loss of blood pressure. Conduction defects may be treated by medications and the use of an artificial pacemaker.

- Premature contraction is an arrhythmia disorder that occurs when an area of the heart known as an ectopic (abnormally placed) pacemaker (not the SA node) sparks and stimulates a contraction of the myocardium. There are three types identified by the area of their location: atrial, ventricular, and AV junctional. Premature atrial contractions (PACs) cause the atria to contract ahead of the anticipated time. Premature junctional contractions (PJCs) have the ectopic pacemaker focused at the junction of the AV node and the bundle of His. Usually PACs and PJCs are of no clinical significance and are caused by stress, nicotine, caffeine, or fatigue. Premature ventricular contractions (PVCs) originate in the ventricles and cause contractions ahead of the next anticipated beat. They can be benign or deadly (ventricular tachycardia). If frequent (5 to 6 per minute) or in pairs, they may require immediate intervention to decrease the irritability of the cardiac muscle and maintain cardiac output.

- In fibrillation the rhythm breaks down and muscle fibers contract at random without coordination. This results in ineffective heart action and is a life-threatening condition. An electrical device called a defibrillator is used to discharge a strong electrical current through the patient's heart through electrode paddles held against the bare chest wall. The shock stops all uncoordinated electrical activity (ventricular fibrillation), allowing the SA node to resume control.

TYPES OF HEART SURGERY

- Angioplasty—a procedure to help open clogged vessels. This may also be referred to as balloon surgery. A small deflated balloon is threaded into the coronary artery; when it reaches the blocked area, the balloon is inflated. The balloon is then opened and closed a few times, until the blockage is pushed against the arterial wall and the area is unblocked. The balloon is then deflated and removed, Figure 13-10.

- Coronary bypass—in coronary artery bypass graft (CABG) surgery a detour or bypass is provided to allow the blood supply to go around the blocked area of the coronary artery. A healthy blood vessel, usually a vein from the leg, is used for this purpose. The vein is inserted before the blocked area and provides another route for the blood supply to the myocardium.

HEART TRANSPLANTS

A heart transplant is needed in cases in which the individual's own heart can no longer function properly. This happens after repeated heart attacks, when there is irreparable damage to the heart muscle, valves, or blood vessels leading to and from the heart. Occasionally a baby or young child might need a heart transplant because of a congenital (present at birth) heart defect.

There are always problems that follow even the most "successful" of heart transplants, however. The problem is one of histocompatibility (matching of tissue type) and organ rejection.

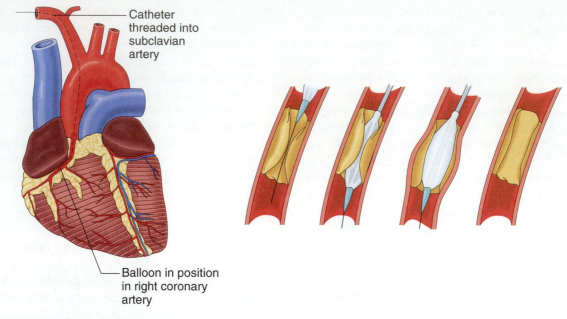

FIGURE 13–10 *Balloon angioplasty.*

Heart transplants that occur between two unrelated people must be monitored carefully. When the heart from the donor is placed into the recipient's body, the recipient's body chemically recognizes the donated heart as a "foreign tissue." Thus the recipient's immune system starts to reject the transplanted heart.

Medical science has counteracted the rejection by developing chemicals called immunosuppressants. These drugs suppress the recipient's immune system so it will not form antibodies to reject the donated heart. Unfortunately the effect of these chemicals is not permanent. Also, suppressing the recipient's immune system indefinitely is not medically wise because he or she will become more susceptible to disease and infection. Often a heart transplant patient dies not from problems arising from the donated heart but from a case of pneumonia. The science and technology of heart transplants is still in its formative stages. However, a heart transplant can perhaps prolong life and maybe even improve the quality of life for an individual with a chronic heart problem.

ARTIFICIAL HEART

The artificial heart was used for the first time on December 3, 1982. The use of the heart has not been as successful as scientists had hoped it would be. Scientists continue to do the necessary research to perfect an artificial heart.

Heart Assist Devices

Physicians are using two devices that help to support the heart's own pumping action. The first device, called an **intra-aortic balloon pump (IABP)**, inflates a gas-filled balloon moments after a heartbeat. The result is improved forward blood flow into the body, as well as improved backflow into the coronary arteries.

The other device, still experimental, is a small in-line pump that helps increase, or augment, the heart's own pumping. Called a **left ventricular assist device**, these micropumps may represent the wave of the future in cardiac care.

MEDICAL HIGHLIGHTS

Pacemakers

The most commonly used artificial pacemaker is the demand pacemaker, which monitors the heart's activity and takes control only when the heart rate falls below a programmed minimum—usually 60 bpm, Figure 13-11. Today, newer types of pacemakers actually monitor a number of physical changes in the body that indicate an increase or decrease in activity. If the heart's own pacing system fails to respond, these rate-responsive pacemakers slowly raise or lower the heartbeat to the appropriate level, from 60 to perhaps 150 bpm.

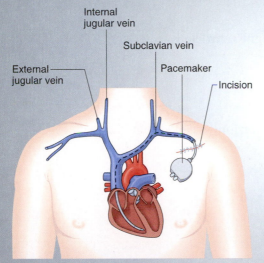

FIGURE 13–11 *Pacemaker.*

Today's modern pacemakers are shielded from stray electromagnetic forces, and people who use pacemakers no longer have to avoid microwave ovens. However, there is some evidence that the use of cellular phones, especially digital ones, can change the pace of pacemakers or speed up people's pulses when used near the heart-regulating devices. Medtronics, Inc., the world's largest developer and manufacturer of pacemakers, recommends that cell phones be kept at least 6 inches away from pacemakers.

Implantable Defibrillators

A defibrillator is a device that can shock the heart back to a regular rhythm. The implantable defibrillator protects patients at risk of severe ventricular tachycardia, a life-threatening arrhythmia. Medication and pacemakers are the most common treatment for arrhythmias, but for a small proportion of patients the implantable defibrillator can save their lives. In May 1996 the Food and Drug Administration also gave approval for the defibrillator to be used on patients who may have had at least one heart attack in the past but who are now without symptoms other than irregular heart rhythms picked up on an ECG. The defibrillator is implanted in the skin of the chest or abdomen and usually needs only one electrode to be routed to the heart through a vein. Through that electrode the tiny computer aboard the defibrillator constantly monitors the heartbeat. If it detects a minor arrhythmia, it activates a built-in conventional pacemaker to reestablish the heart rhythm. If that fails, it delivers a small defibrillating electrical jolt to the heart. The electrical jolt may be startling and a bit uncomfortable; however, the minor annoyance is acceptable to most patients, because they realize that a potentially life-threatening heartbeat irregularity has been detected and corrected.

Angioplasty-Palmaz-Schatz Stent

This stent device is a tiny, expandable, stainless steel tube that holds arteries open following angioplasty. After angioplasty the coronary artery blockage can return within a matter of months if new plaque deposits develop or clot formation occurs. ■

● REVIEW QUESTIONS

Select the letter of the choice that best completes the statement.

1. The organs of the circulatory system include the:
    a. heart, blood vessels, and liver
    b. heart, blood vessels, and lungs
    c. heart, blood vessels, and lymph
    d. heart, blood vessels, and kidneys

2. The outer layer of the heart is called the:
    a. myocardium
    b. endocardium
    c. pericardium
    d. pleural lining

3. The muscle layer of the heart is called the:
    a. myocardium
    b. endocardium
    c. pericardium
    d. pleural lining

4. The valve between the right atrium and the right ventricle is called the:
    a. tricuspid valve
    b. aortic semilunar valve
    c. bicuspid valve
    d. pulmonary semilunar valve

5. The blood vessel that brings blood to the right atrium is called the:
    a. pulmonary vein
    b. aorta
    c. pulmonary artery
    d. vena cava

6. The pacemaker of the heart is the:
    a. SA node
    b. AV node
    c. Bundle branches
    d. Purkinje fibers

7. The heart's electrical impulse follows this path:
    a. bundle branches, AV node, SA node
    b. AV node, bundle branches, SA node
    c. SA node, AV node, bundle branches
    d. bundle branches, SA node, AV node

8. The device used to measure the electrical activity of the heart is called an:
    a. EEG
    b. MRI
    c. ECG
    d. EMG

9. A heart rate below 60 is called:
   a. bradycardia
   b. tachycardia
   c. arrhythmia
   d. murmur

10. An inflammation of the inner layer of the heart is called:
    a. pericarditis
    b. myocarditis
    c. endocarditis
    d. phlebitis

11. The term *heart attack* is another name for:
    a. rheumatic heart disease
    b. myocardial infarction
    c. heart block
    d. congestive heart failure

12. The treatment for a heart attack may include all but:
    a. angioplasty
    b. antibiotics
    c. coronary bypass
    d. anticoagulants

13. Another name for a stationary blood clot is:
    a. embolus
    b. stenosis
    c. thrombus
    d. thrombosis

14. The treatment for heart block may include:
    a. coronary bypass
    b. anticoagulants
    c. insertion of a pacemaker
    d. angioplasty

15. The circulation that carries blood from the heart to lungs and back to heart is the:
    a. coronary
    b. fetal
    c. cardiopulmonary
    d. portal

● LABELING

Locate and label the various structures of the heart. Also include valves, vessels, and nodes. Trace blood from right atrium to aorta.

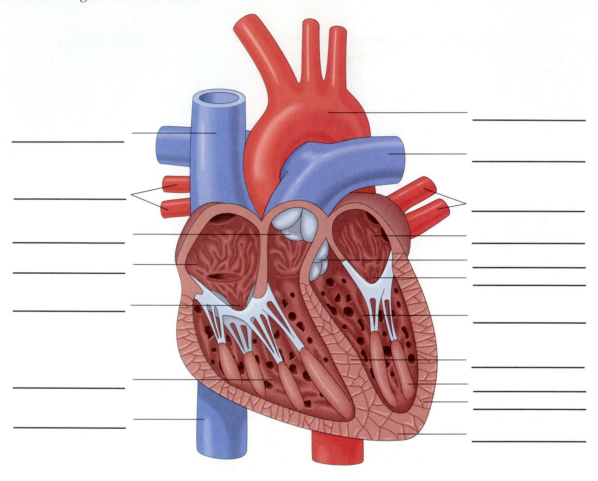

● MATCHING

Match each term in Column A with its correct description or function in Column B.

Column A	Column B
_____ 1. pulmonary artery	a. vein that carries freshly oxygenated blood from the lung to the heart
_____ 2. lymphatic system	
_____ 3. pulmonary vein	b. circulation route that carries blood to and from the heart and lungs
_____ 4. septum	
_____ 5. pulmonary circulation	c. divides the heart into right and left sides
_____ 6. left ventricle	d. artery that carries deoxygenated blood from the heart to the lung
_____ 7. general circulation	
_____ 8. right ventricle	e. system that consists of lymph and tissue fluid derived from the blood
_____ 9. aortae	
	f. blood from the pulmonary vein that reenters the heart through the left atrium
	g. artery that carries blood with nourishment, oxygen, and other materials from the heart to all parts of the body
	h. ventricle from which the aorta receives blood
	i. circulation that carries blood throughout the body
	j. ventricle from which the pulmonary artery leaves the heart

●APPLYING THEORY TO PRACTICE

1. Pretend you are a blood cell that has just arrived in the right atrium. Trace the journey you will take to get to the aorta.

2. A child has chronic strep throat. If this condition is not treated, what heart disease can occur? Describe what happens in the heart. How can this be prevented?

3. When a person has a heart attack, what happens to the cardiac muscle? Describe the types of surgery that can be done to treat this condition. Describe the feelings of the patient and the family.

14

Circulation and Blood Vessels

Objectives

- Trace the path of cardiopulmonary circulation
- Name and describe the specialized circulatory systems
- Trace the blood in fetal circulation
- List the types of blood vessels
- Identify the principal arteries and veins of the body
- Describe some disorders of the blood vessels
- Define the key words that relate to this chapter

Key Words

aneurysm
aortic dissection
arteriole
arteriosclerosis
artery
atherosclerosis
backward failure
brachial artery
capillary
cerebral hemorrhage
cerebrovascular accident (CVA)
claudication
common carotid artery
core organs
decompensated shock
diastolic pressure
dorsalis pedis artery
dysphasia
femoral artery
fetal circulation
gangrene
hemiplegia
hemorrhoids
hepatic vein

hepatic-jugular reflex (HJR)
hypotension
jugular venous distention (JVD)
ligamentum arteriosus
lumen
modified Trendelenburg position
pecking order
pedal edema
perfusion
peripheral edema
peripheral vascular disease
phlebitis
popliteal artery
portal circulation
portal vein
pulmonary edema
pulse pressure
radial artery
sacral edema
shock syndrome
shunting
systolic blood pressure

(continues)

Key Words (continued)

temporal artery	valves
tunica adventitia (externa)	varicose veins
	vasotonia
tunica intima	vein
tunica media	venule

The blood vessels circulate the blood through two major circulatory systems:

1. *Pulmonary circulation*—circulates blood from the heart to the lungs and back to the heart.

2. *Systemic circulation*—circulates blood from the heart to the tissues and cells and back to the heart.

There are two specialized systemic routes:

1. *Portal circulation*—takes blood from the organs of digestion to the liver through the portal vein.

2. *Fetal circulation*—only occurs during pregnancy. The fetus obtains oxygen and nutrients from the mother's blood.

PULMONARY CIRCULATION

Pulmonary circulation takes deoxygenated blood from the heart to the lungs, where carbon dioxide is exchanged for oxygen. The oxygenated blood returns to the heart. As stated in Chapter 13, blood enters the right atrium, which contracts, forcing the blood through the tricuspid valve into the right ventricle.

The right ventricle contracts to push the blood through the pulmonary valve into the pulmonary trunk. The pulmonary trunk bifurcates (divides in two). It branches into the right pulmonary artery, bringing blood to the right lung, and into the left pulmonary artery, bringing blood to the left lung, Figure 14-1.

Inside the lungs, the pulmonary arteries branch into countless small arteries called **arterioles**. The arterioles connect to dense beds of capillaries lying in the alveoli lung tissue. There, gaseous exchange takes place: Carbon dioxide leaves the red blood cells and is discharged into the air in the alveoli, to be excreted from the lungs. Oxygen from air in the alveoli combines with hemoglobin in the red blood cells. From these capillaries the blood travels into small veins or **venules**.

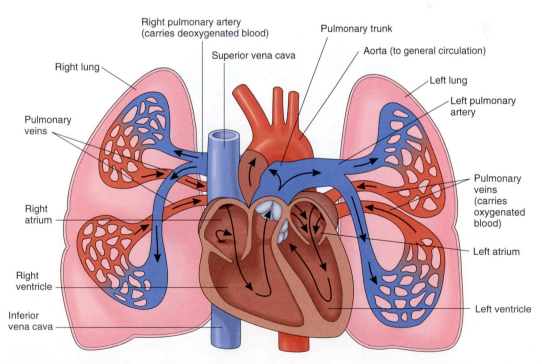

● **FIGURE 14–1**   *Pulmonary circulation.*

Venules from the right and left lung form large pulmonary veins. These veins carry oxygenated blood from the lungs back to the heart and into the left atrium.

The left atrium contracts, sending the blood through the bicuspid, or mitral, valve into the left ventricle. This chamber acts as a pump for newly oxygenated blood. When the left ventricle contracts, it sends oxygenated blood through the aortic semilunar valve and into the aorta.

PATH OF SYSTEMIC/GENERAL CIRCULATION

The function of the general (systemic) circulation is fourfold: It circulates nutrients, oxygen, water, and secretions to the tissues and back to the heart; it carries products such as carbon dioxide and other dissolved wastes away from the tissues; it helps equalize body temperature; and it aids in protecting the body from harmful bacteria.

The aorta is the largest artery in the body. The first branch of the aorta is the coronary artery, which takes blood to the myocardium (cardial muscle). As the aorta emerges (ascending aorta) from the anterior (upper) portion of the heart, it forms the aortic arch. Three branches come from this arch: the brachiocephalic, the left common carotid, and the left subclavian arteries, Figure 14-2. These arteries and their branches carry blood to the arms, neck, and head.

From the aortic arch, the aorta descends along the mid-dorsal wall of the thorax and abdomen. Many arteries branch off from the descending aorta, carrying oxygenated blood throughout the body.

As the descending aorta proceeds posteriorly, it sends off additional branches to the body wall, stomach, intestines, liver, pancreas, spleen, kidneys, reproductive organs, urinary bladder,

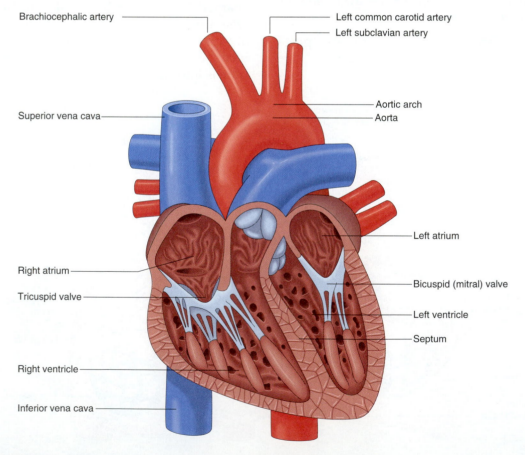

● **FIGURE 14–2** *Blood flow into, around, and out of the heart.*

legs, and so forth. Each of these arteries subdivides into still smaller arteries, then into arterioles, and finally into numerous capillaries embedded in the tissues. This is where hormones, nutrients, oxygen, and other materials are transferred from the blood into the tissue.

In turn, metabolic waste products, such as carbon dioxide and nitrogenous wastes, are picked up by the blood. Hormones secreted by specialized tissues, and nutrients from the small intestines and liver, are also absorbed by the blood. Blood then runs from the capillaries first into tiny veins, through increasingly larger veins, and finally into one (or more) of the veins that exit from the organ. Eventually it empties into one of the two largest veins in the body, see Figure 14-2.

Deoxygenated venous blood, returning from the lower parts of the body, empties into the interior vena cava. Venous blood from the upper body parts (arms, neck, and head) passes into the superior vena cava. Both the inferior and superior vena cava empty their deoxygenated blood into the right atrium.

Portal Circulation

The **portal circulation** is a branch of the general circulation. Veins from the pancreas, stomach, small intestine, colon, and spleen empty their blood into the **portal vein**, which goes to the liver, Figure 14-3.

It is very important that venous blood makes a detour through the liver before returning to the

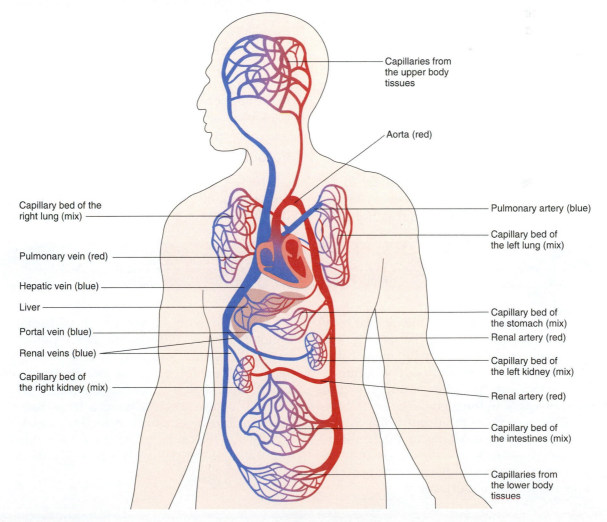

Capillaries from the upper body tissues

Aorta (red)

Capillary bed of the right lung (mix)

Pulmonary vein (red)

Hepatic vein (blue)

Liver

Portal vein (blue)

Renal veins (blue)

Capillary bed of the right kidney (mix)

Pulmonary artery (blue)

Capillary bed of the left lung (mix)

Capillary bed of the stomach (mix)

Renal artery (red)

Capillary bed of the left kidney (mix)

Renal artery (red)

Capillary bed of the intestines (mix)

Capillaries from the lower body tissues

● **FIGURE 14–3**   *The systemic, pulmonary, renal, and portal blood circuits.*

The foramen ovale usually closes during birth, but on rare occasions it fails to close. The result is a "hole in the heart" between the right and left sides of the heart.

As blood flows through either a ventricular-septal defect (VSD) or an atrial-septal defect (ASD), the turbulent blood flow creates a loud machinery-like murmur. The resulting redirection of the blood's flow through the defect, changing some of the blood's flow from right to left to left to right, is called shunting. Shunted blood does not pass through the lungs and thus is not oxygenated. This deoxygenated blood produces cyanosis, a bluish tint to the skin, and the infant is called a "blue baby."

Another fetal structure, called the ductus arteriosus, allows the blood to flow from the pulmonary artery to the aorta. In a fetus the purpose of the blood circulating through the heart is to give the heart and blood vessels oxygen and nutrients to grow. When birth occurs, the foramen ovale closes, the ductus arteriosus collapses, and the normal cardiopulmonary circulation begins. ■

---

heart. After meals, blood reaching the liver contains a higher than normal concentration of glucose. The liver removes the excess glucose, converting it to glycogen. In the event of vigorous exercise, work, or prolonged periods without nourishment, glycogen reserves are changed back into glucose for energy. This detour ensures that the blood's glucose concentration is kept within a relatively narrow range.

The liver also detoxifies (neutralizes) drugs and toxins, breaks down hormones no longer useful to the body, and produces urea during the catabolism of amino acids. The liver also removes worn-out red blood cells from circulation.

Deoxygenated venous blood leaves the liver through the hepatic vein, which carries it to the inferior vena cava. From the inferior vena cava, blood enters the right atrium.

Fetal Circulation

Fetal circulation occurs in the fetus (unborn baby). Instead of using its own lungs and digestive system, the fetus obtains oxygen and

After childbirth the ductus arteriosus closes and the remains of this fetal circulation changes into a ligament called the ligamentum arteriosus. The ligamentum arteriosus stretches from the pulmonary artery to the arch of the aorta.

The ligamentum arteriosus is the only attachment that the heart has to another structure; in effect the heart hangs freely from the great vessels and the only tether the heart has is the ligamentum arteriosus.

In a sudden deceleration, such as during a motor vehicle collision, the heart swings forward violently and is restrained by this ligament. If the force is great enough, the ligament's foundation at the aorta is pulled off the wall of the aorta, leaving a large hole. This aortic tear, or aortic disection, bleeds rapidly into the center of the chest, the mediastinum, and the patient bleeds to death in minutes. ■

nutrients from the mother's blood. The fetal and maternal blood do not mix. The exchange of gases, food, and waste takes place in the structure known as the placenta, located in the pregnant uterus.

In fetal circulation, blood may follow two paths: In the fetal heart there is an opening in the septum called the foramen ovale, which permits blood to flow from the right atrium to the left atrium; also, blood may move from the right ventricle through the pulmonary semilunar valve to the pulmonary artery.

BLOOD VESSELS

The heart pumps the blood to all parts of the body through a remarkable system of three types of blood vessels: arteries, capillaries, and veins.

Arteries

Arteries carry oxygenated blood away from the heart to the capillaries. (There is one exception: the pulmonary arteries carry deoxygenated blood from the heart to the lungs). The arteries transport blood under very high pressure; they are elastic, muscular, and thick walled. The thickness of the arteries makes them the strongest of the three types of blood vessels. Table 14-1 lists the principal arteries and the areas they serve. See also Figure 14-4.

As seen in Figure 14-5, the arterial walls are composed of three layers. The outer layer is called the **tunica adventitia** or **externa**. This layer is composed of fibrous connective tissue with bundles of smooth muscle cells, which lends great elasticity to the arteries. This elasticity allows the arteries to withstand sudden large increases in internal pressure, created by the large volume of blood forced into them during each heart contraction. When arteries become hardened, as in arteriosclerosis, the systolic blood pressure increases greatly.

The **tunica media** is the middle arterial layer. It is composed of muscle cells arranged in a circular pattern. This layer controls the artery's diameter by dilation and constriction, which regulates the flow of blood through the

TABLE 14-1 *Principal Arteries*

PRINCIPAL ARTERIES	AREAS SERVED
Common carotid	Head and face
Internal carotid	Brain
External carotid	Face *(pulse point)*
Vertebral	Spinal column and brain
Brachiocephalic	Right arm and shoulder, head
Subclavian	Shoulder
Axillary	Axilla area
Brachial	Upper arm and elbow area *(pulse point)*
Radial	Arm, wrist *(pulse point)*
Thoracic aorta	Chest cavity
Celiac	Liver, spleen, stomach, and pancreas
Splenic	Spleen
Hepatic	Liver
Superior mesenteric	Small intestines and colon
Renal	Kidney
Common iliac	Lower abdominal area
Internal iliac	Pelvis and bladder
External iliac	Groin and lower leg
Femoral	Groin *(pulse point)*
Popliteal	Knee area *(pulse point)*
Anterior tibialis	Anterior lower leg
Posterior tibialis	Posterior lower leg *(pulse point)*
Dorsalis pedis	Ankle *(pulse point)*

artery. This keeps the blood flow steady and even and reduces the heart's work.

The autonomic nervous system controls the muscles within the artery's tunica media that, in turn, control the internal diameter of the arterial channel, called the artery's **lumen**. It is the function of the arterioles to expand and contract the lumen that changes intermittent blood flow, the pulse from the heart, to a constant stream of blood flow. The function of these vasomotor muscle fibers is to ensure continuous uninterrupted blood flow to the capillary beds. This process is called maintaining **vasotonia**.

Complex control of fluid balance, nervous system function, and blood viscosity by the

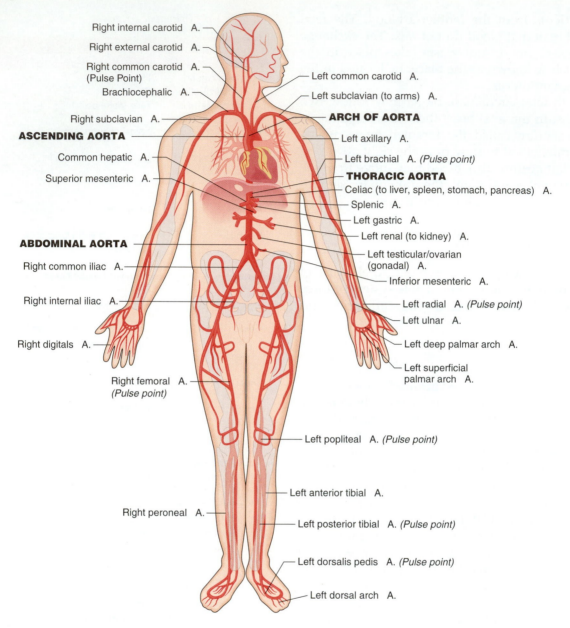

Right internal carotid A.
Right external carotid A.
Right common carotid A.
(Pulse Point)
Brachiocephalic A.
Right subclavian A.
ASCENDING AORTA
Common hepatic A.
Superior mesenteric A.

ABDOMINAL AORTA
Right common iliac A.
Right internal iliac A.
Right digitals A.
Right femoral A.
(Pulse point)

Right peroneal A.

Left common carotid A.
Left subclavian (to arms) A.
ARCH OF AORTA
Left axillary A.
Left brachial A. *(Pulse point)*
THORACIC AORTA
Celiac (to liver, spleen, stomach, pancreas) A.
Splenic A.
Left gastric A.
Left renal (to kidney) A.
Left testicular/ovarian
(gonadal) A.
Inferior mesenteric A.
Left radial A. *(Pulse point)*
Left ulnar A.
Left deep palmar arch A.
Left superficial
palmar arch A.

Left popliteal A. *(Pulse point)*

Left anterior tibial A.

Left posterior tibial A. *(Pulse point)*

Left dorsalis pedis A. *(Pulse point)*

Left dorsal arch A.

● **FIGURE 14–4** *Arterial distribution.*

kidneys, the autonomic nervous system, and the endocrine system helps to ensure this steady flow by modifying arterial lumen size, as well as blood composition.

The autonomic nervous system's control of the arteries thus creates resistance to forward blood flow from the heart, or peripheral/systemic vascular resistance (P/SVR). Specifically, the diameter of the arterial blood vessels creates resistance to the heart's pumping ac-

tion, systole. Smaller arterial lumens equal increased SVR, whereas larger lumens create decreased SVR.

This systemic vascular resistance can be roughly approximated by measuring the blood's pressure during diastole, when the heart is at rest. The pressure measured in a large artery during diastole is called the **diastolic pressure**.

Increased autonomic nervous system activity, particularly the sympathetic nervous sys-

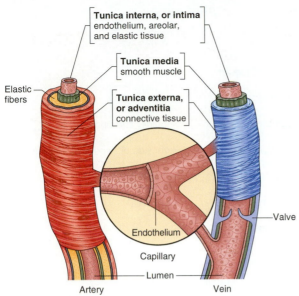

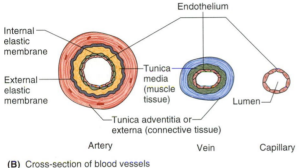

FIGURE 14–5   *Different types of blood vessels and their cross-sectional views.*

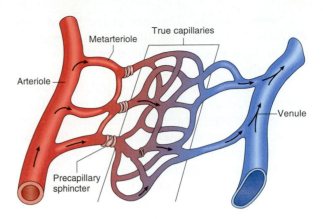

FIGURE 14–6   *Capillary bed connecting an arteriole with a venule.*

tem, as well as excretion of epinephrine (adrenaline) from the kidney's adrenal glands can cause an increased diastolic pressure. This increased diastolic pressure, called hypertension, can be helpful in times of crisis. However, over time the prolonged elevation of the diastolic pressure can create damage to delicate tissues within the kidneys, as well as cause the heart to enlarge, or hypertrophy.

An inner layer (**tunica intima**) consists of three smaller layers: endothelium, areolar, and elastic tissue. The endothelium gives the artery a smooth lining, which allows for the free flow of blood, see Figure 14-5.

The aorta leads away from the heart and branches into smaller arteries. These smaller ar-

teries, in turn, branch into arterioles, which still have some smooth muscle in the walls and are also resistant vessels. Arterioles give rise to the capillaries, Figure 14-6.

Capillaries

Capillaries, which connect the arterioles with venules, are the smallest blood vessels; they can only be seen through a compound microscope. Capillaries are branches of the finest arteriole divisions, known as metarterioles. The metarterioles have lost most of their connective tissue and muscle layers. Eventually the last traces of these two tissues disappear and there remains only a simple endothelial cell layer. This endothelial cell layer constitutes the capillaries.

The capillary walls are extremely thin to allow for the selective permeability of various cells and substances. Nutrient molecules and oxygen pass out of the capillaries and into the surrounding cells and tissues. Metabolic waste products, such as carbon dioxide and nitrogenous wastes, pass back from the cells and tissues into the bloodstream for excretion at their proper sites (e.g., lungs and kidneys).

Tiny openings in the capillary walls allow white blood cells to leave the bloodstream and enter the tissue spaces to help destroy invading bacteria. In the capillaries, some of the plasma diffuses out of the bloodstream and into the tissue spaces. This fluid is called interstitial fluid and is returned to the bloodstream in the form of lymph via the lymphatic vessels.

Sometimes the diameter of red blood cells exceeds that of the capillaries. They become compressed and distorted as they flow through the capillary.

Blood flow through the capillaries can be controlled, despite the fact that muscle cells do not line the capillary walls. This is achieved by the action of small muscular bands called precapillary sphincters.

Although capillaries are ultimately responsible for transporting blood to all tissues, not all capillaries are open simultaneously. This system allows for regulation of blood flow to "active" tissues. In the human brain, for instance, most of the capillaries remain open. However, in a resting muscle, only 1/20 to 1/50 of the capillaries transport blood to the muscle cells. Compare this with an actively contracting muscle, in which as many as 190 capillaries per square millimeter are open. If the same muscle is not active, there may be as few as five capillaries open per square millimeter.

Veins

The **veins** carry deoxygenated blood away from the capillaries to the heart. The smallest vein is hardly larger than a capillary, but it contains a muscular layer that is not present within capillaries. Table 14-2 lists the principal veins and the areas they serve. See also Figure 14-7.

The veins are composed of three layers: the tunica externa, tunica media, and tunica intima. Veins are considerably less elastic and muscular than arteries. The walls of the veins are much thinner than those of the arteries, because they do not have to withstand such high internal pressures. This is because pressure from the heart's contraction is greatly diminished by the time the blood reaches the veins for its return journey. Thus the thinner walled veins can collapse easily when not filled with blood. Finally, veins have **valves** along their length. These valves allow blood to flow only in one direction, toward the heart. This prevents reflux (backflow) of blood toward the capillaries, Figure 14-8. Valves are found in abundance in veins in which there is a greater chance of reflux. There are many valves in the

TABLE 14-2 *Principal Veins*

PRINCIPAL VEINS	AREAS SERVED
External jugular	Face
Internal jugular	Head and neck
Subclavian	Shoulder and upper limbs
Brachiocephalic	Right side of head and shoulder
Left cephalic	Shoulder and axillary
Axillary	Axilla area
Brachial	Upper arm
Radial	Lower arm and wrist
Superior vena cava	Upper part of body
Inferior vena cava	Lower part of body and abdominal area
Hepatic	Liver
Renal	Kidney
Hepatic portal	Organs of digestion
Splenic	Spleen
Superior mesenteric	Small intestine and colon

Common iliac
    Internal iliac
    External iliac
	Lower abdominal and pelvis,
	bladder, and reproductive organs
	Lower limbs

Great saphenous	Upper leg
Femoral	Upper leg and groin area
Popliteal	Knee
Posterior tibialis	Posterior leg
Dorsal venous arch	Foot

lower extremities, where blood has to oppose the force of gravity.

Eventually all the venules converge to make up larger veins, which ultimately form the body's largest veins, the vena cavae. Venous blood from the upper part of the body returns to the right atrium via the superior vena cava; blood from the lower body parts is conducted to the heart via the inferior vena cava.

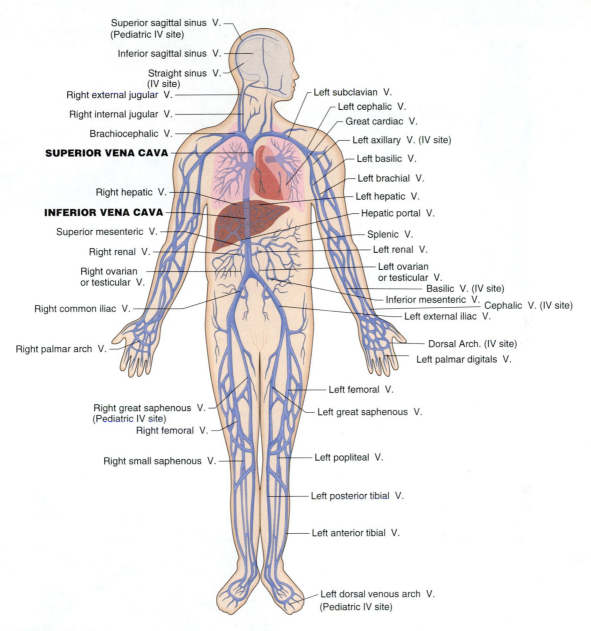

Superior sagittal sinus V.
(Pediatric IV site)

Inferior sagittal sinus V.

Straight sinus V.
(IV site)

Right external jugular V.

Right internal jugular V.

Brachiocephalic V.

SUPERIOR VENA CAVA

Right hepatic V.

INFERIOR VENA CAVA

Superior mesenteric V.

Right renal V.

Right ovarian
or testicular V.

Right common iliac V.

Right palmar arch V.

Right great saphenous V.
(Pediatric IV site)

Right femoral V.

Right small saphenous V.

Left subclavian V.

Left cephalic V.

Great cardiac V.

Left axillary V. (IV site)

Left basilic V.

Left brachial V.

Left hepatic V.

Hepatic portal V.

Splenic V.

Left renal V.

Left ovarian
or testicular V.

Basilic V. (IV site)

Inferior mesenteric V.   Cephalic V. (IV site)

Left external iliac V.

Dorsal Arch. (IV site)

Left palmar digitals V.

Left femoral V.

Left great saphenous V.

Left popliteal V.

Left posterior tibial V.

Left anterior tibial V.

Left dorsal venous arch V.
(Pediatric IV site)

● **FIGURE 14–7**   *Venous distribution.*

● VENOUS RETURN

In addition to valves, the skeletal muscles contract to help push the blood along its path. In the abdominal and thoracic cavity, pressure changes occur when you breathe; this also helps to bring the venous blood back to the heart. Think about sitting for a long period, on a car ride for example. Think how sleepy you start to get. The reason may be that blood isn't getting back to the heart for oxygen. To reduce the drowsiness, you might stop the car and get out and walk around for a while. This improves circulation and the drowsiness usually passes.

When the heart starts to fail as a pump, either because of damage (acute myocardial infarction [AMI]) or overload (overhydration), the blood starts to back up from the heart, causing congestive heart failure (CHF), also called **backward failure**.

Blood flow toward the heart

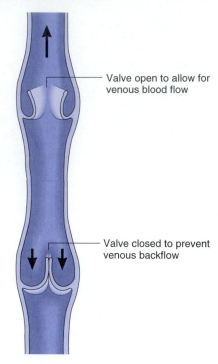

Valve open to allow for venous blood flow

Valve closed to prevent venous backflow

● **FIGURE 14–8** *Valves in the veins.*

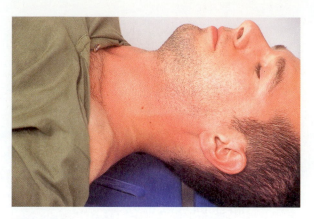

● **FIGURE 14–9** *Jugular venous distention.*

usually settles in a dependent area (the area lowest from the heart). If the patient is seated, the edema settles in the feet; this is called **pedal edema**, Figure 14-10. If the patient is bedridden, the edema settles in the small of the back in the sacral region; this is called **sacral edema**.

In the case of the left side of the heart, the blood backs up into the lungs, causing swelling and edema. This **pulmonary edema** sounds like crackles as air moves through the moist passages during inspiration.

As the blood further backs up, through the lungs and through the right side of the heart, it enters the systemic circulation.

Blood first reaches the jugular veins of the neck, which rapidly become swollen with blood; this **jugular venous distention (JVD)** is markedly visible to the EMS provider, Figure 14-9. JVD should be assessed while the patient is sitting at a 45-degree angle.

Next the blood backs up into the liver, distending the liver. If the EMS provider presses on the liver, at the left upper quadrant of the abdomen, a pressure wave is transmitted to the jugular veins. This reaction is called a **hepatic-jugular reflex (HJR)**.

Blood then backs up and distends the mesentery veins, creating abdominal distention and tenderness. Finally, the blood backs up into the periphery of the body. The swelling created, called **peripheral edema**,

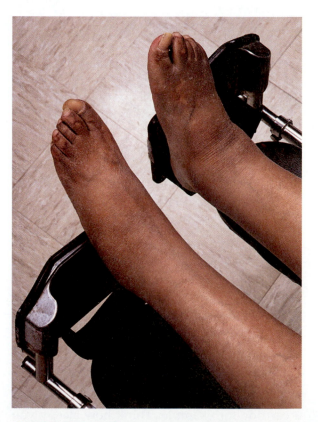

● **FIGURE 14–10** *Swelling is often felt and not seen.*

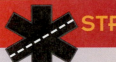

STREET SMART

As a person ages, the skin becomes thinner and there is less subcutaneous fat under the skin. An advanced EMS provider who tries to start an intravenous (IV) line on the patient may experience some difficulty.

In a younger person the subcutaneous fat and associated connective tissue helps stabilize the vein. Without these tissues, the vein is more mobile and may even appear to roll when an IV needle approaches.

Furthermore, as the advanced EMS provider advances the needle, he or she may overshoot and penetrate both sides of the vein, thereby causing the vein to bleed posterior to the IV insertion. This overestimation of depth is in part due to the miscalculation of skin thickness.

The flesh of dark-skinned individuals, outdoor laborers, and farmers tends to be thicker, whereas the flesh of the elderly tends to be thinner. These differences must be taken into account before an IV is attempted. ■

● ARTERIAL BLOOD PRESSURE

When the heart pumps blood into the arteries, the surge of blood filling the vessels creates pressure against their walls. The pressure measured at the moment of contraction is the **systolic blood pressure**. The lessened force of the blood (measured when the ventricles are relaxed) is called diastolic pressure. The pressure in arteries that are closest to the heart is greatest and gradually decreases as the blood travels farther away from the heart.

The average systolic pressure in an adult is 120 millimeters of mercury (mm Hg). The average diastolic pressure in an adult is 80 mm Hg. The blood pressure is recorded as 120/80. **Pulse pressure**, a term associated with blood pressure, is the difference between the systolic and diastolic; if blood pressure is 120/80, the pulse pressure is 40.

● ARTERIAL PULSE

If you touch certain areas (pulse points) of the body, such as the radial artery at the wrist, you will feel alternating, beating throbs. These throbs represent your body's pulse. A pulse is the alternating expansion and contraction of an artery as blood flows through it. The pulse rate usually is the same as the heart rate.

Try this simple demonstration: Place your fingertips (except for the thumb, which has its own pulse) over an artery that is near the surface of the skin and over a bone. There are seven locations where you can conveniently feel your pulse, Figure 14-11.

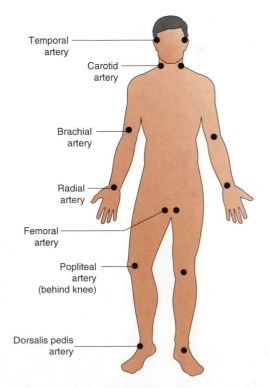

Temporal artery

Carotid artery

Brachial artery

Radial artery

Femoral artery

Popliteal artery (behind knee)

Dorsalis pedis artery

● **FIGURE 14–11**   *Pulse points.*

CHANGES OF AGING

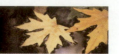

Arteriosclerosis is the disease that occurs when the arterial walls thicken because of a loss of elasticity as persons age. **Atherosclerosis** is the disease that occurs when deposits of fatty substances form along the walls of the arteries. Exercise and a low-fat diet are recommended to prevent this disease. In both arteriosclerosis and atherosclerosis there is a narrowing of the blood vessel opening. This interferes with the blood supply to the body parts and causes hypertension. Symptoms develop where the circulation is impaired; numbness and tingling of the lower extremities or loss of memory indicates interference with circulation, Figure 14-12. ■

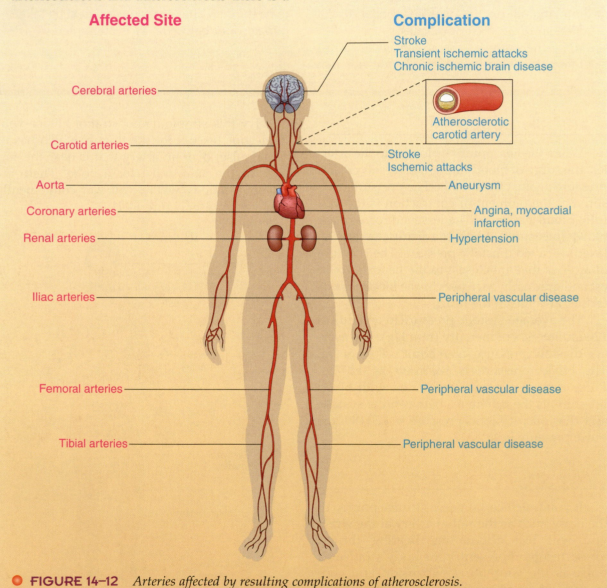

Affected Site

Complication

Stroke
Transient ischemic attacks
Chronic ischemic brain disease

Cerebral arteries

Atherosclerotic
carotid artery

Carotid arteries

Stroke
Ischemic attacks

Aorta — Aneurysm

Coronary arteries — Angina, myocardial infarction

Renal arteries — Hypertension

Iliac arteries — Peripheral vascular disease

Femoral arteries — Peripheral vascular disease

Tibial arteries — Peripheral vascular disease

● **FIGURE 14–12**   *Arteries affected by resulting complications of atherosclerosis.*

1. **Brachial artery**—located at the crook of the elbow, along the inner border of the biceps muscle.

2. **Common carotid artery**—found in the neck, along the front margin of the sternocleidomastoid muscle, near the lower edge of the thyroid cartilage.

3. **Femoral artery**—in the inguinal, or groin, area.

4. **Dorsalis pedis artery**—on the anterior surface of the foot, below the ankle joint.

5. **Popliteal artery**—behind the knee (may be hard to palpate).

6. **Radial artery**—at the wrist, on the same side as the thumb.

7. **Temporal artery**—slightly above the outer edge of the eye.

DISORDERS OF BLOOD VESSELS

Aneurysm is the ballooning out of an artery, accompanied by a thinning arterial wall, caused by a weakening of the blood vessel (almost like having a bubble on a tire). The aneurysm pulsates with each systolic beat. The symptoms are pain and pressure; however, sometimes there are no symptoms. The most common aneurysm site is in the aorta.

Gangrene is death of body tissue resulting from an insufficient blood supply caused by disease or injury.

Phlebitis is an inflammation of the lining of a vein, accompanied by clotting of blood in the vein. Symptoms include edema (swelling) of the affected area, pain, and redness along the length of the vein. Phlebitis can result from complications of an IV line.

Embolism is a traveling blood clot. A pulmonary embolism is a blood clot in the lungs.

Varicose veins are the swollen veins that result from a slowing down of blood flow back to the heart. Blood backs up in the veins if the muscles do not massage them. The weight of the stagnant blood distends the valves; the continued pooling of blood then causes distention and inelasticity of the vein walls. This condition develops as a result of hereditary weakness in vein structure. In addition, poor posture, prolonged periods of standing, and physical exertion can cause valves in the superficial leg veins to enlarge and weaken. Age and pregnancy are other factors responsible for varicose veins.

Hemorrhoids are varicose veins in the walls of the lower rectum and the tissues around the anus.

Cerebral hemorrhage refers to bleeding from blood vessels within the brain. It can be caused by arteriosclerosis, disease, or injury, such as a blow to the head.

Peripheral vascular disease is caused by blockage of the arteries, usually in the legs. Symptoms are pain or cramping in the legs or buttocks while walking. This pain is called **claudication**. As the condition worsens, symptoms may include pain in the toes or feet while at rest, numbness, paleness, and cyanosis in the foot or leg. If the condition is not treated, amputation may be necessary. Treatments include medication to reduce cholesterol, improved or modified diet, and other therapies to improve circulation.

Hypertension (high blood pressure) is frequently called the "silent killer" because there are usually no symptoms of the disease. This condition leads to strokes, heart attacks, and kidney failure. Most people discover that they have the condition during a routine physical. Hypertension means that blood pressure is 140/90 or higher. Incidence of hypertension is higher in African-Americans and postmenopausal women. Risk factors for hypertension are stress, smoking, obesity, diets high in fat, diabetes, and a family history of the disease. Treatment consists of relaxation techniques, reducing fat in the diet, exercise, weight loss, and medication to control blood pressure. Patients often do not understand the disease and its risks, thereby jeopardizing their treatment. They frequently stop taking their medication because of costs and side effects. Health care workers must realize that better education and communication will lead to more effective treatment and a higher level of drug compliance by patients.

Transient ischemic attacks (TIAs) are temporary interruptions of the blood flow (ischemia) to the brain. The cause is usually a narrowing of the carotid artery resulting from an accumulation of fat. Patients may experience strokelike symptoms such as dizziness, weakness, or temporary paralysis that lasts less than 24 hours. Approximately 50% of people who have TIAs have a major stroke within the following year.

Cerebrovascular accident (CVA), or stroke, is the sudden interruption of the blood supply to the brain, Figure 14-13. This results in a loss of oxygen to brain cells, causing impairment of the brain tissue or death. Stroke is the third leading cause of death in the United States. Based on statistics from the American Heart Association, approximately 525,000 persons in the United States suffer from stroke every year, with about 155,000 of these incidents resulting in death.

Risk factors include smoking, hypertension, heart disease, and family history. Approximately 90% of strokes are caused by blood clots. The clots become lodged in the carotid arteries, choking off the blood supply to the brain. The remaining 10% are hemorrhagic strokes, which are caused when blood vessels within the brain rupture, Figure 14-14.

Symptoms depend on which side of the brain has its blood supply interrupted. Loss of blood supply to the right cerebrum results in weakness or **hemiplegia** (paralysis) on the left side of the body. Loss of blood supply to the left side of the brain results in right-sided paralysis. Other symptoms include sudden, severe headache; dizziness; sudden loss of vision in one eye; aphasia (loss of speech); **dysphasia** (inability to say what one wishes); and coma, Figure 14-15. Death can result.

For treatment to be effective, it should begin as soon as possible and within 3 hours after the stroke. On arrival at the hospital, a computed tomography (CT) scan is done to determine if the cause is a blood clot or a ruptured blood vessel. If the cause is a blood clot, a drug such as tPA is used to dissolve the clot, restoring the blood supply to the brain.

Physicians are exploring ways to prevent strokes. Patients who have had TIAs are being examined to check the patency of the carotid artery to see if they would benefit from a balloon angioplasty. In 39% of patients who have had TIA, one aspirin per day seems to help prevent a stroke. Other drugs are currently being tested to determine whether they can prevent or reverse the damage by a stroke. To reduce risk factors, encourage patients to stop smoking, get exercise, and control hyperten-

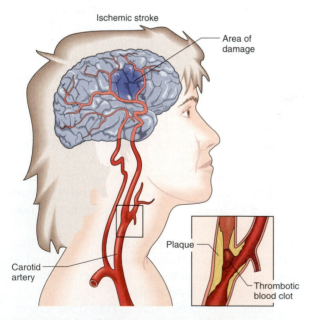

● **FIGURE 14–13** *An ischemic stroke occurs when a cerebral vessel is occluded and the brain cells go without oxygenated blood for a time.*

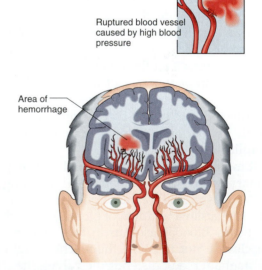

● **FIGURE 14–14** *Rupture of cerebral blood vessel results in damage to surrounding brain tissue.*

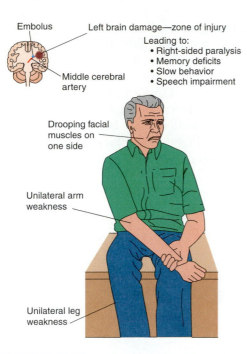

Embolus

Left brain damage—zone of injury

Leading to:
• Right-sided paralysis
• Memory deficits
• Slow behavior
• Speech impairment

Middle cerebral artery

Drooping facial muscles on one side

Unilateral arm weakness

Unilateral leg weakness

● **FIGURE 14–15** *Each area of the brain is responsible for controlling a different part of the body. When one area is affected by a stroke, the patient's symptoms correspond to the area of brain that is affected.*

sion. Be aware of the signs and symptoms of stroke and get to a hospital immediately if they occur. A stroke occurs suddenly, and a patient who wakes up paralyzed and unable to speak will be very frightened. A health care worker must be supportive of the patient.

Shock Syndrome

The body's systemic circulatory system attempts to maintain a blood flow to all the cells of the body, called **perfusion**, and thus maintain hemostasis. Whenever there is a problem, because of pump failure or circulatory problems or a loss of blood resulting from hemorrhage, the circulatory system collapses and the body cannot perfuse all the cells equally.

As a result, certain cells become **hypoperfused**. The selection of cells, tissues, and organs that are deprived of blood is predictable. The process of depriving certain organs of oxygen-rich blood to save other organs is called **shock syndrome**.

The goal of the body is to perfuse certain oxygen-dependent organs, called the **core**

MEDICAL HIGHLIGHTS

Cardiac catheterization is the insertion of a catheter, usually into the femoral artery or vein. The catheter tip is fed into the chambers of the heart. Dye is inserted and pictures are taken as the fluid moves through the chambers of the heart. The patient may experience a warm or flushing sensation as the dye moves through the circulatory system; this lasts only a few seconds. This test is useful to determine patency of the coronary blood vessels, as well as the efficiency of the structures of the heart. Patients must be asked if they have any allergies, especially to shellfish. The procedure usually only takes two hours.

Angiography is a specialized x-ray taken of a blood vessel. The procedure is similar to the cardiac catheterization. A catheter is inserted usually into the femoral artery or vein and guided into the blood vessels to be visualized. X-ray pictures are taken. This test is done to indicate the status of blood flow, collateral circulation, an aneurysm, or a hemorrhage. Patients must be asked if they have any allergies, especially to shellfish.

Stress tests determine how the physiological stress of vigorous exercise affects the heart. The test is done while a patient is exercising on a bicycle or treadmill under careful supervision. Any abnormalities may be seen on an electrocardiogram. Scientists are now reporting, however, that psychological stress may be a better determination of how the heart muscles react to stress. ■

organs, at all costs. These core organs, specifically the heart, lungs, and brain, are essential to life.

Certain other organs, such as the skin, can go without oxygen for prolonged periods. Understandably, when the body is going into shock, the first organ to be deprived of blood is the skin. When the skin is hypoperfused it becomes pale and cool to the touch.

In succession, the capillary beds of certain organ systems are shut down and the blood redirected, or shunted, to the core organs. This process of selective perfusion is called the **pecking order**, Figure 14-16.

To shut down an organ's capillary bed, the muscular bundles at the beginning of the capillaries, called the precapillary sphincter, contract, acting like a dam in a river, see Figure 14-6.

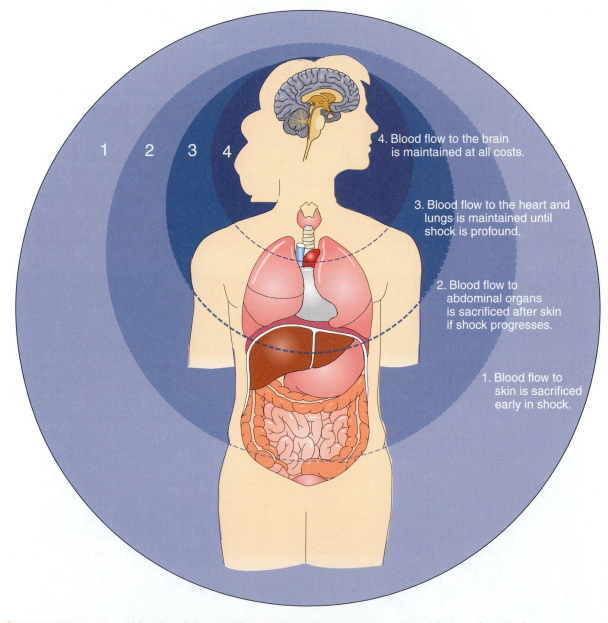

1   2   3   4

4. Blood flow to the brain is maintained at all costs.

3. Blood flow to the heart and lungs is maintained until shock is profound.

2. Blood flow to abdominal organs is sacrificed after skin if shock progresses.

1. Blood flow to skin is sacrificed early in shock.

● **FIGURE 14–16**   *If faced with hypoperfusion, the body will sacrifice the perfusion of particular organs to maintain the blood supply to others.*

STREET SMART

The efforts of EMS providers are intended to support the patient as the body attempts to compensate for hypoperfusion. The administration of high-concentration oxygen to optimize oxygenation, positioning the patient with the legs elevated above the heart (**modified Trendelenburg position**) to increase blood return to the core organs, and a blanket to increase warmth normally provided by blood in the skin are all examples of how the EMS provider can support the shock patient. ■

These precapillary sphincters are sensitive to the autonomic nervous system, as well as acid in the blood.

It is through shunting of blood to the core organs that the body can survive. By compensating for its faults, the body attempts to preserve the heart, lungs, and brain. However, there comes a point when acids in the blood build up to the point that the precapillary sphincters can no longer hold and a massive vasodilation results. The patient's blood pressure drops markedly, called **hypotension**, and the patient's core organs start to fail. This is called **decompensated shock**. Without aggressive medical treatment by the EMS provider and other health care professionals, the patient will rapidly progress to irreversible shock and death.

● REVIEW QUESTIONS

Select the letter of choice that best completes the statement.

1. The name of the blood vessel that supplies the myocardium is the:
   a. coronary artery
   b. brachial artery
   c. aorta
   d. subclavian artery

2. Special circulation that collects blood from the organs of digestion and takes it to the liver is the:
   a. coronary
   b. fetal
   c. cardiopulmonary
   d. portal

3. In fetal circulation the opening between the right atrium and the left atrium is the:
   a. umbilical artery
   b. foramen ovale
   c. umbilical vein
   d. ductus arteriosus

4. The blood vessel that carries blood away from the heart to the lungs is called the:
    a. pulmonary artery
    b. pulmonary vein
    c. coronary sinus
    d. coronary artery

5. The inner layer of the artery is called the:
    a. tunica adventitia
    b. tunica intima
    c. tunica media
    d. externa

6. The blood supply to the brain is carried by which artery?
    a. external carotid
    b. popliteal
    c. internal carotid
    d. coronary

7. The blood supply returns from the legs through which vein?
    a. saphenous
    b. external jugular
    c. superior vena cava
    d. hepatic

8. A buildup of fat in the arterial walls can cause:
    a. gangrene
    b. atherosclerosis
    c. arteriosclerosis
    d. aneurysm

9. An inflammation of the lining of the vein is called:
    a. hemorrhoid
    b. thrombus
    c. embolism
    d. phlebitis

● MATCHING

Match each term in Column A with its correct description in Column B.

Column A	Column B
_____ 1. arteries	a. small arteries that lead to capillaries
_____ 2. capillaries	b. permit blood to flow in only one direction
_____ 3. valves	c. blood vessels that carry blood back to the heart
_____ 4. veins	d. connect arterioles with venules
_____ 5. arterioles	e. large, thick, muscle-walled blood vessels that carry blood
_____ 6. aorta	away from the heart
_____ 7. atria	f. lower chambers of the heart
_____ 8. cardiac	g. loss of elasticity in the artery
_____ 9. coronary	h. referring to the lungs
_____10. hypertension	i. largest artery in body
_____11. atherosclerosis	j. traveling blood clot
_____12. aneurysm	k. upper chambers of heart
_____13. arteriosclerosis	l. enlargement of a blood vessel
_____14. pericardium	m. circulation through kidneys
_____15. portal circulation	n. blood pressure over 140/90
_____16. pulmonary	o. arteries that nourish heart
_____17. embolism	p. largest vein in body; returns to right atrium
_____18. vena cavae	q. deposit of fatty substance in the arteries
(superior and	r. pertaining to the heart
inferior)	s. goes to liver from small intestine
_____19. ventricles	t. covering of heart
	u. membrane that lines the chest cavity

●APPLYING THEORY TO PRACTICE

1. You are a red blood cell and you are leaving the arch of the aorta. Trace your journey to the right great toe. Name all the blood vessels you travel through.

2. You are a red blood cell in the left finger. You need oxygen and you must get to the lungs. Trace your journey from the finger to the lungs. Name all the blood vessels and structures you travel through.

3. You have just heard about a friend's grandmother who has arteriosclerosis of the brain. Your friend asks you to explain the disease and how her grandmother will act.

4. The fetal heart is unique. Why is it different? Describe the structures of the fetal heart that change at birth.

5. Take the pulse and blood pressure of a 20-year-old, a 40-year-old, and a 70-year-old. Compare the results. If they are different, why are they different?

6. You arrive on scene to discover a patient experiencing weakness on his right side. He appears frightened and confused. How do you reassure and help this patient? You suspect the patient is having a CVA. Explain what this means, including symptoms and treatment.

15

The Lymphatic System and Immunity

Objectives

- Describe the lymphatic system
- Define the components of the lymphatic system
- Outline the function of the lymph nodes
- Explain what is meant by *immunity*
- Identify the causative agents of AIDS
- List the symptoms of AIDS
- Describe the modes of AIDS transmission and measures used to prevent its transmission and acquisition
- Describe standard precautions
- Define the key words that relate to this chapter

Key Words

acquired immunity
acquired immuno-
    deficiency syndrome
    (AIDS)
active acquired
    immunity
adenitis
adenoids
allergen
anaphylactic shock
anaphylaxis
artificial acquired
    immunity
autoimmune disorder
autoimmunity
axillary node
barrier devices
bio-weapons
biopsy
direct contact
endotracheal tube (ET)
friable
hepatomegaly
Hodgkin's disease
human immuno-
    deficiency virus (HIV)

hypersensitivity
immunity
immunization
immunoglobulin
immunosuppressed
indirect contact
infectious mononucleosis
interstitial fluid
intubation
Kaposi's sarcoma
lingual
lumpectomy
lymph
lymphadenitis
lymphadenopathy
lymphatic system
lymph nodes
lymphedema
lymphoma
lymph vessels
natural acquired
    immunity
natural immunity
opportunistic infection
passive acquired
    immunity

(continues)

The **lymphatic system** can be considered a supplement to the circulatory system. It is composed of lymph, lymph nodes, lymph vessels, the spleen, the thymus gland, lymphoid tissue in the intestinal tract, and the tonsils. Unlike the circulatory system, it has no muscular pump or heart.

FUNCTIONS OF THE LYMPHATIC SYSTEM

The functions of the lymphatic system are as follows:

1. Lymph fluid acts as an intermediary between the blood in the capillaries and the tissue.

2. Lymph vessels transport the excess tissue fluid back into the circulatory system.

3. Lymph nodes produce lymphocytes and filter out harmful bacteria.

4. The spleen
   - produces lymphocytes and monocytes
   - acts as a reservoir for blood in case of emergency

   - works as a recycling plant, destroying and removing old red blood cells, preserving the hemoglobin

5. The thymus gland produces the T-lymphocytes necessary for the immune system.

LYMPH

Lymph is a straw-colored fluid, similar in composition to blood plasma. Plasma is what diffuses from the capillaries into the tissue spaces. Because lymph bathes the surrounding spaces between tissue cells, it is also referred to as intercellular fluid, **interstitial fluid**, or tissue fluid. Lymph is composed of water, lymphocytes, some granulocytes, oxygen, digested nutrients, hormones, salts, carbon dioxide, and urea. It contains no red blood cells or protein molecules too large to diffuse through the capillaries.

Lymph acts as an intermediary between the blood in the capillaries and the tissues. It carries digested food, oxygen, and hormones to the cells. It also carries metabolic waste products (e.g., carbon dioxide, urea wastes) away from the cells and back into the capillaries for excretion.

Because the lymphatic system has no pump, other factors operate to push lymph through the lymph vessels. The contractions of the skeletal muscles against the lymph vessels cause the lymph to surge forward into larger vessels. The breathing movements of the body also cause lymph to flow. Valves located along the lymph vessels prevent backward lymph flow.

STREET SMART

In years past, a sick patient was encouraged to stay in bed for the duration of an illness. The importance of getting a patient out of bed and moving is now recognized. This physical activity helps to circulate oxygen-enriched blood, improves the flow of disease-fighting lymph, and generally promotes healing. For these reasons many patients are encouraged to ambulate during recovery. ■

● LYMPH VESSELS

The **lymph vessels** accompany and closely parallel the veins. They form an extensive, branchlike system throughout the body that may be considered as an auxiliary to the circulatory system.

Lymph vessels are located in almost all the tissues and organs that have blood vessels. They are not found in the cuticle, nails, or hair. Lymphatic capillaries are not in the cartilage, central nervous system, epidermis, eyeball, inner ear, or spleen.

The lymph surrounding tissue cells enters small lymph vessels, Figure 15-1. These, in turn, join to form larger lymph vessels called lymphatics. They continue to unite, forming larger and larger lymphatics, until the lymph flows into one of two large, main lymphatics. They are the **thoracic duct** and the **right lymphatic duct**.

The thoracic duct, also called the **left lymphatic duct**, receives lymph from the left side of the chest, head, neck, abdominal area, and lower limbs. Lymph in the thoracic duct is carried to the left subclavian vein, and from there to the superior vena cava and the right atrium. In this manner, lymph carrying digested nutrients and other materials can return to the systemic circulation. Lymph from the right arm, right side of the head, and upper trunk enters the right lymphatic duct. From there it enters the right subclavian vein at the right shoulder, then flows into the superior vena cava, Figure 15-2.

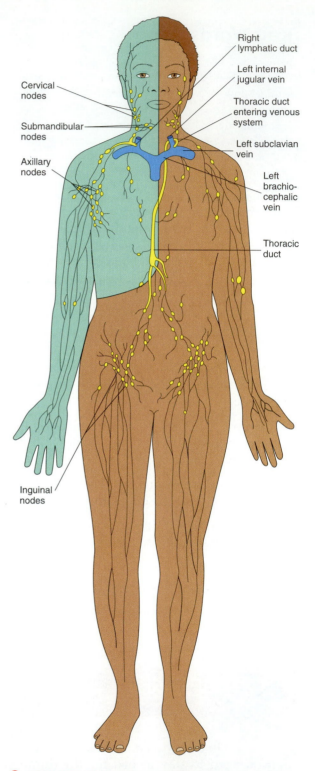

FIGURE 15–2 *Lymphatic trunks pass their lymph into two main collecting ducts, the thoracic duct and the right lymphatic duct. These ducts empty into the left and right subclavian veins, respectively.*

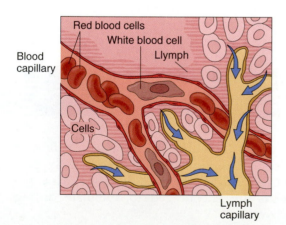

● **FIGURE 15–1** *Lymph circulation.*

Unlike the circulatory system, which travels in closed circuits through the blood vessels, lymph travels in only one direction: from the body organs to the heart. It does not flow continually through vessels forming a closed circular route.

LYMPH NODES

Lymph nodes are tiny oval-shaped structures ranging in size from the head of a pin to an almond, Figure 15-3. They are located alone or grouped in various places along the lymph vessels throughout the body. Their function is to provide a site for lymphocyte production and to serve as a filter for screening out harmful substances (such as bacteria or cancer cells) from the lymph. If the harmful substances occur in such large quantities that they cannot be destroyed by the lymphocytes before the lymph node is injured, the node becomes inflamed. This causes a swelling in the lymph glands, a condition known as **adenitis**.

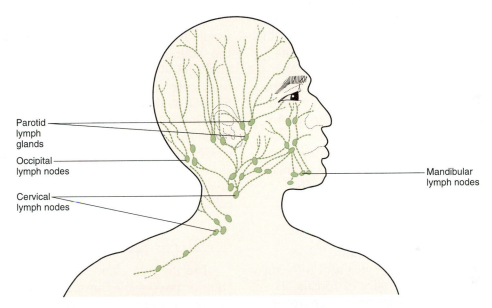

Parotid lymph glands

Occipital lymph nodes

Cervical lymph nodes

Mandibular lymph nodes

● **FIGURE 15–3** *Lymph nodes and lymph vessels found in the head.*

STREET SMART

It is a common surgical practice to remove the lymph nodes immediately adjacent to the breast during surgery for breast cancer. Often it is not apparent that the person had surgery for breast cancer, because only a small portion of the breast is removed, a procedure called a **lumpectomy**.

As a result of the lymph node removal, lymph from the arm may not drain as well and swelling in the arm, called **lymphedema**, may occur.

Advanced EMS providers are usually prohibited from starting an intravenous (IV) line in the affected limb. IV solutions often migrate into the tissue spaces. IV fluids infused into an arm of a patient with lymphedema may swell and create damage of fragile nerves and muscles.

EMS providers should also avoid taking a blood pressure measurement on the affected limb. ■

Knowledge of the location of lymph nodes is important to any health care provider. For example, when giving care to patients with severe infections of the upper leg or thigh, the lymph nodes of the groin (inguinal) and the popliteal area are checked for tenderness and swelling.

Another example of care based on knowledge may be applied to patients with breast cancer. In such cases, lymph nodes under the arms (**axillary nodes**) and near the breasts may contain entrapped cancer cells. These cancer cells are filtered out of the lymph that comes from the breast area. These lymph nodes are called **sentinel nodes**. Sentinel nodes are then examined, in a procedure called a **biopsy**, to see if they contain cancer cells and determine if the cancer has spread (metastasized).

Early detection of unusual lumps in the breast is possible through monthly self-examination and routine mammography. Early detection and treatment are vital. If discovered too late, the cancer cells may have spread (metastasized) to other areas. Cancer cells are spread by the lymphatic vessels.

TONSILS

Tonsils are masses of lymphatic tissues capable of producing lymphocytes and filtering bacteria. There are three pairs of tonsils. The most common are the palatine, which are located on the sides of the soft palate. The tonsils located in the upper part of the throat are more commonly known as **adenoids**. The third pair, **lingual**, may be found at the back of the tongue.

During childhood the tonsils frequently become infected and enlarged, causing difficulty in swallowing, severe sore throat, elevated temperature, and chills. This condition is known as **tonsillitis**. Surgery is done only in extreme cases, because the tonsils have an important role in the line of defense against infection. The tonsils get smaller in size as a person gets older.

SPLEEN

The **spleen** is a saclike mass of lymphatic tissue. It is located near the upper left area of the abdominal cavity, just beneath the diaphragm. The spleen forms lymphocytes and monocytes. Blood passing through the spleen is filtered, as in any lymph node.

The spleen stores large amounts of red blood cells. During excessive bleeding or vigorous exercise, the spleen contracts, forcing the stored red blood cells into circulation. It also destroys and removes old or fragile red blood cells and forms erythrocytes in the embryo.

THYMUS GLAND

The thymus gland is located in the upper anterior part of the thorax, above the heart. Its function is to produce T-lymphocytes. The thymus is often classified with the lymphatic organs because it is composed largely of lymphatic tissue. It is also considered an endocrine

STREET SMART

Advanced EMS providers who can perform a procedure called **intubation**, which involves inserting a plastic tube into the airway, use a tool called a laryngoscope.

The laryngoscope helps to open the airway so that the vocal cords can be visualized and an **endotracheal tube (ET)** can be passed into the lungs.

The laryngoscope is in very close proximity to the tonsils when it is in use. Swollen and infected tonsils are very fragile and the tissue may be torn, or **friable**. Tonsils that are damaged during intubation often bleed freely, making a bad situation worse. ■

gland because it secretes a hormone called thymosin, which stimulates production of lymphoid cells.

DISORDERS OF THE LYMPH SYSTEM

Lymphadenitis is an enlargement of the lymph nodes. This frequently occurs when an infection is present and the body is attempting to fight the infection. The term *swollen glands* is often used to describe this condition.

Hodgkin's disease is a form of cancer of the lymph nodes. The most common early symptom of this disease is painless swelling of the lymph nodes. Treatment of Hodgkin's disease is chemotherapy and radiation, with very good results.

Infectious mononucleosis is a disease caused by the Epstein-Barr virus. It frequently occurs in young adults and children. This disease is spread by oral contact and is frequently called the "kissing disease" or "mono." The symptoms are enlarged lymph nodes, fever, and physical and mental fatigue. There is a marked increase in the number of leukocytes. This illness is treated symptomatically (the symptoms are treated as they appear). Bed rest is essential in the treatment of "mono." In some cases the liver may be affected and hepatitis can result.

IMMUNITY

Sometimes pathogens and foreign materials succeed in penetrating a person's first line of defense, the unbroken skin. The body's ability to resist these invaders and the diseases they cause is called **immunity**. Individuals differ in their ability to resist infection. In addition, an individual's resistance varies at different times.

NATURAL AND ACQUIRED IMMUNITIES

There are two general types of immunity: natural and acquired, Table 15-1. **Natural immunity** is the immunity with which we are born. It is inherited and permanent. This inborn immunity consists of anatomical barriers, such as the unbroken skin, and cellular secretions, such as mucus and tears. Blood phagocytes and local inflammation are also part of one's natural immunity.

When the body encounters an invader, it creates a specific substance to combat and kill it. The body also tries to make itself permanently resistant to these intruders. **Acquired immunity** is the reaction that occurs as a result of exposure to these invaders. This is the immunity developed during an individual's lifetime. It may be passive or active.

Passive acquired immunity is borrowed immunity. It is acquired artificially by injecting antibodies from the blood of other individuals or animals into a person's body to protect him or her from a specific disease. The immunity produced is immediate in its effect. However, it lasts only from 3 to 5 weeks. After this period, the antibodies are inactivated by the individual's own macrophages.

Because it is immediate, passive immunity is used when a person has been exposed to a

TABLE 15-1 *Types of Immunity*

NATURAL IMMUNITY	ACQUIRED IMMUNITY	
Lasts a lifetime	Reaction as a result of exposure	
Born with it	ACTIVE: Lasts a long time.	PASSIVE: Borrowed; lasts a short time.
Inherited	Natural—Get the disease and recover, or get a mild form of disease with no symptoms with no recovery.	Natural—Transmitted from mother's placenta or mother's milk to baby.
	Artificial—Vaccination; immunization.	Artificial—Serum from another; immunoglobulin; antitoxin.

virulent disease, such as measles, tetanus, and infectious hepatitis, and has not acquired active immunity to that disease. The borrowed antibodies confer temporary protection.

A baby has temporary passive immunity derived from the mother's antibodies. These antibodies pass through the placenta to enter the baby's blood. In addition, the mother's milk also offers the baby some passive immunity. Thus a newborn infant may be protected against poliomyelitis, measles, and mumps. Measles and mumps immunity may last for nearly a year. Then the child must develop his or her own active immunity.

Active acquired immunity is preferable to passive immunity because it lasts longer. There are two types of active acquired immunity: natural acquired immunity and artificial acquired immunity. The following explains how these two types of immunity are acquired:

- **Natural acquired immunity** is the result of having had and recovered from the disease. For example, a child who has had measles and has recovered ordinarily does not get it again because the child's body has manufactured antibodies. This form of immunity is also acquired by having a series of unnoticed or mild infections. For example, a person who has had a mild form of a disease one or more times and has fought it off, sometimes unnoticed, is later immune to the disease.

- **Artificial acquired immunity** comes from being inoculated with a suitable vaccine, antigen, or toxoid. For example, a child vaccinated for measles has been given a very mild form of the disease; the child's body will thus be stimulated to manufacture its own antibodies.

Immunization is the process of increasing an individual's resistance to a particular infection by artificial means. An antigen is a substance that is injected to stimulate production of antibodies. For example, toxins produced by live bacteria, dead or weakened bacteria, viruses, and foreign proteins are examples of antigens. Toxin stimulates the body to produce antibodies, whereas the antitoxin weakens or neutralizes the effect of the toxin.

An **immunoglobulin** is a protein that functions specifically as an antibody. There are five classes of immunoglobulins: immunoglobulin G (IgG), IgM, IgA, IgD, and IgE.

Autoimmunity

Autoimmunity results when an individual's immune system goes awry. It causes the immune system to form antibodies to the body's own tissues; the antibodies destroy the tissues. This is also known as an **autoimmune disorder**.

A well-known example of this disorder is rheumatic fever. A person may get a streptococcal infection, as in a "strep" throat, that slightly alters heart tissue. Later streptococcal infections can cause further heart damage. This is because the antibodies formed against the streptococci also attack the altered heart tissue. This type of heart damage is known as rheumatic heart disease.

Hypersensitivity

Hypersensitivity occurs when the body's immune system fails to protect itself against foreign material. Instead the antibodies formed irritate certain body cells. A hypersensitive or allergic individual is generally more sensitive to certain allergens than most people.

An **allergen** is an antigen that causes allergic responses. Examples of allergens include grass, ragweed pollen, ingested food, penicillin and other antibiotics, and bee and wasp stings. Such allergens stimulate antibody formation, some of which are known as the IgE antibodies. Antibodies are found in individuals who are allergic, drug sensitive, or hypersensitive. The antibodies bind to certain cells in the body, causing a characteristic allergic reaction.

In asthma the IgE antibodies bind to the bronchi and bronchioles; in hay fever they bind to the mucous membranes of the respiratory tract and eyes, causing runny nose and itchy eyes. In hives and rashes they bind to the skin cells.

An even more severe and sometimes fatal allergic reaction is called **anaphylaxis**, or **anaphylactic shock**. It is the result of an antigen-antibody reaction that stimulates a massive secretion of histamine. Anaphylaxis can be caused by insect stings and injected drugs such as penicillin. A person suffering from anaphylaxis experiences breathing problems, headache, facial swelling, falling blood pressure, stomach cramps, and vomiting. The antidote is an injection of either adrenaline or antihistamine. If proper care is not given immediately, death may occur in minutes.

EMS providers should always ask patients whether they are allergic to any allergens or drugs. This precaution is necessary to prevent negative and sometimes fatal allergic responses to injected drugs. People with such hypersensitivities should wear a Medic Alert tag around the neck or wrist. This alerts health professionals in the event of an emergency. Such tags have saved the lives of patients rendered unconscious or otherwise unable to communicate.

COMMON DISEASES

It is important that EMS providers be knowledgeable about diseases and, perhaps more importantly, how to prevent them. Diseases are caused by microorganisms that cannot be seen by the naked eye.

These microorganisms exist everywhere in the environment. Some are dangerous to humans and can cause life-threatening illness. These microorganisms are called **pathogens**, which literally means "disease producing." Other microorganisms are harmless (benign) and may actually help prevent pathogens from multiplying.

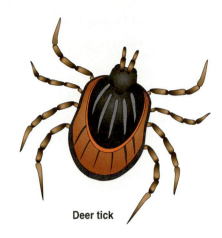

Deer tick

● **FIGURE 15–4** *Disease is spread rapidly with the help of vectors such as the tick.*

Disease can be transmitted by **direct contact**, person-to-person contact, or **indirect contact** via a contaminated object, including animals such as ticks or mosquitoes, Figure 15-4.

In every case of disease, EMS providers can protect themselves from infection by the use of **standard precautions**, described later in the chapter, and specifically with use of **barrier devices**. Barrier devices, such as gloves, gowns and masks, create an impenetrable physical barrier against disease transmission.

EMS providers can further protect themselves from disease by keeping their immunizations up to date. Table 15-2 lists several of the more common diseases that EMS providers may expect to encounter. Vaccines already exist that

STREET SMART ─

Certain antisocial individuals and groups have threatened the widespread use of certain deadly pathogens. The intent of these attacks would be to cause panic and fear among the general population. These terrorists have learned how to take certain pathogens, such as smallpox, and turn them into **bio-weapons**.

The federal government, including the Department of Justice and Department of

Defense, along with the Federal Bureau of Investigation, have developed plans to react in the case of a biological attack by a terrorist.

These plans include EMS providers as the first line of defense. EMS providers should be encouraged to seek training about these **weapons of mass destruction** to prepare. ■

TABLE 15-2 *Common Disease-Causing Organisms and Infectious Illnesses*

ORGANISM/ILLNESS	SIGNS AND SYMPTOMS	MODE OF TRANSMISSION
Adenovirus (the common cold)	Runny nose, cough, sore throat, congestion	Contact with droplets, airborne
Varicella virus (chickenpox and shingles)	Rash (itchy or painful)	Contact with open lesions, airborne
Mycobacterium tuberculosis (tuberculosis)	Cough, sweats, weight loss	Airborne
Hepatitis type A virus	Fever, nausea, vomiting, yellow skin color	Contaminated food or water
Hepatitis types B, C, D viruses	Fever, nausea, vomiting, yellow skin color, abdominal pain	Direct contact with blood or other body fluid
Herpes simplex 1 virus (oral herpes)	Blisters, usually around mouth	Contact with saliva or wound
Herpes simplex 2 virus (genital herpes)	Blisters, usually in genital area	Contact with lesions
Human immunodeficiency virus (cause of AIDS)	Multiple infections such as pneumonia, thrush, herpes	Contact with blood or body fluids
Influenza virus (causes the flu)	Cough, fever, headache, vomiting, diarrhea, general malaise	Airborne
Methicillin-resistant *Staphylococcus aureus* (MRSA)	None (a bacterium that can inhabit a wound or healthy skin)	Contact with contaminated area
Neisseria meningitidis (a bacterium, one cause of meningitis)	Fever, rash, headache, stiff neck	Airborne respiratory secretions

can provide artificial acquired immunity, but EMS providers must get vaccinated *before* the exposure. This process of vaccination, called immunization, can help strengthen EMS providers' resistance to infection from common pathogens.

At present, there is not an immunization against all pathogens. Therefore EMS providers are well advised to practice standard precautions with every patient regardless of their immunization status.

Certain diseases have become resistant to the strongest antibiotics. These "super bugs," such as methicillin-resistant *Staphylococcus* (MRSA), are particularly troublesome. The existence of these pathogens should encourage EMS providers to be even more vigilant against exposures and possible infection.

● AIDS/HIV

Between October 1980 and May 1981, five young, previously healthy homosexual men were treated for a pneumonia caused by a para-site, *Pneumocystis carinii*. Before this, P. carinii pneumonia occurred only in **immunosuppressed** (suppression of the immune system, resulting in decreased ability to fight disease and infections) patients, especially those receiving cancer therapy. At the same time, a rare and unusual blood vessel malignancy called **Kaposi's sarcoma** was being diagnosed with increasing frequency in young homosexual males. In 1981, 26 cases of Kaposi's sarcoma were diagnosed in young homosexual males. These cases were an early indication of an epidemic of a previously unknown disease. Later it was named **acquired immunodeficiency syndrome (AIDS)**. It is said to be the third leading cause of death in young people.

Causative Agent of AIDS

The causative agent of AIDS is human T-lymphotrophic virus type III (HTLV-III). The most common name is **human immunodeficiency virus (HIV)**.

HIV Statistics

HIV has become a worldwide epidemic. The World Health Organization (WHO) estimates that there are 36.1 million people living with HIV, plus another 5.3 million who were infected in the year 2000.

HIV is not just a disease of homosexual males anymore. More than 16.4 million women are infected with HIV, and more than 1.4 million children under the age of 15 are HIV positive. It is further estimated that 13.2 million children have been orphaned because of the HIV/AIDS epidemic, the majority of whom are in sub-Saharan Africa.

As of 2000, more than 21.8 million people had died from the AIDS epidemic since it began, and almost half (9 million) have been women. In 2000 alone, more than 3 million people were estimated to have died from AIDS.

In the United States, the Centers for Disease Control and Prevention (CDC) in Atlanta reported 733,374 cases of AIDS at the end of 1999. Of these cases, 82% were men and 18% were women. In the United States, homosexual white males still compose the majority of AIDS cases (74%), but that is rapidly changing. The AIDS epidemic is steadily shifting its population to heterosexual African-Americans, Hispanics, and women.

Symptoms of AIDS

AIDS is a disease that suppresses the body's natural immune system. A patient with AIDS cannot fight off cancers and most infections. The term AIDS, or acquired immunodeficiency syndrome, stands for the following:

- *A*, Acquired—The disease is not inherited or caused by any form of medication.
- *I*, Immuno—Refers to the body's natural defenses against cancers, disease, and infections.
- *D*, Deficiency—Lacking in cellular immunity.
- *S*, Syndrome—The set of diseases or conditions that are present to signal the diagnosis.

There are three possible outcomes that can result from infection with the HIV virus. One is the actual development of AIDS, the second is the development of a condition called AIDS-related complex (ARC), and the third is known as an asymptomatic infection.

Screening Tests for HIV/AIDS

The HIV antibody test detects the presence of antibodies in the blood. Antibodies to HIV viruses can be detected in the blood as soon as 2 weeks to 3 months after infection. A positive result may indicate that the person has fought off the infection and is now immune to AIDS, the person is carrying the infection but is not sick, or the person may be developing or already have AIDS.

Enzyme-linked immunosorbent (ELISA) test is an AIDS antibody indicator. It can detect antibodies for the AIDS virus but not the virus itself.

Western Blot is a follow-up test to confirm the ELISA test.

The Food and Drug Administration (FDA) has approved the sale of over-the-counter (OTC) at-home HIV testing. These tests utilize either saliva or urine and are extremely easy to use, requiring no refrigeration or special equipment. More importantly, the at-home HIV test can be as accurate as a blood test.

ACQUIRED IMMUNODEFICIENCY SYNDROME

AIDS is the most severe type of HIV infection. When a patient has AIDS, the immune system is severely suppressed. The person becomes highly susceptible to certain cancers and opportunistic infections. (An opportunistic infection can normally be fought off by a healthy individual with a normally functioning immune system but infects a person with immune dysfunction.) The opportunistic conditions include the following:

- Cancers, especially Kaposi's sarcoma and at times primary lymphoma (tumors) of the brain.

- Parasitic infections such as *P. carinii* pneumonia and toxoplasmosis.*

- Fungal infections such as candidiasis and histoplasmosis.†

- Viral infections such as cytomegalovirus (CMV) disease,‡ herpes simplex, hepatitis B, and hepatitis C.

- Persons who are HIV positive are at a higher risk for tuberculosis and syphilis.

- Women who are HIV positive are also at a higher risk for cervical cancer.

The symptoms of AIDS are often nonspecific and similar to illnesses such as the common cold or the flu. Unfortunately, these symptoms usually do not go away. They include the following:

- Prolonged fatigue that is not caused by physical exertion or other disorders

- Persistent fevers or night sweats

- A persistent, unexplained cough

- A thick, whitish hairlike coating in the throat or on the tongue

---

*Toxoplasmosis is caused by a protozoa called *Toxoplasma gondii*. Orally acquired toxoplasmosis seldom causes illness and may often go undetected, marked only by fatigue and muscle pains. Acute toxoplasmosis is rare. Symptoms range from fever, **lymphadenopathy** (lymph node enlargement), muscle fatigue, and pain to cerebral infection. Its symptoms can mimic aseptic meningitis, hepatitis, myocarditis, or pneumonia, depending on the site of the parasite.

†Histoplasmosis is an infection caused by the fungus *Histoplasma capsulatum*. The indications range from a mild respiratory infection to more severe symptoms such as fever, anemia, **hepatomegaly** (liver enlargement), **splenomegaly** (spleen enlargement), leukopenia (reduction of the number of white blood cells in the peripheral blood), pulmonary lesions, gastrointestinal ulcerations, and suprarenal necrosis.

‡CMV is a disease that is particularly severe in immunosuppressed persons, especially those with AIDS. Symptoms range from hepatitis and mononucleosis to pneumonia.

- Easy bruising or unexplained bleeding

- Recent appearance of discolored or purplish lesions of the mucous membranes or skin that do not go away and slowly increase in size

- Chronic diarrhea

- Shortness of breath

- Unexplained lymphadenopathy (swollen glands) that has persisted for more than 3 months

- Unexplained weight loss of 10 or more pounds in less than 2 months

Incubation Period. The incubation period (the period between becoming infected and the actual development of the disease symptoms) for AIDS is quite long, ranging from 1 month to 12 years. The exact number of people who are HIV positive and later develop the disease is still an unknown.

At present, there is no cure for AIDS. However, the opportunistic infections can be treated. Several antiretroviral drugs are being used on persons with AIDS in the United States and Europe. Other doctors and health care professionals are treating patients with only minimal symptoms early in the onset of their disease to see if more serious symptoms can be prevented. There is no known vaccine at present. The most common treatment is with AZT or similar drugs that help to prevent the HIV virus from duplicating itself. They act by slowing down the destruction of T-lymphocytes, producing a stronger immune response from the body. In 1996, clinical trials demonstrated that protease inhibitors used with AZT can reduce the virus to a level that the immune system can handle.

AIDS-Related Complex

An individual can contract the HIV virus and develop other conditions, but not AIDS itself. These conditions are called AIDS-related complex. Symptoms range from chronic diarrhea to chronic lymphadenopathy to unexplained weight loss. Some individuals with ARC develop a life-threatening opportunistic infection; when this occurs, the person is then said to have AIDS.

STREET SMART

Questions regarding breach of patient confidentiality and a patient's right to privacy make documentation of HIV/AIDS status on a patient care report (PCR) inadvisable unless the EMS provider has permission from the patient, medical control, or county and state health authorities.

Although documentation of a patient's symptoms is always important, documentation of HIV/AIDS status is unnecessary as long as all health care providers practice standard precautions. ■

Asymptomatic Infection

Some people who have been infected with the HIV virus do not develop any symptoms. These are known as asymptomatic infections and occur with all viruses; AIDS is no exception. Only long-term follow-up studies of infected, asymptomatic people will show whether or not they will later develop AIDS or ARC.

High-Risk Groups for AIDS

The following individuals are at the highest risk of contracting AIDS:

- Homosexual and bisexual men with multiple sexual partners
- Male and female IV drug users who share needles and syringes
- Infants born to persons who are HIV positive
- Persons who may have received blood or blood products before all blood banks were required to test for the HIV virus

This disease is now more prevalent in heterosexuals, and there has been an increase in the number of teenagers who are HIV positive.

Transmission of AIDS

The transmission of the HIV virus occurs in three ways:

1. Through sexual intercourse in which semen enters the body (about 75% of the adults in the United States who have AIDS contracted it through sexual intercourse)

2. Through sharing of hypodermic needles among IV drug users—infected blood is injected into the body (accounts for 17% to 25% of the AIDS cases in the United States)

3. Through an infected mother to her unborn or newborn infant in utero or at birth

Transmission of the HIV virus through transfusion of blood or blood products has been almost eliminated. This is possible because blood banks now test all blood donors to determine whether they have been exposed to the HIV virus. Also, federal guidelines recommend that individuals in the high-risk group do not donate blood or blood products. So far, it seems unlikely that AIDS can be contracted through casual contact. The virus cannot be contracted through air, feces, food, urine, or water. The virus is fragile outside the body and cannot survive. Even close nonsexual contact such as coughing, sneezing, embracing, shaking hands, and sharing eating utensils cannot spread the virus.

STANDARD PRECAUTIONS

Standard precautions are guidelines to be used during routine patient care and cleaning duties, Table 15-3 and Figure 15-5.

TABLE 15-3 *Standard Precautions for Infection Control*

Wash Hands (plain soap)
Wash after touching **blood, body fluids, secretions, excretions**, and **contaminated items**. Wash immediately **after gloves are removed** and **between patient contacts**. Avoid transfer of microorganisms to other patients or environments.

Wear Gloves
Wear when touching **blood, body fluids, secretions, excretions**, and **contaminated items**. Put on **clean** gloves just **before touching mucous membranes** and **nonintact skin**. Change gloves between tasks and procedures on the same patient after contact with material that may contain high concentrations of microorganisms. Remove gloves promptly after use, before touching noncontaminated items and environmental surfaces, and before going to another patient, and wash hands immediately to avoid transfer of microorganisms to other patients or environments.

Wear Mask and Eye Protection or Face Shield
Protect mucous membranes of the eyes, nose, and mouth during procedures and patient-care activities that are likely to generate **splashes** or **sprays** of **blood, body fluids, secretions**, or **excretions**.

Wear Gown
Protect skin and prevent soiling of clothing during procedures that are likely to generate **splashes** or **sprays** of **blood, body fluids, secretions**, or **excretions**. Remove a soiled gown as promptly as possible and wash hands to avoid transfer of microorganisms to other patients or environments.

Patient Care Equipment
Handle used patient care equipment soiled with **blood, body fluids, secretions**, or **excretions** in a manner that prevents skin and mucous membrane exposures, contamination of clothing, and transfer of microorganisms to other patients or environments. Ensure that reusable equipment is not used for the care of another patient until it has been appropriately cleaned and reprocessed and that single-use items are properly discarded.

Linen
Handle, transport, and process used linen soiled with **blood, body fluids, secretions**, or **excretions** in a manner that prevents exposures and contamination of clothing and avoids transfer of microorganisms to other patients or environments.

Use **resuscitation devices** as an alternative to mouth-to-mouth resuscitation.

(Courtesy of BREVIS Corporation)

Handwashing

Handwashing is the single most effective way to prevent infection.

1. Wash hands after touching blood, body fluids, secretions, excretions, and contaminated items, whether or not gloves are worn.

2. Wash hands immediately after removing gloves, between patient contacts, and when otherwise indicated to avoid transfer of microorganisms to other patients or the surrounding environment.

3. Use a plain soap for handwashing.

4. Wash hands for a minimum of 10 seconds.

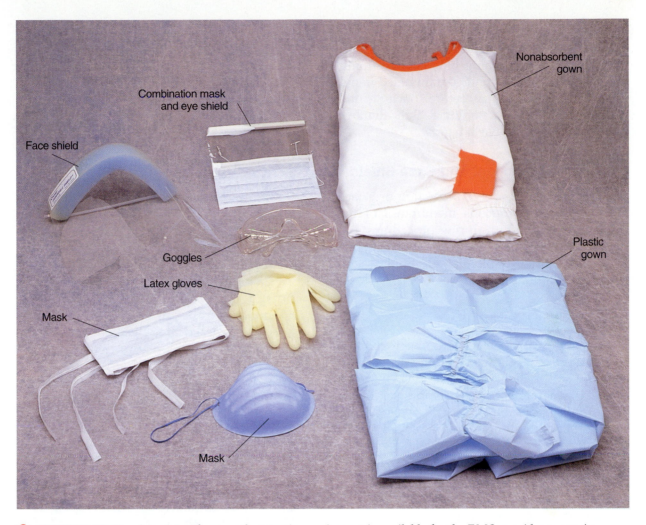

- **FIGURE 15–5** *A variety of personal protective equipment is available for the EMS provider to use in infection control.*

![STREET SMART]

Many EMS providers, after routinely wearing latex gloves, have developed an allergy to the latex. The allergy can be as mild as a skin irritation, called contact dermatitis, or an acute, life-threatening anaphylaxis.

However, EMS providers should *not* give up wearing gloves. There are nonlatex vinyl gloves available that perform as well as latex gloves.

EMS providers should also be aware that some patients are also allergic to latex. Special latex-free equipment, as well as nonlatex gloves, should be used by EMS providers while caring for these patients. ■

Gloves

Wear gloves (clean, nonsterile gloves are adequate) when touching blood, body fluids, secretions, excretions, and contaminated items. Put on clean gloves just before touching mucous membranes and nonintact skin. Remove gloves after use and wash hands.

Mask, Eye Protection, and Face Shield

Wear a mask and eye protection or a face shield to protect mucous membranes of the eyes, nose, and mouth during procedures and patient care activities that are likely to generate splashes or sprays of blood, body fluids, secretions, or excretions.

Gown

Wear a clean, nonsterile gown to protect skin and prevent soiling of clothing during procedures and patient care activities that are likely to generate splashes or sprays of blood, body fluids, secretions, or excretions, or cause soiling of clothing. Remove a soiled gown promptly and wash hands to avoid transfer of microorganisms to other patients or the surrounding environment.

Patient Care Equipment

Handle used patient care equipment soiled with blood, body fluids, secretions, or excretions in a manner that prevents skin and mucous membrane exposures, contamination of clothing, and transfer of microorganisms to other patients and environments. Be certain that reusable equipment is properly cleaned and reprocessed before it is used on another patient. Single-use items must be discarded properly.

Linens

Handle, transport, and process used linen soiled with blood, body fluids, secretions, or excretions in a manner that prevents skin and mucous membrane exposure, contamination of clothing, and transfer of microorganisms to other patients and environments.

Occupational Health and Bloodborne Pathogens

1. Take care to prevent injuries from needles, scalpels, and other sharp instruments or devices when handling them after procedures, when cleaning used instruments, and when disposing of used needles. CAUTION: never recap used needles or use any technique that involves directing the point of the needle toward any part of the body. Place used disposable syringes, needles, scalpels, and other sharp items in appropriate puncture-resistant containers located as close as practical to the area in which the items were used, Figure 15-6.

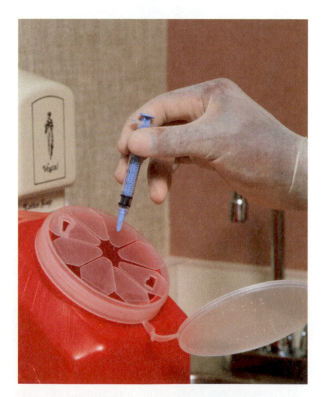

● **FIGURE 15–6**   *Sharp objects, such as IV needles, must be properly disposed of immediately.*

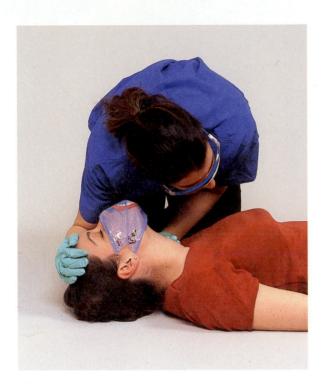

2. Use mouthpieces, resuscitation bags, or other ventilation devices as an alternative to mouth-to-mouth resuscitation methods, Figure 15-7.

Patient Placement

Place a patient who contaminates the environment or who does not assist in maintaining appropriate hygiene or environmental precautions in a private room or other relatively isolated area, Table 15-4 and Table 15-5.

TABLE 15-5 *Common EMS Tasks and Personal Protective Equipment*

TASK	GLOVES	MASK	EYEWEAR	GOWN
Taking pulse rate	X			
Measuring blood pressure	X			
Controlling bleeding (minimal visible blood)	X			
Giving an injection	X			
Inserting oropharyngeal/ nasopharyngeal airway	X	X	X	
Suctioning	X	X	X	
Intubation	X	X	X	
Arterial bleeding control	X	X	X	X
Assisting childbirth	X	X	X	X
Disinfecting equipment	X	X	X	X

● **FIGURE 15–7**   *Barrier devices give the EMS provider another margin of safety when performing CPR.*

TABLE 15-4 *Common Chief Complaints and Personal Protective Equipment*

CHIEF COMPLAINT	GLOVES	MASK	EYEWEAR	GOWN
Fever	X	X		
Rash	X	X		
Seizures	X	X		
Coughing	X	X	X	
Bleeding wounds	X	X	X (if spurting)	X (if spurting)
Neck stiffness	X	X		
Vomiting	X	X		

● REVIEW QUESTIONS

Select the letter of the choice that best completes the statement.

1. Lymph fluid may also be called:
   a. plasma
   b. blood
   c. interstitial
   d. serum

2. The function of the lymph nodes is to produce:
   a. platelets
   b. lymphocytes
   c. basophils
   d. erythrocytes

3. The name of the vessel through which lymph finally rejoins general circulation is the:
   a. thoracic duct
   b. left lymphatic duct
   c. superior vena cava
   d. right lymphatic duct

4. The organ composed of lymphatic tissue that filters blood and produces white blood cells is called the:
   a. spleen
   b. liver
   c. kidney
   d. stomach

5. The ability of the body to resist disease is known as:
   a. sensitivity
   b. resistance
   c. immunity
   d. noninfection

● MATCHING

Match each term in Column A with its correct description in Column B.

Column A	Column B
_____ 1. natural immunity	a. immunization
_____ 2. acquired active immunity	b. immune globulin
_____ 3. acquired passive immunity	c. inherited
_____ 4. acquired active artificial	d. obtained through mother's milk
_____ 5. acquired passive artificial	e. have the disease and recover

● COMPLETION

Complete the following sentences:

1. A person who is highly sensitive to an allergen is said to be _____.

2. An antigen that causes an allergic response is an _____.

3. A fatal allergic response is _____.

4. A cancer of the lymph nodes is called _____.

5. A mass of lymph tissue in the throat is called _____.

●APPLYING THEORY TO PRACTICE

1. A family member is entering school and must have his immunizations complete. Explain to the parent what this means.

2. Your friend says, "I think I have the kissing disease. What is it?" Explain the disease to your friend and how the disease is transmitted and treated.

3. Your agency is putting on an educational forum on AIDS for a local community group. Outline the topic; include description of the disease, causes, high-risk groups, treatment, confidentiality, standard precautions, and how the disease impacts the patient, family, and society.

4. You go to the doctor because you have swollen glands and a temperature of 101° F. The doctor states that the body is fighting an infection, which is causing your swollen glands. What does this mean?

5. A woman is complaining of swelling in her left arm after a mastectomy on her left breast. She also had lymph nodes removed for testing. Explain to the patient why the swelling has occurred.

16 Respiratory System

Objectives

- Describe the functions of the respiratory system
- Describe the structures and functions of the organs of respiration
- Explain breathing and the respiratory process
- Discuss how breathing is controlled by neural and chemical factors
- Discuss respiratory disorders
- Define the key words that relate to this chapter

Key Words

alveolar sacs (alveoli)
anterior nares
agonal respiration
apnea
asphyxia
aspiration
asthma
atelectasis
auscultation
bag-valve-mask (BVM) device
bronchiectasis
bronchitis
bronchoscopy
cancer of the larynx
cancer of the lungs
cellular respiration (oxidation)
Cheyne-Stokes
chronic obstructive pulmonary disease (COPD)
cilia
cricoid cartilage
cricoid pressure

cricothyrotomy
dead space
deep vein thrombosis (DVT)
diphtheria
dyspnea
emphysema
eupnea
expiration
expiratory reserve volume (ERV)
external respiration
functional residual capacity
glottis
Hering-Brewer reflex
hyperpnea
hyperventilation
hypopharynx
hypoxic drive
influenza
inspiration
inspiratory reserve volume (IRV)
internal respiration

(continues)

INTRODUCTION TO THE RESPIRATORY SYSTEM

The countless millions of cells that make up the human body require a constant supply of energy. This energy is required for cells to perform their many chemical activities, which maintain the body's homeostasis. For this to occur, energy-rich nutrient (fuel) molecules must be transported to the cells. Oxygen facilitates the release of energy stored in nutrient molecules. It must be in constant supply to the body. Without oxygen, a human being can live no more than a few minutes.

FUNCTIONS OF THE RESPIRATORY SYSTEM

1. The respiratory system provides the structures for the exchange of oxygen and carbon dioxide in the body through respiration, which is subdivided into external respiration, internal respiration, and cellular respiration, Figure 16-1.

2. The respiratory system is responsible for the production of sound; the larynx contains the vocal cords. When air is expelled from the lungs, it passes over the vocal cords and produces sound.

Respiration

External respiration is also known as breathing, or ventilation. This is the exchange of oxygen and carbon dioxide among the lungs, the body, and the outside environment. The breathing process consists of inspiration (inhalation) and expiration (exhalation). On inspiration, air enters the body and is warmed, moistened, and filtered as it passes to the air sacs of the lungs (alveoli). The concentration of oxygen in the alveoli is greater than in the bloodstream. Oxygen diffuses from the area of greater concentration (the alveoli) to an area of lesser concentration (the bloodstream), then into the red blood cells. At the same time, the concentration of carbon dioxide in the blood is greater than in the alveoli, so it diffuses from the blood to the alveoli. Expiration expels the carbon dioxide from the alveoli of the lungs. Some water vapor is also given off in the process.

Internal respiration includes the exchange of carbon dioxide and oxygen between the cells and the lymph surrounding them, plus the oxidative process of energy in the cells. After inspiration, the alveoli are rich with oxygen and transfer the oxygen into the blood. The resulting greater concentration of oxygen in the blood diffuses the oxygen into the tissue cells. At the same time, the cells build up a higher carbon dioxide concentration. The concentration increases to a point that exceeds the level in the blood. This causes the carbon dioxide to diffuse out of the cells and into the blood, where it is then carried away to be eliminated.

Deoxygenated blood, produced during internal respiration, carries carbon dioxide in the form of bicarbonate ions (HCO_3^-). These ions are transported by both blood plasma and red blood cells. Exhalation expels carbon dioxide

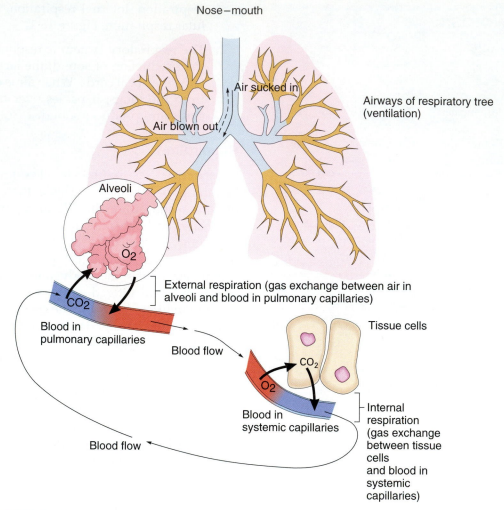

Nose—mouth

Air sucked in

Airways of respiratory tree
(ventilation)

Air blown out

Alveoli

O_2

CO_2

External respiration (gas exchange between air in
alveoli and blood in pulmonary capillaries)

Blood in
pulmonary capillaries

Blood flow

Tissue cells

CO_2

O_2

Blood in
systemic capillaries

Internal
respiration
(gas exchange
between tissue
cells
and blood in
systemic
capillaries)

Blood flow

● **FIGURE 16–1** *Respiration.*

from the red blood cells and the plasma; it is released from the body in the following manner:

$$H_2CO_3 = H_2O + CO_2$$

(Bicarbonate ions decompose
to form water and carbon dioxide)

Cellular respiration, or **oxidation**, involves the use of oxygen to release energy
stored in nutrient molecules such as glucose.
This chemical reaction occurs within the cells.
Just as wood gives off energy in the form of
heat and light when burned (oxidized), so does
food give off energy when it is burned, or oxidized, in the cells. Much of this energy is released in the form of heat to maintain body
temperature. Some of it, however, is used directly by the cells for such work as contraction

of muscle cells. It is also used to carry on other
vital processes.

Food gives off waste products when oxidized, including carbon dioxide and water vapor. These waste products are carried away
through the process of internal respiration.

● RESPIRATORY ORGANS AND STRUCTURES

Figure 16-2 illustrates how air moves into
the lungs through several passageways. The
following structures are included: nasal cavity,
pharynx, larynx, trachea, bronchi, bronchioles,
alveoli, lungs, pleura, and mediastinum.

The loss of an airway, either upper or lower,
is a significant contributing cause in the majority

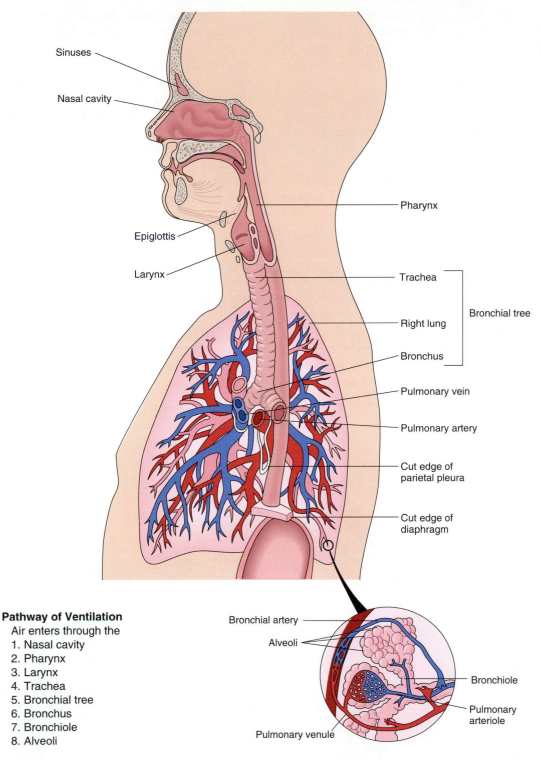

Pathway of Ventilation
Air enters through the
1. Nasal cavity
2. Pharynx
3. Larynx
4. Trachea
5. Bronchial tree
6. Bronchus
7. Bronchiole
8. Alveoli

● **FIGURE 16–2**   *Respiratory organs and structures.*

of deaths. For this reason, the airway has special significance to the EMS provider. Countless hours are spent learning how to open, clear, and maintain the airway; a common mantra is *open, assess, suction, secure.*

Advanced EMS providers learn and practice special airway techniques, including endotracheal intubation, as well as assisting the patient's ventilation with a **bag-valve-mask (BVM) device.**

All this effort is spent trying to ensure adequate airflow from the environment to the lungs.

THE NASAL CAVITY

In humans, air enters the respiratory system through two oval openings in the nose. They are called the nostrils, or **anterior nares**. From there, air enters the nasal cavity, which is divided into right and left chambers, or smaller cavities, by a partition known as the **nasal septum**. Both cavities are lined with mucous membranes.

Protruding into the nasal cavity are three **turbinate**, or nasal conchae bones. These three scroll-like bones (superior, middle, and inferior concha) divide the large nasal cavity into three narrow passageways. The turbinates increase the surface area of the nasal cavity, causing turbulence in the flowing air. This causes the air to move in various directions before exiting the nasal cavity. As it moves through the nasal cavity, dust and dirt particles are filtered from the air by the mucous membranes lining the conchal and nasal cavity. The air is also moistened by the mucus and warmed by blood vessels that supply the nasal cavity. At the front of the nares are small hairs, or **cilia**, which entrap and prevent the entry of larger dirt particles. By the time the air reaches the lungs, it has been warmed, moistened, and filtered. Nerve endings providing the sense of smell (**olfactory nerves**) are located in the mucous membrane, in the upper part of the nasal cavity.

The **sinuses**, named frontal, maxillary, sphenoid, and ethmoid, are cavities of the skull

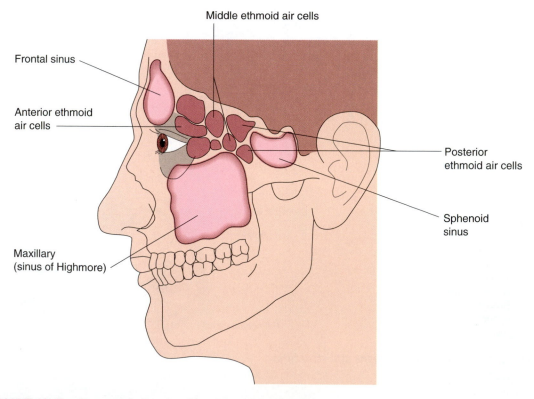

Middle ethmoid air cells

Frontal sinus

Anterior ethmoid air cells

Posterior ethmoid air cells

Sphenoid sinus

Maxillary (sinus of Highmore)

FIGURE 16–3   *Paranasal sinuses, side cross-sectional view.*

in and around the nasal region, Figure 16-3. Short ducts connect the sinuses with the nasal cavity. Mucous membrane lines the sinuses and helps to warm and moisten air passing through them. The sinuses also give resonance to the voice. The unpleasant voice heard in a person suffering from a nasal cold results from the blockage of sinuses.

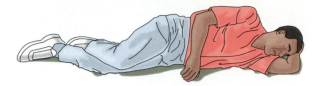

● **FIGURE 16–4** *The recovery position allows natural drainage of airway secretions.*

● THE PHARYNX

After air leaves the nasal cavity it enters the pharynx, commonly known as the throat. The pharynx serves as a common passageway for air and food. It is about 5 inches long and can be subdivided into three sections. The uppermost section, just after the nasal cavity, is the nasopharynx. The left and right eustachian tubes open directly into the nasopharynx, connecting each middle ear with the nasopharynx. Because of this connection, nasopharyngeal inflammation can lead to middle ear infections. The oropharynx lies behind the mouth. The lowest portion is known as the laryngopharynx. Air travels down the pharynx on its way to the lungs; food travels this route on its way to the stomach.

The laryngopharynx, also called the hypopharynx, is the last area that can be seen in the back of the throat without special instrumentation. For this reason, this is the farthest point that a basic EMS provider is allowed to probe.

The gag reflex is located in the posterior wall of the throat in the hypopharynx. Irritation of this area, stimulating the hypoglossal nerve, can cause retching and vomiting. A patient who is stimulated to vomit may accidentally breath in the vomitus, called aspiration.

Aspiration can lead to a total blockage of the airway, or asphyxia. Uncorrected, an aspiration with complete airway obstruction that results in asphyxia can quickly deteriorate into respiratory arrest and then cardiopulmonary arrest.

Aspiration can also lead to an inflammation of the lungs, called pneumonia. Pneumonia, as a disease, is one of the top 10 causes of death in the United States, with almost 92,000 cases in 1998 alone.

However, aspiration-related asphyxia and aspiration pneumonia can be prevented. To prevent this problem, an unconscious patient should be placed in the recovery position, Figure 16-4. The recovery position allows free drainage of the airway with minimum risk of aspiration.

When food is swallowed, a cartilage "lid" called the epiglottis is pushed by the base of the tongue to cover the opening into the larynx. At the same time, the larynx moves up to help close the opening. With the opening to the larynx covered by the epiglottis, food is directed down the esophagus into the stomach, Figure 16-5.

Above the epiglottis and proximal to the hyoid bone is a space called the vallecula. A special tool called a laryngoscope blade is placed in the vallecula to help the advanced

CHANGES OF AGING

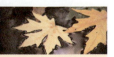

The pediatric epiglottis is different than an adult's. Smaller and relatively more anterior, the pediatric epiglottis is w-shaped, like the Greek letter *omega* (ω). ■

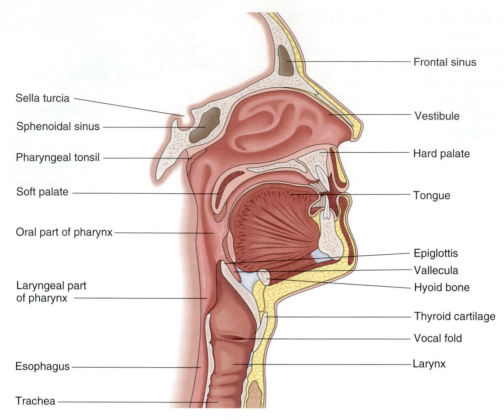

Frontal sinus

Sella turcia

Sphenoidal sinus

Pharyngeal tonsil

Soft palate

Oral part of pharynx

Laryngeal part of pharynx

Esophagus

Trachea

Vestibule

Hard palate

Tongue

Epiglottis

Vallecula

Hyoid bone

Thyroid cartilage

Vocal fold

Larynx

● **FIGURE 16–5** *Sagittal section of the upper airway.*

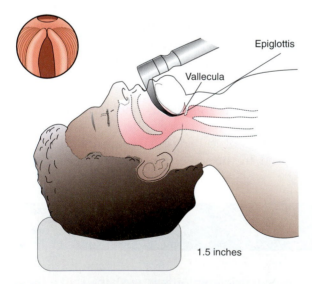

Epiglottis

Vallecula

1.5 inches

● **FIGURE 16–6** *The Macintosh blade is designed to fit into the vallecula and lift the tongue to allow a view of the vocal cords.*

EMS provider visualize the vocal cords before endotracheal intubation, Figure 16-6.

● THE LARYNX

The larynx, or voice box, is a triangular chamber found below the pharynx. The laryngeal walls are composed of nine fibrocartilaginous plates. The largest of these plates is commonly called the "Adam's apple." During puberty, the vocal cords become larger in the male, making the Adam's apple more prominent in men.

The larynx is lined with a mucous membrane, continuous from the pharyngeal lining above to the tracheal lining below. Within the larynx are the characteristic vocal cords. There is a space between the vocal cords known as the glottis. When air is expelled from the lungs, it passes the vocal cords. This sets off a vibration, creating sound. The action of the lips and tongue on this sound produces speech.

STREET SMART

There is one cartilage ring in the airway that is different than the others. The cricoid cartilage, located just inferior to the larynx, is a complete ring.

Because of its unique O shape, the cricoid cartilage can be compressed externally by an EMS provider and it will effectively close off the esophagus, located behind the trachea, Figure 16-7. This procedure, called cricoid pressure, may prevent aspiration after passive vomiting (regurgitation). It may also aid in the visualization of the vocal cords during intubation. ■

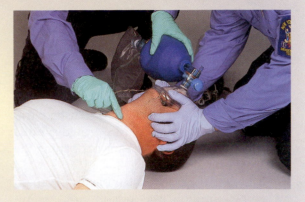

● **FIGURE 16–7** *Notice that the EMS provider ventilating the patient is using a free hand to apply some gentle cricoid pressure to the patient.*

● THE TRACHEA

The trachea, or windpipe, is a tubelike passageway some 11.2 centimeters (about 4.5 inches) in length. It extends from the larynx, passes in front of the esophagus, and continues to form the two bronchi (one for each lung). The walls of the trachea are composed of alternate bands of membranes, and 15 to 20 C-shaped rings of hyaline cartilage. These rings are virtually noncollapsible, keeping the trachea open for the passage of oxygen into the lungs. However, the trachea can be obstructed by large pieces of food, tumorous growths, or the swelling of inflamed lymph nodes in the neck.

The walls of the trachea are lined with both mucous membrane and ciliated epithelium. The function of the mucus is to entrap inhaled dust particles; the cilia then sweep the dust-laden mucus upward to the pharynx. Coughing and expectoration dislodge and eliminate the dust-laden mucus from the pharynx.

An upper airway obstruction, from a tumor, for example, may require that an artificial airway be created for the patient. The surgical procedure in which an opening in made in the trachea is called a tracheostomy. When the tra-

chea must be permanently diverted to the anterior neck, a surgical procedure called a laryngectomy is performed.

In both cases an opening is created in the front of the throat and the patient breathes through that opening instead of through the mouth. The patient with either a tracheostomy or a laryngectomy does not have the protection of the upper airway and is therefore prone to mucous plugs and airway obstructions, Figure 16-8.

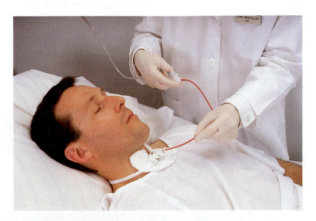

● **FIGURE 16–8** *Tracheostomy tubes often become clogged with mucus and can be suctioned gently, using a French catheter.*

STREET SMART

EMS providers are occasionally confronted with an airway that cannot be controlled by routine measures such as manual external manipulation, for example a head-tilt, chin-lift maneuver, or intubation. Examples include a firmly lodged foreign body airway obstruction or a crushed trachea. In those cases the EMS provider must resort to more dramatic means of opening the airway for breathing.

Access to the trachea is typically obtained by going through the cricothyroid membrane, and an opening is made in the anterior neck for the passage of airway. This procedure is called a cricothyrotomy.

A cricothyrotomy can be performed either with a scalpel, called a surgical cricothyrotomy, or by using a needle, called a needle cricothyrotomy. Most advanced EMS providers prefer to perform a needle cricothyrotomy because of a decreased risk of complications such as bleeding. ■

THE BRONCHI AND THE BRONCHIOLES

The lower end of the trachea divides into the right bronchus and the left bronchus. There is a slight difference between the two bronchi, the right bronchus being somewhat shorter, wider, and more vertical.

As the bronchi enter the lung, they subdivide into bronchial tubes and smaller bronchioles. The divisions are Y-shaped. The two bronchi are similar in structure to the trachea, because their walls are lined with ciliated epithelium and ringed with hyaline cartilage. However, the bronchial tubes and smaller bronchi are ringed with cartilaginous plates instead of incomplete C-shaped rings. The bronchioles lose their cartilaginous plates and fibrous tissue. Their thinner walls are made from smooth muscle and elastic tissue lined with ciliated epithelium. At the end of each bronchiole, there is an alveolar duct, which ends in clusters called alveolar sacs (alveoli).

THE ALVEOLI

The alveolar sacs consist of many alveoli and are composed of a single layer of epithelial tissue. There are approximately 500 million alveoli in the adult lung, about three times the amount necessary to sustain life. Each alveolus forming a part of the alveolar sac possesses a globular shape. Their inner surfaces are covered with a lipid material known as surfactant. The surfactant helps to stabilize the alveoli, preventing their collapse. Each alveolus is encased by a network of blood capillaries.

STREET SMART

Because of the difference in anatomy between the right and left mainstem bronchi, an advanced EMS provider who is performing an endotracheal intubation is more likely to insert the endotracheal tube (ET) into the right mainstem bronchi. Careful assessment with a stethoscope while listening to breath sounds, called auscultation, reveals whether the endotracheal tube is placed too deeply. ■

CHANGES OF AGING

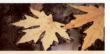

A significant difficulty a premature infant may have to overcome is the lack of surfactant. Without surfactant, the lungs do not expand properly and the infant eventually suffocates. Modern medicine has discovered a source of surfactant from an unlikely source, the cow. By injecting surfactant directly into the premature infant's lungs, the lungs can expand and the infant can breathe naturally. ■

It is through the moist walls of both the alveoli and the capillaries that rapid exchange of carbon dioxide and oxygen occurs. In the blood capillaries, carbon dioxide diffuses from the erythrocytes, through the capillary walls, into the alveoli, and is exhaled through the mouth and nose.

The opposite process occurs with oxygen, which diffuses from the alveoli into the capillaries, and from there into the erythrocytes.

● THE LUNGS

The lungs are fairly large, cone-shaped organs filling up the two lateral chambers of the thoracic cavity. They are separated from each other by the mediastinum and the heart. The upper part of the lung, underneath the collarbone, is the apex; the broad lower part is the base. Each base is concave, allowing it to fit snugly over the convex part of the diaphragm.

Lung tissue is porous and spongy because of the alveoli and the tremendous amount of air it contains. For example, if a specimen of a cow lung were placed into a tankful of water, it would float quite easily.

The right lung is larger and broader than the left because the heart inclines to the left side. The right lung is also shorter as a result of the diaphragm's upward displacement on the right to accommodate the liver. The right lung is divided by fissures (clefts) into three lobes: superior, middle, and inferior.

The left lung is smaller, narrower, and longer than its counterpart. It is subdivided into two lobes: superior and inferior.

● THE PLEURA

The lungs are covered with a thin, moist, slippery membrane made up of tough endothelial cells, or **pleura**. There are two pleural membranes. The membrane lining the lungs and dipping between the lobes is the pulmonary, or visceral pleura. Lining the thoracic cavity and the upper surface of the diaphragm is the parietal pleura. Consequently, each lung is enclosed in a double-walled sac. **Pleurisy** is an inflammation of this lining.

The space between the two pleural membranes is the pleural cavity, filled with serous fluid called **pleural fluid**. This fluid is necessary to prevent friction as the two pleural membranes rub against each other during each breath.

The pleural cavity may on occasion fill up with an enormous quantity of serous fluid. This occurs when there is an inflammation of the pleura. The increased pleural fluid compresses and sometimes even causes parts of the lung to collapse. This obviously makes breathing extremely difficult. To alleviate the pressure, a **thoracentesis** may be performed. This procedure entails the insertion of a hollow, tubelike instrument through the thoracic cavity and into the pleural cavity to drain the excess fluid.

Another disorder that can affect the pleural cavity is **pneumothorax**. This condition occurs if there is a buildup of air within the pleural cavity on one side of the chest. The excess air increases pressure on the lung, causing it to collapse. Breathing is not possible with a collapsed lung, but the unaffected lung can still continue the breathing process.

STREET SMART

Causes of a pneumothorax can roughly be divided into medical and trauma. Medical causes include a spontaneous pneumothorax. Certain people, particularly tall, thin males, have defects on their lung surface, called blebs, that unexpectedly rupture, thereby creating a pneumothorax.

Other people with the lung disease emphysema also develop these imperfections and are therefore prone to a spontaneous pneumothorax.

In cases of severe chest trauma, a broken rib can puncture the lung, resulting in a pneumothorax.

In some cases the steady buildup of air in the chest cavity from a pneumothorax can cause a dangerous condition called a tension pneumothorax.

In a tension pneumothorax the built-up air compresses the heart, as well as kinking off the great vessels, stopping blood flow to the heart in the same way kinking a garden hose stops water flow. The result is that insufficient blood reaches the heart, the heart cannot pump effectively against the pressure surrounding it, and, untreated, the blood flow from the heart is decreased, resulting in hypoperfusion.

Advanced EMS providers are taught a special procedure called a needle decompression that can release the air trapped in the chest cavity and alleviate the pressure crushing the heart and great vessels.

A long hollow needle is placed into the chest cavity and the trapped air is allowed to escape. A needle decompression removes trapped air quickly and allows the injured lung to re-expand and the heart to beat normally again. ■

THE MEDIASTINUM

The mediastinum, also called the inter-pleural space, is situated between the lungs along the median plane of the thorax. It extends from the sternum to the vertebrae. The mediastinum contains the thoracic viscera: the thymus gland, heart, aorta and its branches, pulmonary arteries and veins, superior and inferior vena cava, esophagus, trachea, thoracic duct, and lymph nodes and vessels.

MECHANICS OF BREATHING

Pulmonary ventilation (breathing) of the lungs is due to changes in pressure that occur within the chest cavity. The normal pressure within the pleural space is always negative, less than atmospheric pressure. The negative pressure helps to keep the lungs expanded. The variation in pressure is brought about by cellular respiration and mechanical breathing movements.

THE BREATHING PROCESS

Pulmonary ventilation allows the exchange of oxygen between the alveoli and erythrocyte, and eventually between the erythrocyte and cells.

Inhalation/Inspiration

There are two groups of intercostal muscles: external and internal. Their muscle fibers cross each other at an angle of 90 degrees. During inhalation, or inspiration, the external intercostals lift the ribs upward and outward, Figure 16-9. This increases the volume of the thoracic cavity. Simultaneously the sternum rises, along with the ribs, and the dome-shaped diaphragm contracts and becomes flattened, moving downward. As the diaphragm moves downward, pressure is exerted on the abdominal viscera. This causes the anterior muscles to protrude slightly, increasing the space within the chest cavity in a vertical direction. As a result, there is

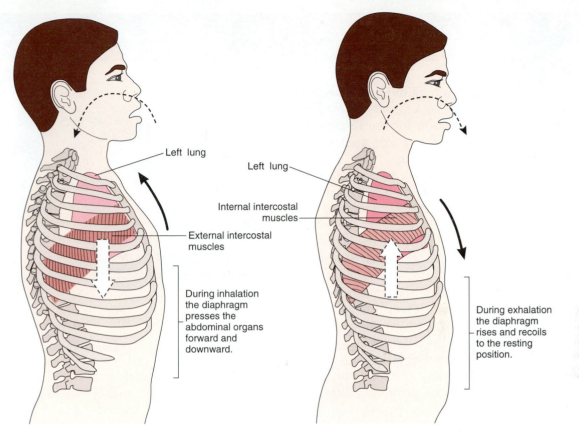

Left lung

Left lung

Internal intercostal muscles

External intercostal muscles

During inhalation the diaphragm presses the abdominal organs forward and downward.

During exhalation the diaphragm rises and recoils to the resting position.

● **FIGURE 16–9** *Mechanics of breathing—inhalation and exhalation.*

a decrease in pressure. Because atmospheric pressure is now greater, air rushes in all the way down to the alveoli, resulting in inhalation.

Exhalation/Expiration

In exhalation, or **expiration**, just the opposite takes place. Expiration is a passive process; all the contracted intercostal muscles and the diaphragm relax. The ribs move down, the diaphragm moves up. In addition, the surface tension of the fluid lining the alveoli reduces the elasticity of the lung tissue and causes the alveoli to collapse. This action, coupled with the relaxation of contracted respiratory muscles, relaxes the lungs; the space within the thoracic cavity decreases, thus increasing the internal pressure. Increased pressure forces air from the lungs, resulting in exhalation.

The lungs are extremely elastic. They are able to change capacity as the size of the thoracic cavity is altered. This ability is known as compliance. When lung tissue becomes dis-

eased and fibrotic, the lung's compliance decreases and ventilation decreases.

Respiratory Movements and Frequency of Respiration

The rhythmic movements of the rib cage when air is drawn in and expelled from the lungs make up the respiratory movements. Inspiration and expiration combined is counted as one respiratory movement. Thus the normal rate in quiet breathing for an adult is about 14 to 20 breaths per minute. This rate is changeable. The respiratory rate can be increased by muscular activity and increased body temperatures and in certain pathological disorders such as hyperthyroidism. It changes with sex, females having the higher rate at 16 to 20 breaths per minute. Age also changes the respiratory rate. For example, at birth the rate is 40 to 60 breaths per minute; at 5 years, 24 to 26 breaths. The body's position also affects the respiration rate. When the body is asleep or

A patient's breathing may become difficult, or labored, for a variety of reasons. Regardless of the reason for the respiratory failure, EMS providers must be prepared to assist the patient's breathing.

Using a bag-valve-mask device, the EMS provider pushes air into the lungs, by positive-pressure ventilation, rather than causing the lung to draw in air by negative inspiratory pressure, Figure 16-10. In both cases the patient's lungs are inflated and internal respiration can occur.

Practice and skill are required to assist a patient with ventilation. Overinflation of the lungs may result in excess air spilling into the esophagus and then the stomach.

If the stomach becomes grossly distended with air, the patient may vomit and aspirate. Use of cricoid pressure can help reduce this risk, but the best method is prevention. A pa-

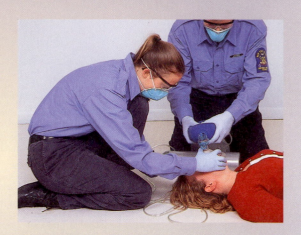

FIGURE 16–10   *The EMS provider should be competent in the use of the bag-valve-mask device to assist with ventilations.*

tient should be ventilated with smaller volumes of air, about 400 to 500 milliliters of air, to prevent accidental gastric inflation. ■

---

prone, the rate is 12 to 14 breaths per minute; in a sitting position, it is 18; and in a standing position, it is 20 to 22 breaths per minute. Emotions play a role in decreasing or increasing the respiratory rate, probably through the hypothalamus and pons. (See Chapter 8, Central Nervous System.)

Other situations that can affect the respiratory rate include the following:

- *Coughing*—a deep breath is taken, followed by a forceful exhalation from the mouth to clear the lower respiratory tract.

- *Hiccoughs* (hiccups)—caused by a spasm of the diaphragm and a spasmodic closure of the glottis. It is believed to be the result of an irritation to the diaphragm or the phrenic nerve.

- *Sneezing*—occurs like a cough except air is forced through the nose to clear the upper respiratory tract.

- *Yawning*—a deep, prolonged breath that fills the lungs, believed to be caused by the need to increase oxygen within the blood.

CONTROL OF BREATHING

The rate of breathing is controlled by neural (nervous) and chemical factors. Although both have the same goal—that of respiratory control—they function independently.

Neural Factors

The respiratory center is located in the medulla oblongata in the brain, Figure 16-11. It is subdivided into two centers: one to regulate inspiration, the other for expiratory control. The upper part of the medulla contains a grouping of cells that is the seat of the respiratory center. An increase of carbon dioxide or a lack of oxygen in the blood triggers the respiratory center.

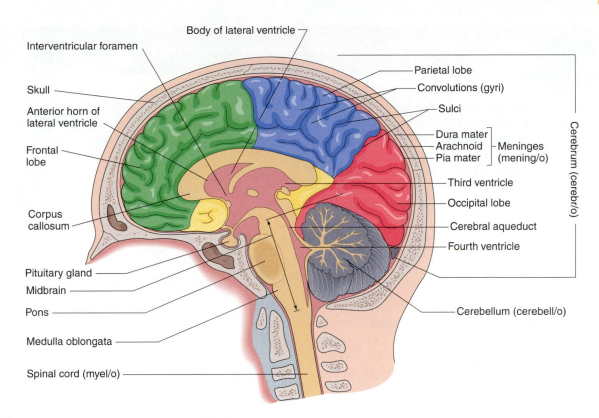

Interventricular foramen
Body of lateral ventricle
Parietal lobe
Convolutions (gyri)
Sulci
Skull
Anterior horn of lateral ventricle
Dura mater
Arachnoid — Meninges (mening/o)
Pia mater
Frontal lobe
Third ventricle
Occipital lobe
Corpus callosum
Cerebral aqueduct
Fourth ventricle
Pituitary gland
Midbrain
Pons
Cerebellum (cerebell/o)
Medulla oblongata
Spinal cord (myel/o)
Cerebrum (cerebr/o)

● **FIGURE 16–11**   *Cross-section of the brain.*

Two neuronal pathways are involved in breathing. One group of motor nerves, called the phrenic nerves, leads to the diaphragm and the intercostal muscles. The other nerve pathway carries sensory impulses from the nose, larynx, lungs, skin, and abdominal organs via the vagus nerve in the medulla.

The phrenic nerve exits the spinal cord between the third, fourth, and fifth cranial nerve. Cervical spine injuries, common in motor vehicle collisions, can cause injury or even permanent damage to the phrenic nerve. Patients with potential cervical spine injury must be handled carefully to avoid injury to the phrenic nerve and possible diaphragmatic paralysis as a result.

The rhythm of breathing can be changed by stimuli originating within the body's surface membranes. For example, a sudden drenching with cold water can make us gasp, whereas irritation to the nose or larynx can make us sneeze or cough.

Although the medulla's respiratory center is primarily responsible for respiratory control, it is not the only part of the brain that controls breathing. The **Hering-Brewer reflex*** helps to prevent the overstretching of the lungs. When the lungs are inflated, the nerve endings in the walls are stimulated. A nerve message is sent from the lungs to the medulla by way of the vagus nerve, inhibiting inspiration and stimulating expiration. This mechanism prevents overinflation of the lungs, keeping them from being ripped apart like an overinflated balloon. Also it prevents the lungs from taking up too much blood and so depriving the left side of the heart of its blood supply.

Chemical Factors

Chemical control of respiration depends on the level of carbon dioxide in the blood. When blood circulates through active tissue, it receives

---

*Named for Karl Hering (1834–1918), a German physiologist, and Josef Brewer (1842–1925), an Austrian psychiatrist.

STREET SMART ------------------------------------

An increase in the level of carbon dioxide in the blood is the normal stimulus to breath. However, patients with lung diseases such as emphysema have chronically high levels of carbon dioxide in the blood. These patients depend on low levels of oxygen to stimulate breathing. This impetus to breathe is called **hypoxic drive**.

For a time EMS providers were concerned that administering oxygen to a patient with lung disease, in effect blunting the hypoxic drive, would cause the patient to stop breathing entirely, or go into **respiratory arrest**.

Although this can occur, for the duration of care provided by an EMS provider it is better to provide oxygen and possibly deal with the consequence (respiratory arrest) than allow the patient to continue to be hypoxic and suffer further harm. ■

carbon dioxide and other metabolic waste products of cellular respiration. As blood circulates through the respiratory center, the respiratory center senses the increased carbon dioxide in the blood and increases the respiratory rate. For example, a person performing vigorous exercise or physical labor breathes more deeply and quickly to cope with the need for more oxygen and the production of extra carbon dioxide.

Other chemical regulators of respiration are the chemoreceptors, which are found in carotid arteries and the aorta. These chemoreceptors are sensitive to the amount of the blood oxygen levels. As the arterial blood flows around these carotid and aortic bodies, the chemoreceptors are particularly sensitive to the amount of oxygen present. If oxygen declines to very low levels, impulses are sent from the carotid and aortic bodies to the respiratory center, which stimulates the rate and depth of respiration. The respiratory center can be affected by drugs such as depressants, barbiturates, and morphine.

LUNG CAPACITY AND VOLUME

Have you ever held your breath for so long that you thought you would burst? To measure how much air you can hold (your lung capacity), use a device called a **spirometer**. A spirometer measures the volume and flow of air during inspiration and expiration. By comparing the reading with the norm for a person's age, height, weight, and sex, it can be determined if any deficiencies exist. Disease processes such as chronic obstructive pulmonary disease affect lung capacity, Figure 16-12.

- **Tidal volume** is the amount of air that moves in and out of the lungs with each breath. The normal amount is about 500 milliliters.

TOTAL LUNG CAPACITY (6000 ml or 6 L)	Tidal volume 500 ml	500 ml	Vital lung capacity 4500 ml
	Inspiratory reserve volume (IRV)	3000 ml	
	Expiratory reserve volume (ERV)	1000 ml	
	Functional residual capacity	2500 ml	
	Residual air	1500 ml	

FIGURE 16–12 *Lung capacity and volume.*

- **Inspiratory reserve volume (IRV)** is the amount of air a person can be forced to take in above the tidal volume. The normal amount is 2100 to 3000 milliliters.

- **Expiratory reserve volume (ERV)** is the amount of air a person can be forced to exhale above the tidal volume. The normal amount is 1000 milliliters.

- **Vital lung capacity** is the total amount of air involved with tidal volume, inspiratory reserve volume, and expiratory reserve volume. The normal vital capacity is 4500 milliliters.

- **Residual volume** is the amount of air that cannot be voluntarily expelled in the lungs. It allows for the continuous exchange of gases between breaths. The normal residual volume is 1500 milliliters.

- **Functional residual capacity** is the sum of the expiratory reserve volume plus the residual volume. The normal amount is 2500 milliliters.

- **Total lung capacity** includes tidal volume, inspiratory reserve, expiratory reserve, and residual air. The normal amount is 6000 milliliters.

- **Dead space** is the space from the opening of the mouth to the bronchioles. Normally about 100 to 150 milliliters, there is no gas exchange in the dead space.

⬤ TYPES OF RESPIRATION

The EMS provider should be aware of the various changes to the respiratory rate and sounds of human respiration. These changes can alert an EMS provider to an abnormal respiratory condition in a patient. The following conditions describe various kinds of respiration.

In the majority of cases an altered breathing pattern is the result of disease. In fact, certain breathing patterns are characteristic of certain diseases. For example, Kussmaul's respiration, described later in this chapter, is most often seen in patients with diabetic ketoacidosis/coma.

To understand alterations in breathing, it is important to understand the mechanism of breathing. The act of breathing is under the control of the respiratory center in the medulla oblongata and the amount of carbon dioxide (the primary mechanism) or oxygen (the backup mechanism) in the blood.

Therefore any medical condition that affects either the brain and its nerves or the amount of respiratory gases in the blood causes a change in the patient's rate or pattern of breathing.

For example, a loss of red blood cells as a result of bleeding (hemorrhage) decreases the body's ability to transport oxygen and carbon dioxide and, if unstopped, starts a series of events that can lead to a syndrome called shock. In fact, the first sign of shock is an increase in the respiratory rate.

Another example is a head injury. Increasing intracranial pressure (ICP) that may be the result of a head injury compresses the medulla oblongata, causing it to malfunction. At first the patient's breathing becomes very rapid, called central neurogenic hyperventilation, then very irregular (called Cheyne-Stokes respiration, described in the following bulleted list), and finally the patient's breathing becomes agonal.

- **Apnea** is the temporary stoppage of breathing movements.

- **Dyspnea** is difficult, labored, or painful breathing, usually accompanied by discomfort and breathlessness.

- **Eupnea** is normal or easy breathing with the usual quiet inhalations and exhalations.

- **Hyperpnea** is an increase in the depth and rate of breathing, accompanied by abnormal exaggeration of respiratory movements.

- **Orthopnea** is difficult or labored breathing when the body is in a horizontal position. It is usually corrected by assuming a sitting or standing position.

- **Tachypnea** is an abnormally rapid and shallow rate of breathing.

- **Cheyne-Stokes** is an erratic waxing and waning of the depth and rate of breathing. It is commonly a result of a head injury, when increasing ICP presses down on the brainstem and the medulla oblongata.

STREET SMART

There are many causes of hyperventilation, and perhaps one of the most common is a panic attack. In the past EMS providers were told to have the patient breathe into a brown paper bag. This approach is effective, provided the source of the hyperventilation is psychotic.

If the source of the hyperventilation is a medical condition, such as a head injury, a brain tumor, or drug overdose from a drug such as aspirin for example, then the use of a brown paper bag deprives the patient of much-needed oxygen. For this reason, the practice of using a brown paper bag to treat hyperventilation without further information should not be encouraged. ■

- **Kussmaul's breathing** is an abnormally deep and almost gasping type of breathing frequently seen in diabetic ketoacidosis. The deep sighing respiration of Kussmaul's breathing is the body's effort to rid itself of excess acid and reduce the blood's pH to normal levels.

- **Agonal respiration**, also called the death gasp, is an extremely irregular series of gasping breaths punctuated with periods of apnea. An agonal respiration usually indicates that respiratory arrest is imminent.

- **Hyperventilation** is a condition that can be caused by disease or stress. Rapid breathing causes the body to lose carbon dioxide too quickly. The blood level of carbon dioxide is lowered, which leads to alkalosis. Symptoms are dizziness and possibly fainting.

DISORDERS OF THE RESPIRATORY SYSTEM

The majority of the disorders of the respiratory system involve some defect or problem that prevents outside air from reaching the alveoli. In many cases the cause of the problem is an infection within either the upper or lower airway. In the rest of the cases the problem is usually a mechanical obstruction of the airway.

Infectious Causes

The respiratory system is subject to various infections and inflammations caused by bacteria, viruses, and irritants.

The greatest loss in production hours each year is caused by the common cold. This respiratory infection spreads quickly through the classroom, factory, or business office. It is often the basis for more serious respiratory disease. It lowers the body's resistance, making it subject to infection. The direct cause of a cold is usually a virus. Indirect causes include chilling, fatigue, lack of proper food, and lack of sleep. A person who has a cold should stay in bed, drink warm liquids and fruit juice, and eat wholesome, nourishing foods.

Pharyngitis is a red, inflamed throat that may be caused by one of several bacteria or viruses. It also occurs as a result of irritants such as too much smoking or speaking. It is characterized by painful swallowing and extreme dryness of the throat.

Laryngitis is an inflammation of the larynx, or voice box. It is often secondary to other respiratory infections. It can be recognized by the incidence of hoarseness or loss of voice. The most common form is chronic catarrhal laryngitis, which is characterized by dryness, hoarseness, sore throat, coughing, and dysphagia (difficulty in swallowing).

Sinusitis is an infection of the mucous membrane that lines the sinus cavities. One or several of the cavities may be infected. Pain and nasal discharge are symptoms of this infection, which, if severe, may lead to more serious complications. The ethmoid, frontal, sphenoid, and maxillary sinuses can be affected.

Bronchitis is an inflammation of the mucous membrane of the trachea and the bronchial tubes that produces excessive mucus. It may be acute or chronic and often follows infections of the upper respiratory tract. Acute bronchitis can be caused by the spreading of an inflammation from the nasopharynx or by inhalation of irritating vapors. This condition is characterized by a cough, fever, substernal pain, and **rhonchi** (raspy breath sounds).

Chronic bronchitis usually occurs in middle or old age. Cigarette smoking is the most common cause of chronic bronchitis. Acute bronchitis may become chronic after many episodes. Symptoms include a severe and persistent cough and large amounts of discolored sputum. To be considered chronic, the cough must last for 3 months and have occurred for 2 consecutive years. Treatment is symptomatic; the patient must stop smoking.

Influenza, or "flu," is a viral infection characterized by inflammation of the mucous membrane of the respiratory system. The infection is accompanied by fever, a mucopurulent discharge, muscular pain, and extreme exhaustion. Complications such as bronchopneumonia, neuritis, otitis media (middle ear infection), and pleurisy often follow influenza. Treatment is symptomatic.

Pneumonia is an infection of the lung. It may be caused by a bacteria or virus. In this condition the alveoli become filled with a thick fluid called exudates, which contains both pus and red blood cells. The symptoms of pneumonia are chest pain, fever, chills, and dyspnea. Treatment may require the administration of oxygen and antibiotics.

Tuberculosis (TB) is an infectious disease of the lungs caused by the bacillus, *Mycobacterium tuberculosis*. The organs usually most affected in TB are the lungs; however, the organism may also affect the kidney, bones, and lymphs. In pulmonary TB, lesions called tuberculum form within the lung tissue. Symptoms

of TB are cough, low-grade fever in the afternoon, weight loss, and night sweats. The diagnostic test for TB is the Mantoux test—a skin test that is read within 48 to 72 hours by a health care professional. A positive skin test indicating a possible exposure to TB is usually followed by a chest x-ray and sputum sample.

The incidence of TB had been declining because of early detection, treatment with drugs, and patient education. The Centers for Disease Control and Prevention (CDC), however, now reports an increase in the number of cases. The reasons for the increase include illegal immigration,* an increase in the number of homeless and poor, and the spread of AIDS. In addition, there is a new strain of the TB bacteria that is resistant to treatment. People with TB must stay on isoniazid (INH) therapy for a long time. Many people stop taking the drug, which then leads to drug-resistant organisms. There is concern that tuberculosis will once again be widespread.

Diphtheria is a highly infectious disease caused by *Corynebacterium diphtheria*. Children receive a vaccine that is effective against diphtheria as part of the normal immunization process.

Pertussis (whooping cough) is characterized by severe coughing attacks that end in a "whooping" sound and dyspnea. The widespread use of the pertussis vaccine limits the number of cases in the United States to about 4000 each year; worldwide, pertussis attacks 50 million children. In August 1996 the Food and Drug Administration (FDA) gave their approval for a new vaccine called Tripedia, which contains diphtheria and tetanus toxoids and acellular pertussis vaccine. Safety data shows that acellular pertussis vaccines cause fewer adverse reactions than whole cell vaccines.

Noninfectious Causes

Some respiratory ailments are unrelated to infectious causes.

Rhinitis is the inflammation of the nasal mucous membrane; it causes swelling and increased

---

*Illegal immigrants do not go through a screening process for tuberculosis.

secretions. Various forms include acute rhinitis and allergic rhinitis, more commonly known as hay fever, which is caused by any allergen.

Asthma is a disease in which the airway becomes obstructed because of an inflammatory response to a stimuli. It was previously thought that the obstruction was due primarily to bronchoconstriction. The stimuli may be an allergen or psychological stress. Approximately 5% of the U.S. population has asthma, which is an increase over the past 10 years. The symptoms include difficulty in exhaling, dyspnea, **wheezing** (a sound produced by a rush of air through a narrowed passageway), and tightness in the chest. Treatment is with antiinflammatory drugs. An inhaled bronchodilator may be used as supplemental therapy.

Asthma is the number one respiratory disease of children. Severe difficulty in breathing is a frequent reason why EMS providers are summoned. Most EMS providers in the United States are trained to either assist or provide the patient a breathing treatment. These treatments consist of medications that are turned into mist and then inhaled.

One method of medication delivery is by **metered-dose inhaler (MDI)**, Figure 16-13. These handheld devices make carrying the medication convenient and practical. Some EMS providers utilize a **small-volume nebulizer (SVN)** to administer the medication. An SVN requires a compressed air source and therefore is reserved for special circumstances.

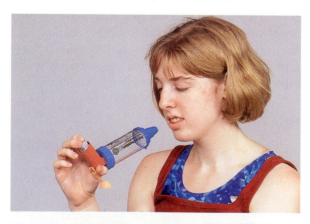

● **FIGURE 16–13**   *A spacer is a device that is commonly used in conjunction with an inhaler, especially by children.*

Atelectasis is a condition in which the lungs fail to expand normally because of bronchial occlusion.

Bronchiectasis is the dilation of a bronchus caused by an inflammation, accompanied by heavy pus secretion.

Silicosis is caused by breathing dust containing silicon dioxide over a long period. The lungs become fibrosed, which results in a reduced capacity for expansion. Silicosis is also called chalicosis, lithosis, miner's asthma, and miner's disease.

Nasal polyps are growths that sometimes occur in the sinus cavity and cause an obstruction of the air pathway. The polyps may be surgically removed, which corrects the condition.

Chronic obstructive pulmonary disease (COPD) is a term that health care professionals use to indicate chronic lung conditions, especially emphysema and chronic bronchitis.

In **emphysema** the alveoli of the lung become overdilated, lose their elasticity, and cannot rebound. The alveoli may eventually rupture. In this process, air becomes trapped and is difficult to exhale; forced exhalation is required, and there is a reduced exchange of carbon dioxide and oxygen. The patient with emphysema experiences dyspnea, which becomes more severe as the disease progresses.

The goal of treatment in COPD is to alleviate the symptoms as much as possible. Persons with COPD need to reduce their exposure to respiratory irritants, prevent infections, and restructure their activity to minimize their need for oxygen.

Cancer of the lungs is caused by a small cell (known as an oat cell) that spreads rapidly to other organs. This type is found mainly in people who are smokers. The other types of lung cancer are squamous cell or adenocarcinoma, which do not spread as rapidly. Symptoms include cough and weight loss. Diagnosis is made by x-ray and white-light **bronchoscopy**. A small, flexible tube is passed through the mouth or nose into the bronchi and the lung. The area is flooded with a white light to find abnormal tissue; then a piece of tissue is obtained for study. It is important for the heath care worker to know that the throat may be anesthetized for this procedure and that the cough reflex must

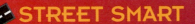
STREET SMART

Many times the source for a pulmonary embolism is a clot in the lower legs called a **deep vein thrombosis (DVT)**. A leg with a DVT is usually warm, swollen, and painful. The cause of a DVT is thought to be prolonged compression of the space behind the knee, as when seated, which prevents blood return.

When the DVT is released, it floats upstream, into the legs, and may become a pulmonary embolism. The patient may complain of sudden severe difficulty in breathing and chest pain.

Because the capillary beds around the alveoli are no longer receiving blood, the patient becomes hypoxic and cyanotic. A telltale sign of a pulmonary embolism is the presence of cyanosis even after high-concentration oxygen has been administered. ■

have returned before the person can have fluid or food. Treatment of the cancer may be surgery, chemotherapy, or radiation.

Cancer of the larynx is curable if the disorder is detected early. It is found most frequently in men over 50.

Pulmonary embolism occurs when a blood clot (embolism) breaks off and travels to the lung. This condition may occur after surgery or if a person has been on bed rest. Symptoms include a sudden severe pain in the chest and dyspnea. Diagnosis is confirmed by a lung scan. Treatment includes anticoagulant therapy. To prevent this, early ambulation (walking) after surgery is important.

Sudden infant death syndrome (SIDS) is also known as "crib death"; it usually occurs between 2 weeks and 1 year of age. The infant stops breathing during sleep. The exact cause of SIDS is unknown; however, evidence suggests that there is a disturbance of the respiratory control center in the brain. If there is any indication that SIDS may occur, the infant is monitored so that an alarm sounds if the infant stops breathing.

Emergency care in many of these respiratory ailments is directed toward maintaining ventilation while making the patient as comfortable as possible. In addition, sufficient rest and proper nourishment are essential.

● REVIEW QUESTIONS

Select the letter of the choice that best completes the statement.

1. The exchange of oxygen and carbon dioxide between the body and the air we breathe in is called:
   a. cellular respiration
   b. external respiration
   c. internal respiration
   d. breathing

2. Oxygen moves from an area of higher concentration through a process called:
   a. active transport
   b. osmosis
   c. diffusion
   d. filtration

3. When air travels through the nose it is filtered and:
   a. warmed and moistened
   b. warmed and exchanged for carbon dioxide
   c. cooled and exchanged for carbon dioxide
   d. cooled and moistened

4. The structure responsible for giving tone to the voice is:
   a. nares
   b. nasal septum
   c. glottis
   d. conchae

5. The structure that contains 15 to 20 cartilage rings and serves as a passageway for air is known as the:
   a. nasopharynx
   b. trachea
   c. pharynx
   d. larynx

6. The structure at the end of the bronchial tree where the exchange between oxygen and carbon dioxide occurs is the:
   a. alveolar ducts
   b. alveoli
   c. bronchiole
   d. bronchial tree

7. Collapse of the lung is called:
   a. pleurisy
   b. pneumonia
   c. pneumothorax
   d. thoracentesis

8. The rate of breathing is affected by which part of the brain?
   a. cerebrum
   b. medulla
   c. cerebellum
   d. frontal lobe

9. Difficult or labored breathing is known as:
   a. eupnea
   b. dyspnea
   c. orthopnea
   d. hyperpnea

10. Pharyngitis is the inflammation of the:
    a. throat
    b. voice box
    c. windpipe
    d. upper nose

11. An inflammation of the lining of the lung is called:
    a. pneumonia
    b. pleurisy
    c. sinusitis
    d. tuberculosis

12. The vaccine used to protect children against "whooping cough" is:
    a. MMR
    b. Mantoux
    c. Tripedia
    d. Salk

13. *Chronic obstructive pulmonary disease* means the person has:
    a. asthma
    b. pneumonia
    c. bronchiectasis
    d. emphysema

14. A respiratory disorder with wheezing and dyspnea is known as:
    a. acute bronchitis
    b. atelectasis
    c. asthma
    d. SIDS

15. A respiratory disease that has shown a marked increase in the past few years is:
    a. asthma
    b. cancer of the lung
    c. tuberculosis
    d. COPD

● MATCHING

Match each term in Column A with its function or description in Column B.

Column A	Column B
_____ 1. respiratory control center	a. opposite of inhalation
_____ 2. inspiration and expiration	b. measures of the ability to inspire and expire air
_____ 3. vagus nerve	c. complemental air
_____ 4. exhalation	d. located in the medulla
_____ 5. increased respiratory rate	e. occur from 16 to 24 times a minute
_____ 6. diaphragm	f. result of increase in carbon dioxide content of the blood
_____ 7. intercostal muscles	g. becomes flattened and moves downward during inhalation
_____ 8. tidal air	h. air that cannot be forcibly expelled from the lungs
_____ 9. residual volume	i. less than atmospheric pressure
_____ 10. pressure in pleural space	j. air inhaled and exhaled during rest
	k. muscles between the ribs that contract during inhalation
	l. inhibits inspiration and stimulates expiration

●APPLYING THEORY TO PRACTICE

1A. You are a little molecule of oxygen, floating in the air. Suddenly you feel a whoosh, and you are in this dark tube with little hairs tickling you. Is this that thing called the nose? Trace your journey from here to the alveoli of the lung; you will recognize it when you get there. It looks like a bunch of grapes. Name the structures along the way.

1B. To go even further, after you arrive at the alveoli, squeeze into the capillary around the alveolus and get to the pulmonary vein. You can now begin a new journey to the left knee; trace that journey. Name the structures and vessels you go through.

2. You have a cold, sinusitis, and you talk funny. What is happening? How do you explain it?

3. Take a breath; now breathe deeper, deeper, deeper. Name the process you have just experienced. Let the breath out; force more and more air out until you gasp. Name the process you have experienced.

4. Tuberculosis is a disease that has been with humankind for a long time. Scientists thought that it was a disease that responded to treatment. However, in the past few years there has been an increase in the number of cases of tuberculosis. Explain the reason for this increase.

5. Breathe on a mirror. Note the moisture that appears from the exhaled air. Discuss the fact that carbon dioxide, heat, and water vapor are given off in exhalation.

6. Jog in place. Note the effect of body activity on the rate of breathing. How does exercise change breathing? Why?

7. Why does a young child breathe more rapidly than an aged person?

Digestive System

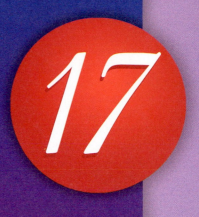

17

Objectives

- Describe the general function of the digestive system
- List the structures and the functions of the digestive system
- Describe the action of the enzymes on carbohydrates, fats, and protein
- Trace food from the beginning of the digestive process to the end
- Describe common disorders of the digestive system
- Define the key words that relate to this chapter

Key Words

absorption
adhesion
alimentary canal
amylase
amylopsin
anus
appendicitis
ascending colon
bicuspids
bile
bilirubin
bolus
buccal cavity
canines
caput medusa
cardiac sphincter
cecum
cholecystitis
chyme
cirrhosis
colitis (IBS)
colon
colostomy
common bile duct
constipation
crown

cystic duct
deciduous
defecation
deglutition
dental caries
dentin
descending colon
diarrhea
digestion
diverticulitis
duodenum
enamel
enteral
enteritis
enzymes
esophageal varices
esophagus
feces
flatulence
gallstones
gastric distention
gastritis
gastroenteritis
gastroesophageal reflux
  disease (GERD)
gingivae

(continues)

Key Words (continued)

glycogen	phototherapy
greater omentum	portal hypertension
halitosis	protease
heartburn	ptyalin
Hemoccult	pulp cavity
hepatic duct	pyloric sphincter
hepatitis	pyloric stenosis
histamine	pylorospasm
hyperbilirubinemia	rebound tenderness
ileocecal valve	rectum
ileum	reflexive emptying
incarceration	root
incisors	rugae
incontinence	salivary glands
intestinal bowel	parotid
obstruction	sublingual
jejunum	submandibular
lipase	segmented movement
mastication	sigmoid colon
McBurney's point	steapsin
mesentery	stomach
molars	stomatitis
neck of tooth	suppository
papillae	taste buds
pancreatitis	transverse colon
parenteral	trypsin
peptic ulcer	ulcer
periodontal membrane	uvula
peristalsis	vermiform appendix
peritoneum	villi
peritonitis	wisdom teeth

All food that is eaten must be changed into a soluble, absorbable form within the body before it can be used by the cells. This means that certain physical and chemical changes must take place to change the insoluble complex food molecules into simpler soluble ones. These can then be transported by the blood to the cells and be absorbed through the cell membranes. The process of changing complex solid foods into simpler soluble forms that can be absorbed by the body cells is called **digestion**. It is accomplished by the action of various digestive juices containing enzymes. **Enzymes** are chemical substances that promote chemical reactions in living things, although they themselves are unaffected by the chemical reactions.

Digestion is performed by the digestive system, which includes the alimentary canal and accessory digestive organs. The **alimentary canal** is also known as the digestive tract or gastrointestinal (GI) tract. The alimentary canal consists of the mouth (oral cavity), pharynx (throat), esophagus (gullet), stomach, small intestine, large intestine (colon), and anus, Figure 17-1. Stretched out, the alimentary canal is a continuous tube some 30 feet (9 meters) in length, from the mouth to anus. However, inside the body, the length of the alimentary canal is much shorter (12 to 15 feet) because muscle tone causes it to contract, much like a collapsed accordion. The accessory organs of digestion directly associated with the GI tract are the tongue, teeth, salivary glands, pancreas, liver, and gallbladder.

The walls of the alimentary canal are composed of four layers: (1) The innermost lining, called the mucosa, is made of epithelial cells; (2) the submucosa consists of connective tissue with fibers, blood vessels, and nerve endings; (3) the third layer is composed of circular muscle; and (4) the fourth has longitudinal muscle. The mucosa secretes slimy mucus. In some areas it also produces digestive juices. This slimy mucus lubricates the alimentary canal, aiding in the passage of food. It also insulates the digestive tract from the effects of powerful enzymes while protecting the delicate epithelial cells from abrasive substances within the food.

● LINING OF THE DIGESTIVE SYSTEM

The abdominal cavity is lined with a serous membrane called the **peritoneum**. This is a two-layered membrane, with the outer, or parietal, side lining the abdominal cavity and the inner, or visceral, side covering the outside of each organ in the abdominal cavity. An inflammation of the lining of this cavity caused by disease-producing organisms is called **peritonitis**.

There are two specialized layers of peritoneum. The peritoneum that attaches to the posterior wall of the abdominal cavity is called the **mesentery**. The small intestines are attached to this layer. In the anterior portion of the abdominal cavity a double fold of peri-

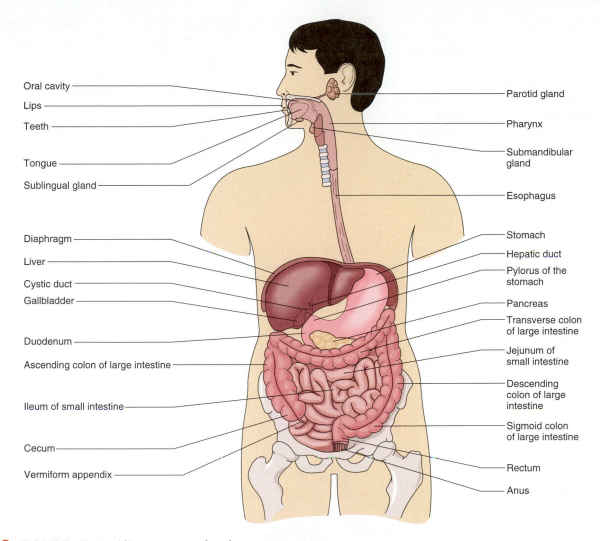

Oral cavity
Lips
Teeth
Tongue
Sublingual gland

Diaphragm
Liver
Cystic duct
Gallbladder

Duodenum
Ascending colon of large intestine

Ileum of small intestine

Cecum

Vermiform appendix

Parotid gland
Pharynx
Submandibular gland
Esophagus

Stomach
Hepatic duct
Pylorus of the stomach
Pancreas
Transverse colon of large intestine
Jejunum of small intestine
Descending colon of large intestine
Sigmoid colon of large intestine
Rectum
Anus

FIGURE 17–1   *Alimentary canal and accessory organs.*

toneum extends down from the greater curvature of the stomach. This hangs over the abdominal organs like a protective apron. This layer contains large amounts of fat and is called the **greater omentum**. The peritoneal structure between the liver and stomach is called the lesser omentum.

FUNCTIONS OF THE DIGESTIVE SYSTEM

The functions of the digestive system include the following:

1. To physically break food down into smaller pieces.

2. To chemically change food by digestive juices into the end products of fat, carbohydrates, and protein.

3. To absorb the nutrients into the blood capillaries of the small intestines for use in the body.

4. To eliminate the waste products of digestion.

STRUCTURE OF ORGANS OF DIGESTION

There are many organs that contribute to digestion. Each serves a specific function as described below.

Mouth

Food enters the digestive tract through the mouth (oral or **buccal cavity**). The lips (labia) protect the opening to the mouth. The inside of the mouth is covered with a mucous membrane. Its roof consists of a hard and soft palate. The hard palate is formed from the maxillary and palatine bones, which are covered by mucous membrane. Behind the hard palate is the soft palate, which is made from a movable mucous membrane fold. It encloses blood vessels, muscle fibers, nerves, lymphatic tissue, and mucous glands. The soft palate is an arch-shaped structure separating the mouth from the nasopharynx. Hanging from the middle of the soft palate is a cone-shaped flap of tissue called the **uvula**. This prevents food from entering the nasal cavity when swallowing, Figure 17-2.

The buccinator muscle, also called the trumpeter's muscle, is located within the cheeks. The buccinator muscle is used when chewing food (**mastication**). The buccal pockets lie on either side of the tongue and are where chewable tobacco is kept in the mouth. This tobacco product is thought to be one of the causes of mouth cancer.

Tongue/Accessory Organ of Digestion

The tongue and its muscles are attached to the floor of the mouth, helping in both chewing and swallowing. The tongue is made from skeletal muscles that lie in many different planes. Because of this, the tongue can be moved in various directions. It is attached to four bones: the hyoid, the mandible, and two temporal bones. On the tongue's epithelial surface are projections called **papillae**, Figure 17-3. There are nerve endings located in many of these papillae, forming the sense organs of taste, or **taste buds**. These taste buds respond

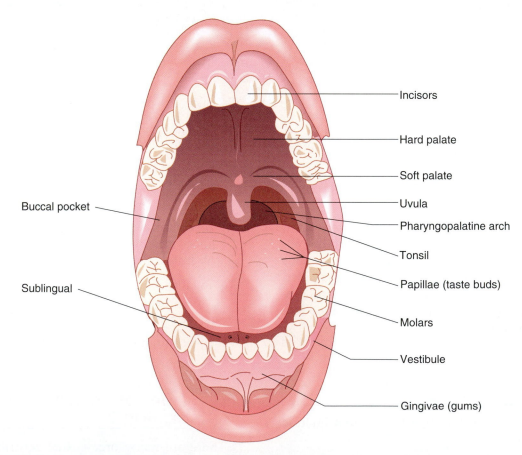

● **FIGURE 17–2**   *The mouth and its structures.*

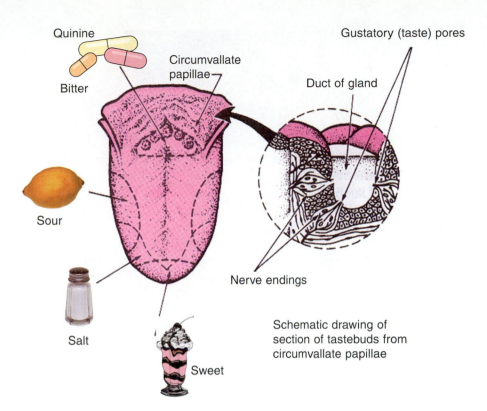

Quinine

Bitter

Circumvallate papillae

Gustatory (taste) pores

Duct of gland

Sour

Nerve endings

Salt

Schematic drawing of section of tastebuds from circumvallate papillae

Sweet

● **FIGURE 17–3**   *There are about 9000 taste buds on the tongue, contained in knoblike elevations called papillae. The taste buds are sensitive to four basic tastes: sweet, sour, salty, and bitter.*

to bitterness, saltiness, sweetness, and sourness in foods, see Figure 17-3. They are also sensitive to cold, heat, and pressure.

For food to be tasted, the chemicals that give it "flavor" must be dissolved in solution. The solution passes through the taste bud openings, stimulating the nerve endings in the taste cells.

The sensation of taste is coupled with the sense of smell. When we experience an odor, it stimulates the olfactory nerve endings in the upper part of the nasal cavity. We may confuse the odor of a food with its flavor when it is simultaneously present in the mouth. A bad cold with nasal congestion frequently impedes the ability to taste the flavor of foods. This is because increased mucous secretions cover the olfactory nerve endings.

Salivary Glands

Saliva is secreted into the oral cavity by three pairs of salivary glands: the parotid, the submandibular, and the sublingual, Figure 17-4. The **parotid salivary glands** are found on both sides of the face, in front of and below the ears. They are the largest salivary glands, the ones that become inflamed during an attack of mumps. Chewing at such times is painful because the motion squeezes these tender, inflamed glands. A parotid duct carries its secretion (almost entirely salivary amylase, a food-dissolving enzyme) into the mouth. It opens on the inner surface of the cheeks, opposite the second molar of the upper jaw.

Below the parotid salivary gland and near the angle of the lower jaw is a **submandibular gland**. This gland is about the size of a walnut, and its secretions contain both mucin and ptyalin. The secretions enter the buccal cavity via the submandibular duct at the anterior base of the tongue.

The final pair of salivary glands are the **sublingual glands**, the smallest of the three. They are found under the sides of the tongue. Their secretion consists mainly of mucus and

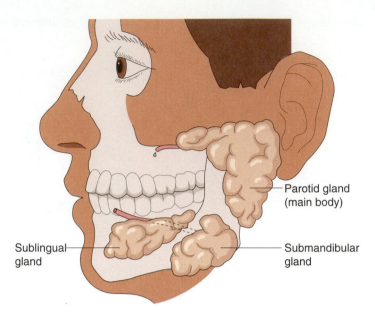

Parotid gland
(main body)

Sublingual
gland

Submandibular
gland

● **FIGURE 17–4** *Salivary glands.*

contains no ptyalin. The mucus from the sublingual glands can help dissolve medications like nitroglycerin that are then absorbed directly into the mucous membrane on the floor of the mouth.

Teeth/Accessory Organ of Digestion

The **gingivae**, or gums, support and protect the teeth. They are made of fleshy tissue covered with mucous membrane. This membrane surrounds the narrow portions of the teeth (also called the cervix or neck) and covers the structures in the upper and lower jaws.

Food ingested by the mouth must be thoroughly chewed, or masticated, by the teeth. Teeth help break food down into very small morsels, increasing the food's surface area. This activity enables the digestive enzymes to digest the food more efficiently and quickly than if it were swallowed without being chewed. During normal growth and development, the human mouth develops two sets of teeth: (1) the deciduous or milk teeth, which are later replaced by (2) the permanent teeth.

Deciduous teeth start to erupt at approximately 6 months and continue until approximately 2 years of age. In total, 20 deciduous teeth are cut during the first 2 years—10 in the upper and 10 in the lower jaw. There are four incisors, two canines, and four molars. This relationship is expressed in the dentition formula shown in Figure 17-5. The **incisors** have sharp edges for biting, the **canines** are pointed for

STREET SMART

The sublingual area below the tongue is richly supplied with blood vessels and is therefore often utilized for rapid medication administration. Certain rapidly dissolving medications, like nitroglycerin tablets and oral glucose paste, are frequently given via this route of administration. However, for these medications to dissolve and be absorbed, there must be an adequate amount of saliva present from the sublingual glands. ■

Dentition Formula for Deciduous Teeth

	Molars	Canine	Incisors	Canine	Molars
Upper jaw	2	1	4	1	2
Lower jaw	2	1	4	1	2

Dentition Formula for Permanent Teeth

	Molars	Premolars	Canine	Incisors	Canine	Premolars	Molars
Upper jaw	3	2	1	4	1	2	3
Lower jaw	3	2	1	4	1	2	3

● **FIGURE 17–5** *Dentition formulas for deciduous and permanent teeth.*

tearing, and the molars have ridges, designed for crushing and grinding. There are no premolars among the deciduous teeth. Deciduous teeth may last up to the age of 12.

Permanent teeth begin developing at this point, pushing out their deciduous predecessors. The first molars lead the way between the fifth and seventh years. The last to emerge are the third molars, or **wisdom teeth**, which may appear anytime from 17 to 25 years of age. In total, the adult mouth develops 32 teeth, 16 in each jaw, Figure 17-5.

Based on the dentition formula, the adult mouth has eight premolars, or **bicuspids**: four in the upper and four in the lower jaw. Bicuspids are broad, with two ridges on each crown, and have only two roots. Their design is ideal for grinding food. Figure 17-6 shows the arrangement of the deciduous and permanent teeth and the years during which they normally erupt.

Structure of a Tooth

Each tooth may be divided into three major parts: the crown, the neck, and the root, Figure 17-7. The **crown** portion is the part of the tooth that is visible; the **neck** is where the tooth enters the gumline; and the **root** is embedded in the alveolar processes of the jaw. Helping to anchor the tooth in place is the **periodontal membrane**.

Inside the tooth is the **pulp cavity**, which contains the nerves and blood supply. The pulp cavity is surrounded by calcified tissue called **dentin**. In the crown portion the dentin is covered by **enamel**. Enamel is the hardest substance in the body. If the enamel wears down on the surface of the tooth, bacteria may enter and caries, or cavities, will develop.

Esophagus

The esophagus connects the mouth with the stomach and serves as a conduit for food. The area around the opening of the esophagus is called the glottis.

When food is swallowed, it enters the upper portion of the esophagus. The **esophagus** is a muscular tube about 25 centimeters (10 inches) long. It begins at the lower end of the pharynx, behind the trachea. It continues downward

STREET SMART

Bad breath, also called **halitosis**, is often a sign that indicates the patient may have dental decay, or **dental caries**. Good dentition is important for health and proper nutrition. Loss of teeth, as sometimes occurs with old age, can precede a general decline in health. ■

(A) PERMANENT TEETH

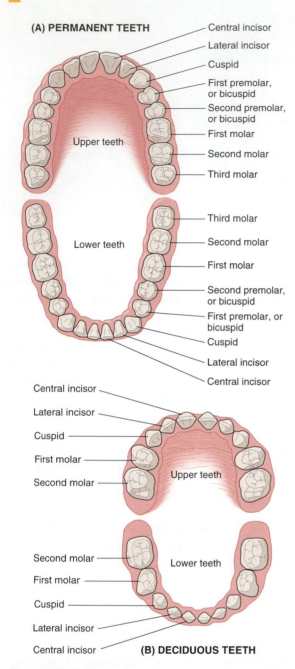

Central incisor
Lateral incisor
Cuspid
First premolar, or bicuspid
Second premolar, or bicuspid
First molar
Second molar
Third molar

Upper teeth

Third molar
Second molar
First molar
Second premolar, or bicuspid
First premolar, or bicuspid
Cuspid
Lateral incisor
Central incisor

Lower teeth

Central incisor
Lateral incisor
Cuspid
First molar
Second molar

Upper teeth

Second molar
First molar
Cuspid
Lateral incisor
Central incisor

Lower teeth

(B) DECIDUOUS TEETH

● **FIGURE 17–6**   *Teeth and their eruption times.*

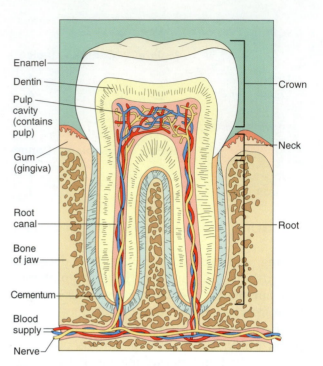

Enamel
Dentin
Pulp cavity (contains pulp)
Gum (gingiva)
Root canal
Bone of jaw
Cementum
Blood supply
Nerve

Crown
Neck
Root

● **FIGURE 17–7**   *Structure of the tooth.*

untary and the lower portion is smooth muscle, or involuntary.

Stomach

The **stomach** is found in the upper part of the abdominal cavity, just to the left of and below the diaphragm. The shape and position are determined by several factors. These include the amount of food contained within the stomach, the stage of digestion, the position of a person's body, and the pressure exerted on the stomach from the intestines below.

The stomach is divided into three portions: the upper part, or fundus; the middle section, called the body or greater curvature; and the lower portion, called the pylorus. At the opening into the stomach is a circular layer of muscle, the **cardiac sphincter** or lower esophageal sphincter, which controls passage of food into the stomach. It is called the cardiac sphincter because of its proximity to the heart. Toward the other end of the stomach lies the **pyloric sphincter** valve, which regulates entrance of food into the **duodenum** (the first part of the small intestine). Sometimes the pyloric sphincter valve fails to relax in infants. In such cases, food remaining in

through the mediastinum, in front of the vertebral column, and passes through the diaphragm. From there the esophagus enters the upper part, or cardiac portion, of the stomach. This point can be located at the end of the sternum, near the level of the xiphoid process.

The esophageal walls have four layers: the mucosa, submucosa, muscular, and external serosa. The muscles in the upper third are vol-

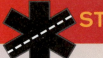

STREET SMART

When a patient is being manually ventilated using a bag-valve-mask (BVM) device, excessive airway pressures as a result of vigorous overventilation can open the sphincters in the esophagus leading to the stomach and force air into the stomach. Excessive air in the stomach leads to **gastric distention**, regurgitation, and possible aspiration into the trachea. Careful attention while ventilating a patient is important to prevent gastric distention and possible risk of aspiration. ■

the stomach is not completely digested and eventually is vomited. This condition is called **pylorospasm**. Another abnormal condition is **pyloric stenosis**, a narrowing of the pyloric sphincter that occurs most often in infants.

The stomach wall consists of four layers: mucous, submucous, muscular, and serous.

1. The mucous coat is the innermost layer. It is a thick layer made up of small gastric glands embedded in connective tissue. When the stomach is not distended with food, the gastric mucosa is thrown into folds called **rugae**, Figure 17-8 (A).

2. The submucous coat is made of loose areolar connective tissue.

3. The muscular coat consists of three layers of smooth muscle: the outer, longitudinal layer; a middle, circular layer; and an inner, oblique layer, Figure 17-8 (A). These muscles help the stomach perform peristalsis, which pushes food into the small intestine.

4. The serosa is the thick outer layer covering the stomach. It is continuous with the peritoneum. The serosa and peritoneum meet at certain points, surrounding the organs around the stomach and holding them in a kind of sling.

Gastric Glands

The gastric mucosa contains millions of gastric glands that secrete the gastric juice necessary for digestion, Figure 17-8 (B).

- Enteroendocrine glands secrete gastrin, which in turn stimulates cells to produce hydrochloric acid (HCl) and pepsinogen.

- Parietal cells produce HCl, which converts pepsinogen into pepsin and destroys bacteria and microorganisms that enter the stomach. It is the body's natural sterilizer.

- Parietal cells also produce the intrinsic factor, an element necessary for the absorption of vitamin B_{12}; without it, a condition known as pernicious anemia exists.

STREET SMART

An advanced EMS provider's failure to correctly differentiate between the trachea and the esophagus or use of a blind intubation technique can result in an accidental intubation of the esophagus.

This all too common error is not a problem as long the missed intubation is realized and the patient is extubated and ventilated. However, an unrecognized esophageal intubation can result in profound hypoxia and even death. ■

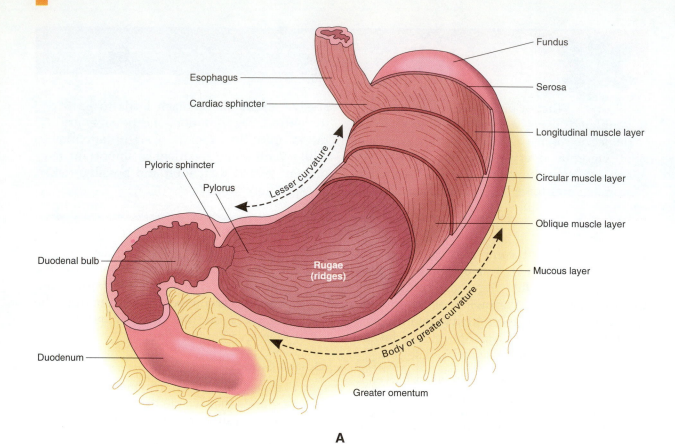

A

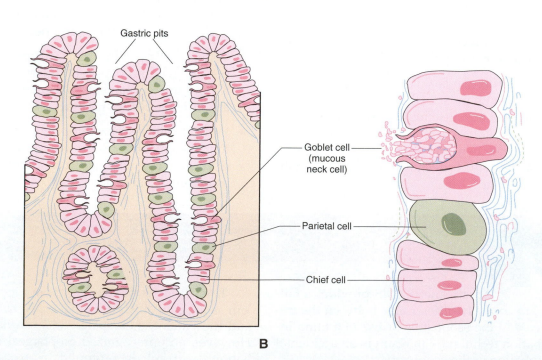

B

● **FIGURE 17–8**   *(A) Parts of the stomach. (B) Three types of gastric gland cells make up the gastric glands that line the stomach.*

- Chief type cells produce pepsinogen, which converts to pepsin. The enzyme pepsin breaks down protein into smaller pieces called protease and peptone.

- Mucous cells secrete alkaline mucus, which helps neutralize the effects of HCl and the other digestive juices.

- Rennin is found in infants and children but not adults. It prepares milk proteins for digestion by other enzymes.

Small Intestine

The small intestine has the same four layers as the stomach: the mucosa, submucosa, muscular, and serosas, Figure 17-9 (A).

The final preparation of food to be absorbed occurs in the small intestine. This coiled portion of the alimentary canal can be as long as 20 feet. The small intestine is divided into three sections: the duodenum, the **jejunum**, and the **ileum**. The small intestine is held in place by the mesentery. The small intestine lining secretes digestive juices and is covered with villi that absorb the end products of digestion, Figures 17-9 (B & C).

The first segment of the small intestine is the duodenum. This 12-inch structure curves around the head of the pancreas. A few inches into the duodenum is the ampulla of Vater, which is where the pancreatic duct and the common bile duct of the liver enter. The pancreatic duct empties the digestive juices of the pancreas, and the common bile duct empties bile from the liver.

The next section of the small intestine is the jejunum, which is about 8 feet long, and the ileum, which is 10 to 12 feet long.

Digestive Juices in the Small Intestines

Digestive juices in the small intestines include the following:

- Enzymes, secretin, and cholecystokinin stimulate the digestive juices of the pancreas, liver, and gallbladder.

- Pancreatic juices, namely **protease** or **trypsin**, which breaks down protein to amino acids, amylase or **amylopsin**, which breaks down starches to glucose, and **lipase** or **steapsin**, which breaks down fats to fatty acids and glycerol. The pancreatic juices also contain sodium bicarbonate, which neutralizes the highly acidic food contents of the stomach.

- **Bile** is necessary to break down or emulsify fat into smaller fat globules to be digested by lipase.

- Intestinal juices secreted by the cells of the small intestine including maltase, lactase, and sucrase, which change starch into glucose; peptidase changes protease and peptone into amino acids; and steapsin changes fat into fatty acids and glycerol.

The combined action of pancreatic juice, bile, and intestinal juice completes the process of changing carbohydrates first into starch and then into glucose, protein into amino acids, and fats into fatty acids and glycerol, Figure 17-10. The end products of digestion are now ready for absorption, Table 17-1.

Absorption in the Small Intestine

Absorption is possible because the lining of the small intestine is not smooth. It is covered with millions of tiny projections called **villi**. Each microscopic villus contains a network of blood and lymph capillaries, see Figure 17-9 (B). The digested portion of the food passes through the villi into the bloodstream and on to the body cells. The indigestible portion passes on to the large intestine.

Pancreas

The pancreas is a feather-shaped organ located behind the stomach, Figure 17-11. It functions both as an exocrine gland, meaning it has a duct that carries away its secretion, and as an endocrine gland, meaning it is ductless and the secretions are emptied directly into the bloodstream. The digestive juices are carried by the pancreatic duct into the duodenum.

Liver

The liver is the largest organ in the body. It is located below the diaphragm, in the

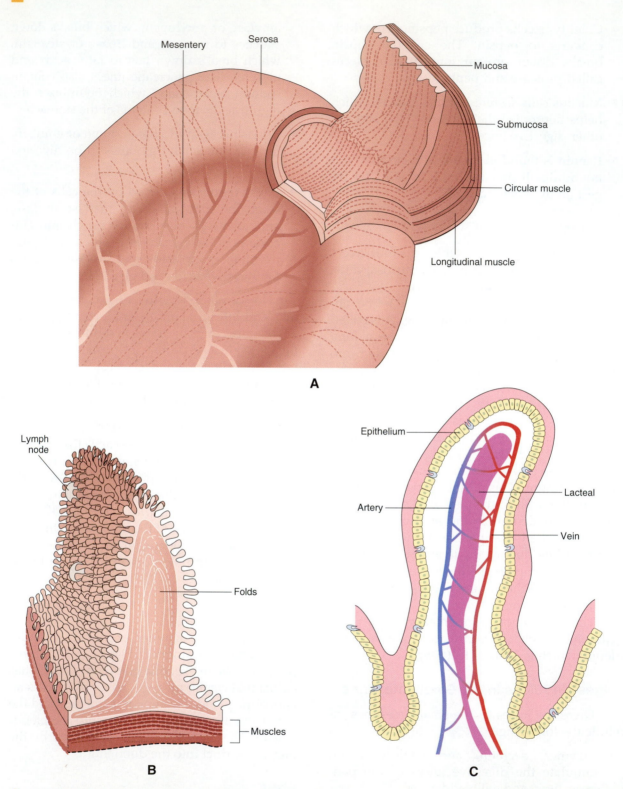

A

B

C

● **FIGURE 17–9**   *(A) Portion of the jejunum showing the inner structure of the small intestine. (B) Diagram of the wall of a portion of the small intestine showing the villi arrangement. (C) Magnification of a single villus.*

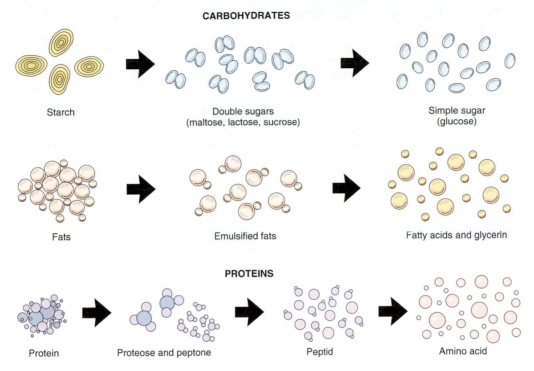

CARBOHYDRATES

Starch → Double sugars (maltose, lactose, sucrose) → Simple sugar (glucose)

Fats → Emulsified fats → Fatty acids and glycerin

PROTEINS

Protein → Proteose and peptone → Peptid → Amino acid

● **FIGURE 17–10**   *Phases in the digestion of starch, fat, and protein.*

upper right quadrant of the abdomen, see Figure 17-11. The portal vein carries the products of digestion from the small intestine to the liver. Some of the liver's many functions include the following:

- Manufacturing bile, a yellow to green fluid, which is necessary for the digestion of fat. The liver produces approximately 800 to 1000 milliliters of bile daily. Bile contains bile salts, bile pigments (mainly **bilirubin**, which comes from the breakdown of the hemoglobin molecule), cholesterol, phospholipids, and some electrolytes. The **hepatic duct** from the liver joins with the **cystic duct** of the gallbladder to form the **common bile duct**, which carries the bile to the duodenum. If this duct is blocked, bile may then enter the bloodstream, causing jaundice, which gives the skin and sclera of the eyes a yellow color.

- Producing and storing glucose in the form of **glycogen**.

- Detoxifying alcohol, drugs, and other harmful substances.

- Manufacturing blood proteins such as fibrinogen and prothrombin, which are necessary for blood clotting; albumin, which is needed for fluid balance in the cells; and globulin, which is necessary for immunity.

- Preparing urea, the chief waste product of protein metabolism from the breakdown of amino acids.

- Storing vitamins A, D, and B complex.

Gallbladder

The gallbladder is a small green organ in the inferior surface of the liver, see Figure 17-11. It stores and concentrates bile when it is not needed by the body. When food high in fat content enters the duodenum, bile is released by the gallbladder through the cystic duct to help digest the fat.

Large Intestine

The ileum empties its intestinal chyme (semiliquid food) into the side wall of the large intestine through an opening called the **ileocecal**

TABLE 17-1 *Summary of Digestive Enzymes Involved in Human Digestion*

ORGAN	JUICE	GLAND	ENZYME(S)	ACTION	ADDITIONAL FACTS
Mouth	Saliva	Salivary	Amylase found in ptyalin	Starch → maltose	Physical, as well as chemical, hydrolysis Mucus flow starts here and continues throughout digestive tract
Esophagus	Mucus	Mucous	None	Lubrication of food	Peristalsis begins here
Stomach	Gastric juice and HCl acid	Gastric	Protease, pepsin	Proteins → peptones and proteoses	Gastrin activates the gastric glands HCl supplies an acidic medium and kills bacteria Temporary food storage
Small intestine	Intestinal	Intestinal	Peptidases	Peptones and proteoses into amino acids	Absorption of end products occurs in small intestine
			Maltase	Maltose → glucose	
			Lactase	Lactose → glucose and galactose	Villi facilitates absorption
			Sucrase	Sucrose → glucose and fructose	
			Lipase	Fats → fatty acids and glycerol	
	Bile	Liver	None	Emulsifies fat	Neutralizes stomach acid
	Pancreatic	Pancreas	Protease (trypsin)	Proteins → peptones and amino acids	
			Amylase (amylopsin)	Starch → maltose	Secretin stimulates the flow of pancreatic juice
			Lipase (steapsin)	Fats → fatty acids and glycerol	
			Nucleases	Nucleic acids (DNA/RNA) nucleotides	

CHANGES OF AGING

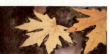

The immature liver of a newborn sometimes has difficulty breaking down and excreting bilirubin. The result is an accumulation of bilirubin, or **hyperbilirubinemia**, in the blood, causing physiological jaundice. Physiological jaundice occurs in about 50% of newborns, usually within 24 hours, and is treated with **phototherapy**. A newborn infant is placed under a white light source, called a bililight, that helps the body break down the excess bilirubin. ■

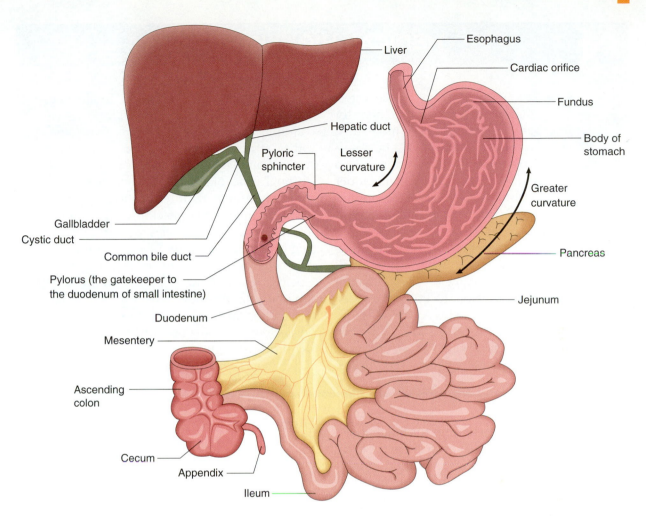

Liver
Esophagus
Cardiac orifice
Fundus
Body of stomach
Hepatic duct
Pyloric sphincter
Lesser curvature
Greater curvature
Gallbladder
Cystic duct
Common bile duct
Pylorus (the gatekeeper to the duodenum of small intestine)
Duodenum
Mesentery
Ascending colon
Cecum
Appendix
Ileum
Pancreas
Jejunum

● **FIGURE 17–11**   *Stomach, liver, gallbladder, pancreas, small intestine, and large intestine.*

valve. This valve permits passage of the chyme to the large intestine and prevents the backflow of chyme into the ileum. The large intestine is about 5 feet long and approximately 2 inches in diameter. The **colon**, as it is also called, frames the abdomen, Figure 17-12.

Cecum and Appendix

Located slightly below the ileocecal valve, in the lower right portion of the abdomen, is a blind pouch called the **cecum**.

Just below the ileocecal valve, to the lower left of the cecum, is the **vermiform appendix**. The appendix is a wormlike projection protruding into the abdominal cavity, see Figure 17-12. It has no digestive function. Because the appendix is a blind sac, it fills up easily but drains quite slowly; substances can remain within the appendix for prolonged periods. Irritation of the lining of the appendix can make it a suitable area for bacterial growth. This often leads to the painful inflammatory condition known as **appendicitis**.

Ascending, Transverse, and Descending Colon

The colon continues upward, along the right side of the abdominal cavity, to the underside of the liver (hepatic flexure), forming the **ascending colon**. Then it veers to the left of the abdominal cavity, across the abdominal cavity, to a point below the spleen (splenic flexure), forming the **transverse colon**. The **descending colon** travels down from the splenic flexure on the left side of the abdominal cavity.

MEDICAL HIGHLIGHTS

Gallbladder surgery, or cholecystectomy, is the most common method for treating gallstones. Each year more than 500,000 Americans have gallbladder surgery. Laparoscopic cholecystectomy is a new alternative procedure for gallbladder removal. About 80% of cholecystectomies are performed using this technique. In this procedure, several small incisions are made into the abdomen to allow the insertion of surgical instruments and a small video camera. The camera sends a magnified image from inside the body to a video monitor, giving the surgeon a close-up view of the organs and tissues. The surgeon watches the monitor and performs the operation by manipulating the surgical instruments through separate small incisions. The gallbladder is identified and carefully separated from the liver and other structures. Finally, the cystic duct is cut and the gallbladder is removed through one of the small incisions. This type of surgery requires meticulous skill. Laparoscopic cholecystectomy does not require the stomach muscles to be cut, resulting in less pain, quicker healing, improved cosmetic results, and fewer complications such as infection. Recovery is usually only a night in a hospital and several days' recuperation at home. The standard cholecystectomy is a major abdominal surgery requiring a week's stay in the hospital and several weeks at home for recuperation. ■

As the descending colon reaches the left iliac region, it enters the pelvis in an S-shaped bend. This section is known as the sigmoid colon, which extends some 7 or 8 inches as the rectum. The rectum opens exteriorly into the anus, see Figure 17-12.

Anal Canal

The anal canal is the last portion of the large intestine; its external opening is the anus. The anus is guarded by two anal sphincter muscles. One is an internal sphincter of smooth, involuntary muscle, the other an external sphincter of

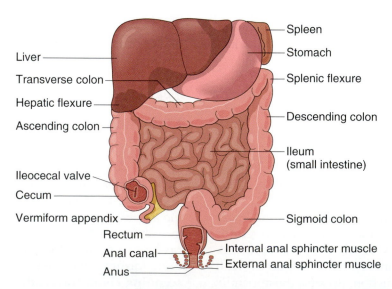

Liver

Transverse colon

Hepatic flexure

Ascending colon

Ileocecal valve

Cecum

Vermiform appendix

Rectum

Anal canal

Anus

Spleen

Stomach

Splenic flexure

Descending colon

Ileum
(small intestine)

Sigmoid colon

Internal anal sphincter muscle

External anal sphincter muscle

● **FIGURE 17–12** *Accessory organs of digestion: pancreas, liver, and gallbladder.*

The anus is rich with blood from the internal and external hemorrhoidal veins. Under special circumstances, medications can be administered via the anus. By placing the medication in a medium such as wax that dissolves with body heat, called a **suppository**, the medication is deposited next to the vein and can be absorbed. This method of medication administration is called per rectum (PR). This method is often used to administer acetaminophen (Tylenol) to children who cannot or will not swallow the tablets. ■

striated, voluntary muscle. Both of these remain contracted to close the anal opening until defecation takes place. The mucous membrane lining the anal canal is folded into vertical folds called rectal columns. Within each rectal column is an artery and a vein. The condition leading to inflammation or enlargement of the rectal column veins is known as hemorrhoids.

GENERAL OVERVIEW OF DIGESTION

Food enters the gastrointestinal tract via the mouth. In the oral cavity the food is mechanically digested by the cutting, ripping, and grinding action of the teeth. Chemical digestion of carbohydrates is initiated by the secretion of saliva containing a digestive enzyme. Then the action of the saliva and rolling motion of the tongue turn the food into a soft, pliable ball called a **bolus**. The bolus slides down to the throat (pharynx) to be swallowed. Next it travels through the esophagus into the stomach. Food is pushed along the esophagus by rhythmic, muscular contractions called **peristalsis**. From the stomach, peristaltic contractions continue to push the food into the small intestine. The nervous system stimulates gland activity and peristalsis.

Each part of the alimentary canal contributes to the overall digestive process. Protein digestion, for instance, is initiated by the stomach. Then the small intestine starts and finishes fat digestion, as well as completes the digestion of carbohydrates and proteins. Numerous digestive glands are located in the stomach and small intestine, which secrete digestive juices containing powerful enzymes to chemically digest the food. As a result of digestion, insoluble food becomes a soluble fluid substance. This substance is then transported across the small intestinal wall into the bloodstream.

Circulated and absorbed through the blood capillaries into the interstitial fluid and finally into the body cells, the soluble food molecules are utilized for energy, repair, and production of new cells. The remaining undigested substances (**feces**) pass into the large intestine and leave the alimentary canal via the anus, Figure 17-13.

ACTION IN THE MOUTH

Food enters the mouth and is broken down into smaller pieces by the cutting, ripping, and grinding action of the teeth. The salivary glands fill the mouth with a watery substance called saliva, which softens and lubricates the food making it easy to swallow.

Saliva contains salivary amylase, also known as **ptyalin**, which converts the starches in carbohydrates into simple sugars. For example, if you place a cracker in your mouth for a few minutes, it will have no taste because it is being broken down into glucose. Saliva is affected by the nervous system; just thinking of food causes your mouth to water, or the opposite effect can occur—a dry mouth when you are nervous or frightened.

ACTION IN THE PHARYNX

Food leaves the mouth and travels to the pharynx, or throat. This structure serves as the

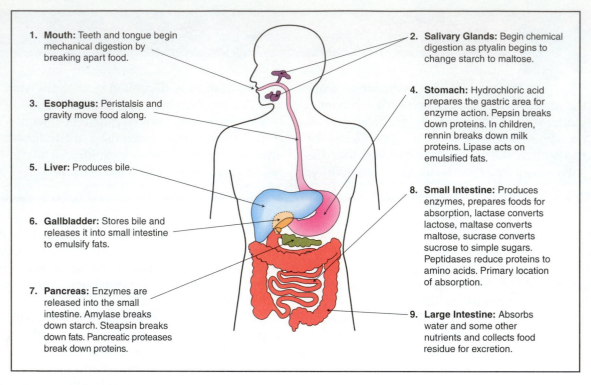

1. **Mouth:** Teeth and tongue begin mechanical digestion by breaking apart food.

3. **Esophagus:** Peristalsis and gravity move food along.

5. **Liver:** Produces bile.

6. **Gallbladder:** Stores bile and releases it into small intestine to emulsify fats.

7. **Pancreas:** Enzymes are released into the small intestine. Amylase breaks down starch. Steapsin breaks down fats. Pancreatic proteases break down proteins.

2. **Salivary Glands:** Begin chemical digestion as ptyalin begins to change starch to maltose.

4. **Stomach:** Hydrochloric acid prepares the gastric area for enzyme action. Pepsin breaks down proteins. In children, rennin breaks down milk proteins. Lipase acts on emulsified fats.

8. **Small Intestine:** Produces enzymes, prepares foods for absorption, lactase converts lactose, maltase converts maltose, sucrase converts sucrose to simple sugars. Peptidases reduce proteins to amino acids. Primary location of absorption.

9. **Large Intestine:** Absorbs water and some other nutrients and collects food residue for excretion.

● **FIGURE 17–13** *Overview of digestion.*

common passageway for food and air. See Chapter 12 for a complete description of the pharynx.

● ACTION IN THE PHARYNX/ SWALLOWING

Swallowing, or **deglutition**, is a complex process involving the constrictor muscles of the pharynx. It begins as a voluntary process, changing to an involuntary process as the food enters the esophagus. When we swallow, the tip of the tongue arches slightly and moves backward and upward. This action forces the food against the hard palate; simultaneously, the soft palate and the uvula shut off the opening to the nasopharynx. Food is thus prevented from entering the nasopharynx.

In swallowing, the constrictor muscles of the pharynx contract, pushing food into the upper part of the esophagus. At the same time, other pharyngeal muscles raise the larynx, causing the epiglottis to cover the trachea

(windpipe) to prevent food from entering it. If we talk while eating, the epiglottis may not close and food may enter the trachea.

The act of swallowing is voluntary. But as a bolus of food passes over the posterior part of the tongue and stimulates receptors in the walls of the pharynx, swallowing becomes an involuntary reflex action. With the contraction of the pharyngeal muscles, followed by the contraction of the muscles lining the esophagus, food passes down into the stomach. (When you swallow, place your fingers near the trachea; you can feel the structure move upward.)

● ACTION IN THE ESOPHAGUS

Food is pushed through the esophagus by the wavelike contractions of the alimentary canal, also called peristalsis. This action explains why you can swallow even while standing on your head; once food enters the esophagus, it goes to the stomach and it is not affected by gravity.

STREET SMART

The term *cardiac* actually refers to an area of the anterior chest proximal to the insertion of the esophagus into the stomach and at the base of the heart. Pain in the cardiac area of the chest is often dismissed as being gastric in origin, "heartburn," when it is actually a significant coronary event. This misinterpretation of the nature and origin of the pain can lead to serious complications such as heart attack (myocardial infarction) or sudden cardiac death (ventricular fibrillation).

Conversely, a person may think he is having a heart attack (myocardial infarction) because of severe chest pain, when in fact a spasm of the esophagus is the cause of the pain. Complicating matters, the treatment for an acute coronary event, sublingual (SL) nitroglycerin, can also relieve esophageal spasm.

Whenever a patient is in doubt as to the cause of chest pain, it is safer to assume that it is a coronary event rather than risk the potentially deadly outcomes that can result from an incorrect decision. All patients with chest pain should seek emergency medical attention from EMS providers immediately. ■

ACTION IN THE STOMACH

When the food reaches the stomach, the cardiac sphincter relaxes and allows food to enter. About 2 to 3 quarts of digestive juices are produced daily, which may explain the gurgling noises you hear at times. When food enters, the gastric juices are released and begin to work on proteins. Salivary amylase continues its work in the stomach.

The action of the gastric juices is helped by the churning of the stomach walls. The semiliquid food is called **chyme**. The chyme leaves the stomach through the pyloric sphincter, which acts as a gatekeeper. This action allows a small squirt of chyme into the duodenum from time to time. Food takes about 2 to 4 hours to leave the stomach. Food moves through the stomach by peristalsis; vomiting occurs because of reverse peristalsis. The only known substances to be absorbed in the stomach are alcohol, small amounts of water, and some medications.

ACTION IN THE SMALL INTESTINE

The small intestine is the main area of the digestive system. It is in this location that the process of digestion is completed and absorption occurs. Bile emulsifies fat to prepare it for digestion by pancreatic and intestinal juices. Pancreatic juices neutralize the acid chyme and complete the digestion of carbohydrates, fats, and proteins, see Figure 17-10. Following are the end products of digestion:

- Carbohydrates are converted to simple sugars such as glucose.

- Proteins are broken down into amino acids.

- Fats are changed into fatty acids and glycerol.

The glucose, amino acids, fatty acids, and glycerol are then absorbed through the villi of the small intestine into the blood and lymph capillaries. The portal vein transports the blood from the small intestine and takes it to the liver, where it is distributed to the organs of the body.

The passage of food through the small intestine occurs because of peristalsis and **segmented movement**. Segmented movement is when single segments of the intestine alternate between contraction and relaxation. Because inactive segments exist between active ones, the food is moved forward and backward—it is mixed, as well as propelled. It takes about 6 to 8 hours for food to go through the small intestine; undigested foods then reach the ileocecal valve and enter the large intestine.

● ACTION IN THE LARGE INTESTINE

The large intestine is concerned with water absorption, bacterial action, fecal formation, gas formation, and defecation. The purpose of these functions is to regulate the body's water balance while storing and excreting waste products of digestion.

Absorption

The large intestine aids in the regulation of the body's water balance by absorbing large quantities of water back into the bloodstream. The water is drawn from the undigested food and indigestible material (like cellulose) that pass through the colon. The large intestine absorbs vitamins B complex and K.

Bacterial Action

A few hours after the birth of an infant, the lining of the colon starts to accumulate bacteria. These bacteria persist throughout the person's lifetime. The bacteria multiply rapidly to form the bacterial population, or flora, of the colon. The intestinal bacteria are harmless (nonpathogenic) to their host. They act on undigested food remains, turning them into acids, amines, gases, and other waste products. These decomposed products are excreted through the colon. Another benefit of the bacterial action is the synthesis (formation) of moderate amounts of B-complex vitamins and vitamin K (needed for blood clotting).

Gas Formation

Most people produce 1 to 3 pints of gas per day and pass it through the rectum (**flatulence**) about 14 times a day. Gas is produced by swallowed air and the normal breakdown of food. The unpleasant odor of flatulence comes from bacteria in the large intestine, which produces gas containing sulfur or methane. Swallowed air usually remains in the stomach and is relieved by burping and belching.

Research has not shown why some foods produce gas in one person and not another or why some people produce methane gas. Some gas-producing foods are beans, vegetables such as broccoli and cabbage, fruit, whole grains, milk and milk products, and foods containing the artificial sweetener sorbitol.

Lactose is the natural sugar found in milk and milk products. Some people have low levels of the enzyme lactase, which is necessary to digest lactose. As people age, their level of lactase decreases, which may explain why older people experience discomfort after using milk products.

Diet modification may reduce the amount of gas produced; however, it is important to remember that some of the foods that produce gas are also essential nutrients.

Fecal Formation

Initially the undigested or indigestible material in the colon contains a lot of water and is in a liquid state. Water absorption and bacterial

STREET SMART

Any medication administered orally, or per os (PO), or using suppositories, per rectum, is absorbed in the digestive system. The route of administration in this case is called the **enteral** route. To prevent medications from being acted on by stomach acids, the medication may be covered with a special enteric coating. For example, enteric-coated aspirin helps prevent the stomach upset sometimes caused by regular aspirin. Most medications are given via the digestive tract.

Any medication not administered via the digestive tract, such as an intramuscular (IM) injection, is said to be administered via a **parenteral** route, or around the intestines. ■

action subsequently converts the undigested material into a semisolid form, called feces.

Feces consist of bacteria, waste products from the blood, acids, amines, inorganic salts, gases, mucous, and cellulose. Amines are waste products of amino acids. The gases are ammonia, carbon dioxide, hydrogen, hydrogen sulfide, and methane. The characteristically foul odor of feces derives from these substances.

Cellulose is the fibrous part of plants that humans are unable to digest. It contributes to the bulk of the feces. This bulk stimulates the muscular activity of the colon, resulting in defecation. Regular defecation (regularity) can be promoted by exercising daily and eating foods containing bulk, such as whole-grain cereals, fruits, and vegetables. These foods supply the necessary roughage to initiate bowel movements.

Defecation

Once approximately every 12 hours the fecal material moves into the lower bowel (lower colon and rectum) by means of a series of long contractions called mass peristalsis. However, frequency of bowel movements in healthy people varies from three movements a day to three a week. When the rectum becomes distended with the accumulation of feces, a defecation reflex is triggered. Nerve endings in the rectum are stimulated, and a nerve impulse is transmitted to the spinal cord. From the spinal cord, nerve impulses are sent to the colon, rectum, and internal anal sphincter. This causes the colon and rectal muscles to contract and the internal sphincter to relax, resulting in emptying of the bowels.

For defecation to occur, the external anal sphincter must also be relaxed. The external anal sphincter surrounds and guards the outer opening of the anus and is under conscious control. This control allows a person to prevent defecation when inconvenient, despite the defecation reflex. However, if this urge is continually ignored, it lessens or disappears totally, resulting in constipation. Temporary relief from constipation may be obtained with the use of laxatives and cathartics. (A laxative is a substance that induces gentle bowel movement; a cathartic stimulates more vigorous movement, which may eventually reduce the bowel's muscle tone.)

COMMON DISORDERS OF THE DIGESTIVE SYSTEM

In times of stress it is not unusual to have "butterflies" in the stomach, nausea, or another type of distress associated with the digestive system. Diseases of the digestive system are responsible for the hospitalization of more people in the United States than any other group of diseases. In recent years, researchers have begun to shed some light on the puzzling aspects of digestive diseases. Diseases once thought to be caused by emotional problems may in fact be caused by viruses interacting with the body's immune system. Some of these diseases are briefly discussed in this unit.

Stomatitis

Stomatitis is an inflammation of the soft tissues of the mouth cavity. Pain and salivation may occur also.

Gastroesophageal Reflux Disease

Gastroesophageal reflux disease (GERD) is a disorder that affects the lower sphincter muscle connecting the esophagus with the stomach. In GERD the sphincter muscle is weak or relaxes inappropriately allowing the stomach's contents to flow up into the esophagus. This is a common occurrence in people who suffer from hiatal hernia or heartburn.

Hiatal Hernia

Hiatal hernia occurs when the stomach protrudes above the diaphragm through the esophagus opening. Hiatal hernia is not uncommon in people over the age of 50. Changes in the diet may relieve the heartburn; surgery is not usually required.

Heartburn

Heartburn, or acid indigestion, results from a backflow of the highly acidic gastric juice into the lower end of the esophagus. This irritates the lining of the esophagus, causing a burning sensation. Heartburn may be experienced on a daily basis by some people, and 25% of all pregnant women experience heartburn.

Temporary relief from heartburn can be obtained by the following:

- Avoiding chocolate and peppermints, which may cause the sphincter to relax

- Stopping smoking

- Taking nonprescription antacids to provide temporary relief

- Avoiding lying down for 2 to 3 hours after eating

- Avoiding coffee, citrus fruits and juices, fried and fatty foods, and tomato products

Pyloric Stenosis

Pyloric stenosis is a narrowing of the pyloric sphincter at the lower end of the stomach. It is often found in infants. Projectile vomiting may result; surgery is often necessary.

Gastritis

Gastritis is an acute or chronic inflammation on the stomach lining.

Gastroenteritis

Gastroenteritis is the inflammation of the mucous membrane lining the stomach and intestinal tract. A common cause is a virus that causes diarrhea and vomiting for 24 to 36 hours. If this condition persists, dehydration may occur. Treatment is symptomatic.

Enteritis

Enteritis is an inflammation of the intestine that may be caused by a bacterial, viral, or protozoan infection. Enteritis can also be caused by an allergic reaction to certain foods or food poisoning.

Peptic Ulcer

An **ulcer** is a sore or lesion that forms in the mucosal lining of the stomach or duodenum, where acid and pepsin are present. Ulcers found in the stomach are called gastric ulcers; those in the duodenum are called duodenal ulcers. In general, both types are referred to as **peptic ulcers**.

For almost a century, doctors believed that lifestyle factors such as stress and diet caused ulcers. Today research shows that most ulcers develop as a result of an infection with bacteria called *Helicobacter pylori (H. pylori)*. Other factors associated with ulcers include lifestyle, acid, and pepsin; however, *H. pylori* is now considered the primary cause.

Lifestyle factors include cigarette smoking, intake of food and beverages containing caffeine, alcohol consumption, and physical stress associated with major injuries or illness. Researchers believe that the stomach's inability to defend itself against the powerful digestive fluids acid and pepsin contribute to ulcer formation. Nonsteroidal antiinflammatory drugs make the stomach vulnerable to the harmful effects of acid and pepsin.

The most common symptom of an ulcer is a burning pain in the abdomen between the sternum and navel. The pain occurs between meals and in the early hours of the morning. It may be relieved by eating or taking an antacid.

Ulcers are diagnosed by x-ray studies of the stomach and laboratory testing for the *H. pylori* bacteria. Treatment depends on the cause. If the cause is *H. pylori*, antibiotics is the treatment. Elimination of the bacteria means that the ulcer will heal and not recur.

Treatment for ulcers from other causes include the use of histamine (H_2) blockers. These drugs reduce the amount of acid the stomach produces by blocking **histamine**, a powerful stimulant of acid secretion. Initially, treatment with H_2 blockers lasts about 6 to 8 weeks. However, because this type of ulcer recurs in about 50% to 80% of cases, many people must continue therapy for years.

Additional treatment includes the use of drugs that stop the stomach's acid pumps, mucosal protective medications, and lifestyle changes.

Bowel Obstruction

Entrapment of a loop of small bowel in the muscular abdominal wall, called an **incarceration** of a hernia, an abdominal tumor, or a growth of extra tissue after abdominal surgery, called an **adhesion**, can all block the large or small intestine.

The resulting **intestinal bowel obstruction** does not allow feces to pass. The bowel distal to the obstruction collapses, while the bowel proximal to the obstruction becomes distended, swollen (edematous), and painful. The abdomen quickly appears bloated and is tender to the touch.

Without prompt medical intervention, blood supply to portions of the bowel may become compromised and the bowel may die (infarct). A small bowel obstruction (SBO) can infarct tissue that then becomes infected with gangrene and may perforate in as little as 6 hours. A perforated bowel can quickly infect the entire abdomen and lead to a massive infection called septicemia.

Colitis or Irritable Bowel Syndrome

Colitis, or irritable bowel syndrome (**IBS**), is a condition in which the large intestine or bowel may be inflamed. The exact cause of this disorder is not known. Researchers speculate that IBD may be a viral or bacterial agent that affects the immune system. The person may experience episodes of either constipation or diarrhea. The chronic diarrhea may lead to dehydration and ulceration of the bowel. This is an extremely frustrating disorder. Medication can be given to quiet bowel activity and reduce anxiety.

Irritable bowel syndrome may also be referred to as Crohn's disease.

Appendicitis

Appendicitis occurs when the vermiform appendix becomes inflamed. If it ruptures, the bacteria from the appendix can spread to the peritoneal cavity, causing peritonitis.

Hepatitis

Hepatitis is an inflammation of the liver. Clinical symptoms are fever, nausea, anorexia, and jaundice.

Hepatitis A

Infectious hepatitis, hepatitis A, is a viral infection of the liver often spread through contaminated water or food. Standard precautions are followed.

Hepatitis B or Serum Hepatitis

Serum hepatitis, hepatitis B, is caused by a virus found only in the blood. It is transmitted by a blood transfusion contaminated with the virus or through the use of inadequately sterilized syringes, needles, or surgical equipment. It is prevalent in drug addicts who use dirty hypodermic needles.

The health care worker is at risk for contracting serum hepatitis; standard precautions must be taken at all times (see Chapter 11). A vaccine is now available for hepatitis B, and it is recommended that health care workers be vaccinated.

STREET SMART ----------------------------------

Appendicitis is sometimes called the "great pretender" because it can first present with many different patterns. In fact, fewer than 50% of patients with appendicitis present with "typical" symptoms. As a rule in emergency medicine, any sudden, severe abdominal pain is first thought to be appendicitis until it can be proven otherwise.

The typical symptoms of appendicitis include periumbilical pain that shifts to the right lower quadrant of the abdomen. Pain when the abdominal wall is compressed and released, called **rebound tenderness**, is another symptom of acute appendicitis.

The pain of acute appendicitis is usually greatest at **McBurney's point**, which is found at the middle of a triangle drawn between the symphysis pubis, the iliac crest, and the umbilicus.

Emergency care and transportation by EMS providers and prompt surgical intervention markedly improve survival and decrease illness severity. ■

Over the past two decades other strains of the hepatitis virus have been identified:

- *Hepatitis C* accounts for 20% to 40% of acute hepatitis. Most patients have a history of intravenous (IV) drug abuse. Standard precautions are followed. Some cases may be treated with the drug interferon-α.

- *Hepatitis D* requires coinfection with type B.

- *Hepatitis E* is transmitted through intestinal excretions.

Cirrhosis

Cirrhosis is a chronic, progressive inflammatory disease of the liver characterized by replacement of normal tissue with fibrous connective tissue. Three fourths of cirrhosis is caused by excessive alcohol consumption. Where viral hepatitis is common, hepatitis causes cirrhosis.

Esophageal Varices

When the liver becomes inflamed, or cirrhotic, it prevents blood from easily passing through the liver. As a result, blood backs up the portal vein, called **portal hypertension**, into the mesenteric veins and the esophageal veins.

When blood backs up into the mesenteric veins, the abdomen becomes distended and the distended veins become visible under the skin, a condition called **caput medusa**, which trans-

---

STREET SMART ----------------------------------

Hepatitis C, formerly known as hepatitis non-A, non-B, is rapidly becoming an epidemic among EMS providers. Although there is no vaccination yet for hepatitis C, infection can be prevented if EMS providers follow standard precautions.

Hepatitis B and hepatitis C are the leading causes of chronic hepatitis, liver failure, and liver cancer. ■

lated means the "head of medusa," the mythical Greek figure who had snakes for hair.

As the esophageal veins start to distend inside the throat, they begin to appear like the varicose veins found on the lower legs. These veins, called **esophageal varices**, are fragile and tend to rupture easily, bleeding vigorously in the process. The bleeding can be life threatening.

Cholecystitis

Cholecystitis is the inflammation of the gallbladder. This condition may cause blockage of the cystic duct, which inhibits the release of stored bile.

Gallstones/Enteric

Bile is normally stored in the gallbladder and secreted into the small intestine where fat is emulsified. Sometimes collections of crystallized cholesterol form in the gallbladder. These are combined with bile salts and bile pigments to form **gallstones**, or cholelithiasis. Gallstones can block the bile duct, causing pain and digestive disorders. Pain may occur in the back between the shoulder blades. In such cases, bile cannot flow into the small intestine to help in fat emulsification, digestion, and absorption. Most gallstones are small and pass with undigested food. However, the larger and obstructive gallstones must be surgically removed.

Pancreatitis

Pancreatitis is the inflammation of the pancreas. The pancreas can become edematous, hemorrhagic, or necrotic. One third of pancreatitis cases are due to unknown causes. Some may be associated with chronic alcoholism.

Diverticulosis

Diverticulosis is a condition in which little sacs (diverticula) develop in the wall of the colon. The majority of people over the age of 60 in the United States have this condition. Most people have no symptoms and would not know they had diverticulosis without an x-ray or intestinal examination. About 20% of people

with this condition may develop **diverticulitis**, which is an inflammation in the wall of the colon.

Diarrhea

If the feces are passed along the colon too rapidly, insufficient water is reabsorbed and the feces become watery. **Diarrhea** is characterized by loose, watery, and frequent bowel movements. It may result from irritation of the colon's lining by dysentery bacteria, poor diet, nervousness, toxic substances, or irritants in food (such as in prunes, which stimulate intestinal peristalsis).

Chronic Constipation

Feces eliminated through the rectum are normally in a semisolid state. When defecation is delayed, however, the colon absorbs excessive water from the feces, rendering them dry and hard. When this occurs, defecation (or evacuation) becomes difficult.

For this reason, suppressing the need to defecate at normal times can lead to **constipation**. Constipation can also be caused by emotions such as anxiety, fear, or fright. Headaches and other symptoms that frequently accompany constipation result from the distention of the rectum, as opposed to toxins from the feces.

Treatment usually consists of eating proper foods, especially cereals, fruits, and vegetables; drinking plenty of fluids; getting enough exercise; developing regular bowel habits; and avoiding tension as much as possible.

Stomach Cancer

The initial cancer cells that develop in the stomach quickly grow into masses of tissue known as tumors.

Malignant stomach cancer cells can spread to other body parts, forming new growths, or metastases. Even if the original tumor is surgically removed, the cancer may recur when malignant cancer cells have spread.

The initial symptoms of stomach cancer are much like those of other digestive disorders: heartburn, loss of appetite, persistent indigestion, slight nausea, a feeling of bloated discomfort after eating, and occasional mild stomach pain. Later symptoms include traces of blood in the feces, pain, weight loss, and vomiting.

Treatment involves surgical removal of the stomach tumor as soon as possible. Depending on the size and the extent of growth of the tumor, part or all of the stomach may have to be removed.

If the cancer has spread, chemotherapy (treatment with anticancer drugs) is prescribed. These drugs are administered into the bloodstream, circulating through the body to kill cancerous cells in any location.

Radiation therapy plays a limited role in the treatment of stomach cancer. Very strong radiation doses are needed to kill the cancer cells, and they might also seriously damage neighboring healthy cells.

Cancer of the Colon

Colon cancer is believed to arise from a polypoid lesion. Early detection is critical. The following procedures are recommended for early detection:

- After the age of 40, an annual digital rectal examination is prescribed.

- After the age of 50, a stool slide specimen is obtained to look for hidden blood (**Hemoccult**).

A colon resection may be performed in a patient with colon cancer. Sometimes it may be necessary to perform a **colostomy**. In this procedure an opening is made through the abdomen into the colon, the cancerous tissue is removed, and the healthy tissue is brought out through the opening onto the skin. A pouch is worn to collect the body's wastes. This procedure causes stress and anxiety.

● REVIEW QUESTIONS

Select the letter of the choice that best completes the statement.

1. The process of changing complex foods into simpler substances to be absorbed is called:
   a. metabolism
   b. cellular respiration
   c. peristalsis
   d. digestion

2. The walls of the digestive tube that contain mucus are called:
   a. submucosa
   b. mucosa
   c. circular muscle
   d. visceral peritoneum

3. The accessory organs of the alimentary canal are the tongue, teeth, salivary glands, pancreas, liver, and:
   a. stomach
   b. esophagus
   c. gallbladder
   d. colon

4. The taste buds are found on projections called:
   a. papillae
   b. parotid
   c. palatine
   d. pharynx

5. The involuntary muscle action of the alimentary canal is called:
   a. pushing
   b. peristalsis
   c. stenosis
   d. contraction

6. Semiliquid food entering the small intestine is called:
   a. pepsin
   b. ptyalin
   c. chyme
   d. bolus

7. The lining of the abdominal cavity is:
   a. pleural
   b. peritoneal
   c. submucosal
   d. epithelial

8. The pancreatic enzyme that breaks down starches is called:
   a. trypsin
   b. steapsin
   c. secretion
   d. amylopsin

9. The enzyme that stimulates the liver to produce bile is called:
   a. protease
   b. steapsin
   c. secretin
   d. trypsin

10. Food is absorbed in the small intestine in the:
    a. villi
    b. submucosa
    c. peritoneal lining
    d. colon

● MATCHING

Match each of the terms in Column A with its correct description in Column B:

Column A	Column B
_____ 1. papillae	a. substances that promote chemical reactions in living things
_____ 2. enzyme	b. bleeding gums
_____ 3. digestion	c. small soft structure suspended from the soft palate
_____ 4. teeth	d. gums that protect the teeth
_____ 5. enamel	e. tract consisting of the mouth, stomach, and intestines
_____ 6. gingivae	f. aids in chewing and swallowing
_____ 7. accessory organs and structures of digestion	g. teeth, tongue, salivary glands, pancreas, liver, gallbladder, and appendix
	h. hardest substance in the body

_____ 8. salivary amylase

_____ 9. uvula

_____ 10. alimentary canal

_____ 11. cirrhosis

_____ 12. gastroenteritis

_____ 13. peptic ulcers

_____ 14. hiatal hernia

_____ 15. heartburn

_____ 16. diarrhea

_____ 17. cholecystitis

_____ 18. infectious hepatitis

_____ 19. pyloric stenosis

_____ 20. peritonitis

i. projections on the surface of the tongue containing the taste buds

j. process of changing complex solid foods into soluble forms to be absorbed by cells

k. enzyme manufactured by the salivary glands

l. frequent liquid bowel movements

m. chronic liver disease

n. protrusion of the stomach into the esophagus

o. viral infection of the liver

p. inflammation of the abdominal cavity

q. obstruction of the hepatic duct

r. inflammation of the stomach and intestinal lining

s. inflammation of the gallbladder

t. narrowing of sphincter in the stomach

u. cardiospasm

v. lesions that may result from acid secretion

w. common symptoms characterized by a burning sensation

● TRUE OR FALSE

Read each statement carefully and determine if it is true or false. Circle the letter *T* for true or *F* for false.

T   F   1. The large intestine is called the colon.

T   F   2. The large intestine is 20 feet long and 2 inches wide.

T   F   3. The cecum is located where the small intestine joins the large intestine.

T   F   4. The function of the appendix is unknown.

T   F   5. The large intestine stores and eliminates the waste products of digestion.

T   F   6. Regulation of water balance occurs in the large intestine because its lining absorbs water.

T   F   7. Constipation may be overcome by intensive and long periods of work and exercise.

T   F   8. Bulk foods such as whole-grain cereals, fruits, and vegetables may help avoid constipation.

T   F   9. The rectum is an extension of the descending colon.

T   F   10. The transverse colon lies between the ascending and the descending colon.

● LABELING

Label the teeth on the following diagram. (The teeth on the left are deciduous; those on the right are permanent teeth.)

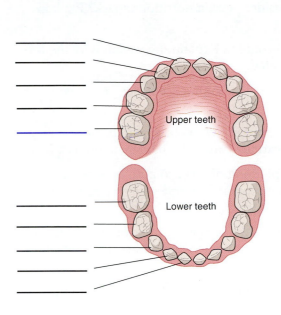
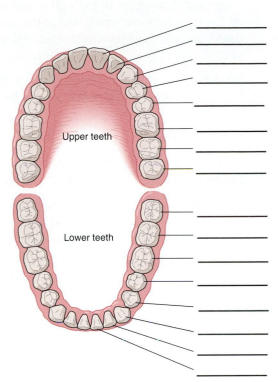

○APPLYING THEORY TO PRACTICE

1. You have just eaten a slice of pizza for lunch. In about 12 hours, that slice of pizza will be ready for absorption in the villi of the small intestine. Trace the journey of the pizza, naming all the enzymes involved, where the action takes place, and the end products of carbohydrate, protein, and fat metabolism. Would you consider pizza a nutritious snack? Explain your answer.

2. Enzymes secreted by the stomach are high in acid content. Explain the reason why the lining of the digestive system does not become ulcerated.

3. Dental checkups make you nervous. Why is it a good health practice to see your dentist at least once a year?

4. A pregnant woman states, "I have so much heartburn, I know my baby will be born with a full head of hair." Explain to her the reasons for heartburn and why her statement is a myth.

5. In the emergency room a woman, age 40, is complaining of a sharp pain between her shoulder blades on the right side. What is this symptomatic of and what type of treatment is necessary for this condition?

6. You must explain to a patient's family members what the necessary precautions are when caring for patients with hepatitis B. The family wants you to explain what a liver infection is and how it affects a person.

7. Your friend states, "All this stress is going to give me an ulcer." Explain to your friend why this is not an accurate statement.

Nutrition

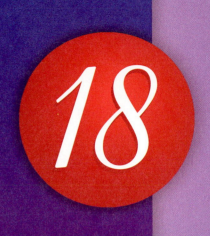

18

Objectives

- Define the term *nutrient*
- Describe the functions of the different types of nutrients
- Differentiate between the fat-soluble and water-soluble vitamins
- Describe the concept of Recommended Daily Dietary Allowances
- List the Dietary Guidelines for Americans
- Define the key words that relate to this chapter

Key Words

adipose tissue
anorexia nervosa
body mass index (BMI)
bulimia
calorie
cholesterol
complete proteins
essential amino acids
fiber
HDL
incomplete proteins
kilocalorie

LDL
mineral
nutrient
obesity
Recommended Dietary
   Allowances (RDA)
trace element
vitamin
VLDL
Wernicke's
   encephalopathy

The pace of an active daily life can at times be hectic and stress filled. This can occasionally cause one to eat on the run, to grab a bite at a fast food restaurant, or to forget to eat nutritiously.

The food one eats and drinks may or may not be nutritious. For food to be nutritious, it must contain the materials needed by the individual cells for proper cell functioning. These materials, or **nutrients**, include the following:

- Water
- Carbohydrates
- Lipids
- Proteins
- Minerals
- Vitamins
- Fiber

● WATER

Water is an essential component of all body tissues. It has several important functions in the human body:

- Acts as a solvent for all biochemical reactions
- Serves as a transport medium for substances
- Functions as a lubricant for joint movement and the digestive tract
- Controls body temperature by evaporation from the pores of the skin
- Serves as a cushion for body organs, such as the lungs and brain

Water makes up 55% to 65% of our total body weight. The body is continually losing water through evaporation, excretion, and respiration. This water loss must be replaced. We supply some of this need by drinking plain water. However, most of the body's water comes from the food we eat (including liquids). Practically all the foods we eat contain water, even those that seem to be dry. Water is the only nutrient for which the body can sense a need. When the body needs water, we experience thirst.

● CARBOHYDRATES

Carbohydrates include simple sugars, such as monosaccharides like glucose ($C_6H_{12}O_6$). Depending on the number of simple sugars found in the carbohydrate, they are classified as monosaccharides, disaccharides, or polysaccharides. Only the monosaccharides are small enough to be absorbed and eventually taken into the cells. The other carbohydrates are broken down by digestion in the digestive tract into the smallest possible molecular subunits before absorption.

Carbohydrates are the main source of energy for the body. Excess carbohydrates are converted into fat and stored in fat tissue. Nutritionists recommend that carbohydrates compose between 50% and 60% of the daily intake of calories.

A **calorie** is a unit that measures the amount of energy contained within the chemical bonds of different foods. The small calorie is defined as the amount of heat required to raise the temperature of 1 gram of water by 1° Celsius. A **kilocalorie** or large calorie is equal to 1000 small

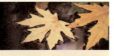

CHANGES OF AGING

Babies have more water in their bodies than adults. The older an adult gets, the less body weight is made up of water. The elderly, who can have as little as 45% body weight from water, are especially prone to the ill effects of water loss, or dehydration.

Cracked lips, skin that tents, and a dry, furrowed tongue are all signs of dehydration in the elderly. Some physicians postulate that the elderly person's sense of thirst is dulled, leading to less fluid intake and eventual dehydration. ■

calories. The calorie content of food is determined by measuring the amount of heat released when food is burned. The energy content of fat (9 kilocalories per gram) is slightly more than twice that of carbohydrate (4 kilocalories per gram) or protein (4 kilocalories per gram).

A normal adult usually requires between 1600 and 3000 kilocalories a day, depending on age, sex, body weight, and degree of physical activity. Newborn infants and young children have higher energy requirements per unit of body weight than adults because of the high energy expenditure of growth. See Table 18-1 for daily recommended energy intakes.

An excess intake of calories, in the form of either fats or carbohydrates, is transformed in the body to stored energy in the form of **adipose tissue**, commonly referred to as body fat.

An abundance of adipose tissue can lead to a serious medical condition called **obesity**. Formerly, health care professionals referred to the Metropolitan Life Insurance tables, first created in 1959, as a reference of normal body weight. Today health care professionals refer to the patient's **body mass index (BMI)**. The BMI is calculated using weight and height. The lowest mortality has been associated with those patients whose BMI is 19 to 22 kilograms per meter squared (kg/m^2). Patients with a BMI greater than 27 kg/m^2 are considered overweight, and those with a BMI greater than 30 kg/m^2 are considered obese. More than 50% of U.S. men and women are obese by definition. Patients more than 60% over their ideal weight double their risk of mortality from all causes.

TABLE 18-1 *Median Heights and Weights and Recommended Energy Intake*

Category	Age (years) or Condition	WEIGHT (kg)	WEIGHT (lb)	HEIGHT (cm)	HEIGHT (in)	REE[a] (Kcal/day)	Multiples of REE	AVERAGE ENERGY ALLOWANCE (kcal)[b] Per kg	Per day[c]
Infants	0.0-0.5	6	13	60	24	320		108	650
	0.5-1.0	9	20	71	28	500		98	850
Children	1-3	13	29	90	35	740		102	1,300
	4-6	20	44	112	44	950		90	1,800
	7-10	28	62	132	52	1,130		70	2,000
Males	11-14	45	99	157	62	1,440	1.70	55	2,500
	15-18	66	145	176	69	1,760	1.67	45	3,000
	19-24	72	160	177	70	1,780	1.67	40	2,900
	25-50	79	174	176	70	1,800	1.60	37	2,900
	51+	77	170	173	68	1,530	1.50	30	2,300
Females	11-14	46	101	157	62	1,310	1.67	47	2,200
	15-18	55	120	163	64	1,370	1.60	40	2,200
	19-24	58	128	164	65	1,350	1.60	38	2,200
	25-50	63	138	163	64	1,380	1.55	36	2,200
	51+	65	143	160	63	1,280	1.50	30	1,900
Pregnant	1st trimester								+0
	2nd trimester								+300
	3rd trimester								+500
Lactating	1st 6 months								+500
	2nd 6 months								+500

[a]*Calculation based on FAO equations, then rounded.*
[b]*In the range of light to moderate activity, the coefficient of variation is ± 20%.*
[c]*Figure is rounded.*
(Reprinted with permission from Recommended Dietary Allowances, 10th edition, *1989, by the National Academy of Sciences. Published by National Academy Press, Washington, D.C.)*

● LIPIDS

Lipids are a group of compounds containing fatty acids combined with an alcohol. They can be subdivided into two groups: simple lipids (fats, oils, waxes) and compound lipids (phospholipids, glycolipids, sterols). Like carbohydrates, fats are a source of energy. The same amount of fat can release more than twice as many calories as the same amount of carbohydrate or protein. The human body stores reserves of energy as fat in fat cells. Likewise, any excess carbohydrate and protein in the diet is transformed into fat and stored along with any excess fat.

Fats are an essential nutrient to the maintenance of the human body. Stored fats provide a supply of energy during emergencies such as sickness or during deficient caloric intakes. Fats also cushion the internal organs and serve as an insulation against the cold. Fats are components of the cell membrane and contribute to the formation of bile and steroid hormones, such as the sex hormones. Fats also contain fat-soluble vitamins, which are an important part of our daily diet. It is therefore essential to have a diet containing fats without exceeding the body's calorie needs. Total daily dietary fat intake should not exceed 25% to 30% of the daily caloric intake.

● CHOLESTEROL

Cholesterol is a fat found in animal products such as meat, eggs, cheese, and ice cream. Cholesterol is a white, waxlike substance used to build cells and make hormones. It is also manufactured by the liver. The cholesterol that you eat is not digested. There are no calories in cholesterol, but once in the body, it is difficult to eliminate. Fats and oils in food are called triglycerides. Your body turns excess calories into triglycerides, which are stored throughout the body as adipose tissue.

Because oil and water do not mix and blood is mostly water, triglycerides and cholesterol must be carried through blood cells by special proteins called lipoprotein: **HDL**, **LDL**, and **VLDL**. The lipoproteins LDL and VLDL carry fats to the cells; HDL, or high-density lipoprotein, is sometimes referred to as the "heavenly"

or "good" kind because it removes excess cholesterol from cells and carries it back to the liver to be broken down or eliminated.

Over the years, if more cholesterol is carried by the LDL than can be removed by HDL or used up in the cells, it builds up inside the artery walls, causing atherosclerosis. A condition called dyslipidemia, a disorder of fat in the blood (i.e., "high blood cholesterol"), exists.

The recommended level of blood cholesterol for people age 40 and over is under 200 milligrams per deciliter (mg/dl); any level over 200 mg/dl is considered too high for the long-term health of the heart.

The two most important steps you can take to lower your blood cholesterol are to reduce your intake of foods high in saturated fat and to lose weight if you are overweight. There are three general kinds of dietary fat:

- Saturated fat—oil from animal products that are solid at room temperature, such as butter, cheese, and meat fat.

- Polyunsaturated fat—oil from vegetable products; liquid at room temperature; used in moderation it lowers blood cholesterol. This type includes safflower oil and sunflower oil.

- Monounsaturated fat—oil from other vegetable products; liquid at room temperature; lowers blood cholesterol. This type includes olive oil and peanut oil.

If a label says "cholesterol free," it does not necessarily mean it is good for you. Look carefully: Many products with no cholesterol contain saturated fats.

Foods to substitute for saturated fat include skim milk, low-fat cheese, poultry, margarine, and low-fat ice cream. Some of the foods that help lower cholesterol include garlic, fresh fruit and vegetables, oat bran, wheat bran, and prunes. The Food and Drug Administration (FDA) has approved the use of Olestra as a fat substitute; it is currently being used in some snack foods.

● PROTEINS

Proteins are structurally more complex than carbohydrates and lipids and contain an amino (NH_2) group. They are synthesized in the cell cytoplasm from constituent molecules called amino acids.

Proteins serve many different functions in the body. Some are enzymes and regulate the rate of chemical reactions; others are important in growth and repair of tissues. When necessary, proteins can also be used as a source of energy. In addition, contractile systems (muscles), hormonal systems, plasma transport systems, clotting mechanisms, and defense systems (antibodies) all depend on proteins.

The body can synthesize some amino acids, but not all. The amino acids that cannot be made in the body are **essential amino acids**. Proteins that contain all the essential amino acids are known as **complete proteins**. Sources of such complete proteins are eggs, meat, milk, and milk products. Proteins that do not contain all the essential amino acids are called **incomplete proteins**. Vegetables contain incomplete proteins. However, a varied diet including vegetables supplies all the necessary complete proteins. For example, beans eaten alone and wheat eaten alone do not provide all the necessary complete proteins. However, when eaten together, they complement each other and supply the necessary complete proteins.

Unlike fats, the human body is unable to store excess amino acids. Any unused amino acids are broken down by the liver, and the amino group is excreted as a nitrogenous waste product called urea. The remainder of the amino acid may be burned for immediate energy or stored as fat or glycogen, a polysaccharide.

Protein synthesis cannot occur without all the essential amino acids present at the same time. Therefore it is important to include some source of complete protein in the various foods we eat during the day. The daily intake of calories from proteins should be no more than 15% to 20%.

Most adults in the United States eat a daily intake of protein in excess of the Recommended Dietary Allowance. This practice puts an extra burden on the liver and kidneys, which must eliminate the urea from the body.

● MINERALS AND TRACE ELEMENTS

A **mineral** is a chemical element that is obtained from inorganic compounds in food. Our knowledge of the role of the essential minerals and trace elements is incomplete. Many are notably necessary for normal human growth and maintenance. Among the most important of these nutrients are sodium, potassium, calcium, iron, phosphorous, and zinc.

Trace elements are present in the body in very small amounts. These include zinc, copper, iodine, cobalt, manganese, selenium, chromium, molybdenum, and fluorine.

The toxic limits of some trace elements are extremely close to the required dosages. This means that there is a critical difference among toxicity, health, and deficiency. Most of the essential minerals and trace elements are already present in the average normal U.S. diet in sufficient concentrations, and supplementation is only indicated for special conditions of disease, during pregnancy, and in old age. However, governmental surveys indicate that females in the United States might be consuming less than optimum daily intakes of calcium and iron.

Age-related osteoporosis is one of the most severely debilitating diseases in the United States and the most prevalent bone disease in

STREET SMART

In the past, certain populations of people living in land-locked areas frequently suffered from a condition called goiter. A person with a goiter had a very large neck caused by an enlarged thyroid gland.

Physicians identified that lack of a trace element, iodine, missing from the diet, was the cause of goiter. Today iodine is added to common table salt and goiter is relatively uncommon. ■

CHANGES OF AGING

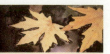

As a person ages, the bones lose calcium in a process called osteoporosis. Osteoporosis leads to lower bone density and bone weakening. The consequences of osteoporosis include more easily fractured bones, such as the hip, and an increasing curvature of the thoracic spine, called kyphosis. Hip fractures, accompanied by the debilitating effects of prolonged bed rest, can be devastating to an elderly person's health. Loss of lung capacity as a result of kyphosis further compromises the patient's health. ■

the world. Although the question of whether osteoporosis is a nutritional disorder remains unanswered, there is much convincing evidence that calcium deficiency accelerates the age-related loss of bone. The hormonal consequences of female menopause result in diminished calcium absorption in the intestines. This physiological consequence of reduced estrogen, along with lower bone density in females than in males during young adulthood, requires that proper attention be paid to calcium intake throughout the life cycle to maximize peak bone density before menopause.

Women of childbearing age tend to have low iron levels because of blood loss during the menstrual flow. Fatigue and iron deficiency anemia in these women can usually be ameliorated by iron supplementation. Table 18-2 summarizes the most important minerals and trace elements in the human diet.

● VITAMINS

A **vitamin** is defined as a biologically active organic compound, often functioning as a coenzyme, that is necessary for normal health and growth. Most enzymatic activity relies on the presence of coenzymes. A dietary vitamin deficiency results in a subclinical or obvious specific disorder. The term *vitamin* usually implies that the substance is not synthesized within the organism and, as a result, must be obtained from the diet. Vitamins are transported by the circulatory system to all the tissues of the body.

Recent evidence indicates that certain vitamins actually behave like hormones physiologically. For instance, both vitamin D and niacin are synthesized in the human (in inadequate amounts), conferring on them hormonal qualities, since hormones are produced in the body. The fat-soluble vitamins A, D, E, and K are readily stored in the body, and within the cell they demonstrate many similarities to the steroid hormones (estrogen, testosterone, cortisol). The water-soluble vitamins are B_1, B_2, B_3, B_6, B_{12}, pantothenic acid, folic acid, biotin, and vitamin C. An excessive intake of water-soluble vitamins results in increased excretion rather than additional storage.

Certain conditions, such as pregnancy, disease, emotional stress, old age, and vitamin de-

STREET SMART

Certain medications, called diuretics, help the body rid itself of excess fluid. Unfortunately these medications also cause a loss of potassium, an important intracellular mineral. To help replace this important mineral, patients on diuretics are encouraged to eat foods high in potassium, such as bananas and tomatoes. ■

TABLE 18-2 *Summary of Essential Minerals and Trace Elements Needed for Health*

MINERAL	FOOD SOURCES	FUNCTION	DEFICIENCY DISEASES
Calcium	Milk, cheese, dark green vegetables, dried legumes, sardines, shellfish	Bone and tooth formation Blood clotting Nerve transmission	Stunted growth Rickets Osteoporosis Convulsions
Chlorine	Common table salt, seafood, milk, meat, eggs	Formation of gastric juices Acid-base balance	Muscle cramps Mental apathy Poor appetite
Chromium	Fats, vegetables oils, meats, clams, whole-grain cereals	Involved in energy and glucose metabolism	Impaired ability to metabolize glucose
Copper	Drinking water, liver, shellfish whole grains, cherries, legumes, kidney, poultry, oysters, nuts, chocolate	Constituent of enzymes Involved with iron transport	Anemia
Fluorine	Drinking water, tea, coffee, seafood, rice, spinach, onions, lettuce	Maintenance of bone and tooth structure	Greater frequency of tooth decay
Iodine	Marine fish and shellfish, dairy products, many vegetables, iodized salt	Constituent of thyroid hormones	Goiter (enlarged thyroid)
Iron	Liver, lean meats, legumes, whole grains, dark green vegetables, eggs, dark molasses, shrimp, oysters	Constituent of hemoglobin Involved in energy metabolism	Iron deficiency anemia
Magnesium	Whole grains, green leafy vegetables, nuts, meats, milk, legumes	Involved in energy conversions and enzyme function	Growth failure Behavioral disturbances Weakness Spasms
Phosphorus	Milk, cheese, meat, fish, poultry, whole grains, legumes, nuts	Bone and tooth formation Acid-base balance Involved in energy metabolism	Weakness Demineralization of bone
Potassium	Meats, milk, fruits, legumes, vegetables	Acid-base balance Body water balance Nerve transmission	Muscular weakness Paralysis
Selenium	Fish, poultry, meats, grains milk, vegetables (depending on amount in soil)	Necessary for vitamin E function	Anemia Increased mortality?
Sodium	Common table salt, seafood, most other foods except fruit	Acid-base balance Body water balance Nerve transmission	Muscle cramps Mental apathy
Sulfur	Meat, fish, poultry, eggs, milk, cheese, legumes, nuts	Constituent of certain tissue proteins	Related to deficiencies of sulfur-containing amino acids
Zinc	Milk, liver, shellfish, herring, wheat bran	Involved in many enzyme systems Necessary for vitamin A metabolism	Growth failure Lack of sexual maturity Impaired wound healing Poor appetite

struction caused by methods of processing, storage, and preparing of foods, must be considered when determining daily individual vitamin requirements. Table 18-3 summarizes the major vitamins needed in the human diet.

● FIBER

Fiber is found only in plant foods, such as whole-grain breads, cereals, beans, and peas, and other vegetables and fruits. Eating a variety of fiber-containing plant foods is important

TABLE 18-3 *Summary of Major Vitamins Needed in the Human Diet*

VITAMIN	FOOD SOURCES	FUNCTION	DEFICIENCY DISEASES
A (Fat soluble)	Butter, fortified margarine, green and yellow vegetables, milk, eggs, liver	Night vision Healthy skin Proper growth and repair of body tissues	Night blindness Dry skin Slow growth Poor gums and teeth
B_1 (thiamine) (Water soluble)	Chicken, fish, meat, eggs, enriched bread, whole-grain cereals	Promotes normal appetite and digestion Needed by nervous system	Loss of appetite Nervous disorders Fatigue Severe deficiency causes beriberi
B_2 (riboflavin) (Water soluble)	Cheese, eggs, fish, meat, liver, milk, cereals, enriched bread	Needed in cellular respiration	Eye problems Sores on skin and lips General fatigue
B_3 (niacin) (Water soluble)	Eggs, fish, liver, meat, milk, potatoes, enriched bread	Needed for normal metabolism Growth Proper skin health	Indigestion Diarrhea Headaches Mental disturbances Skin disorders
B_{12} (Cyanocobalamin) (Water soluble)	Milk, liver, brain, beef, egg yolk, clams, oysters, sardines, salmon	Red blood cell synthesis Nucleic acid synthesis Nerve cell maintenance	Pernicious anemia Nerve cell malfunction
Folic acid (Water soluble)	Liver, yeast, green vegetables, peanuts, mushrooms, beef, veal, egg yolk	Nucleic acid synthesis Needed for normal metabolism and growth	Anemia Growth retardation
C (ascorbic acid) (Water soluble)	Citrus fruits, cabbage, green vegetables, tomatoes, potatoes	Needed for maintenance of normal bones, gums, teeth, and blood vessels	Weak bones Sore and bleeding gums Poor teeth Bleeding in skin Painful joints Severe deficiency results in scurvy
D (Fat soluble)	Beef, butter, eggs, milk	Needed for normal bone and teeth development Controls calcium and phosphorus metabolism	Poor bone and teeth structure Soft bones Rickets
E (tocopherol) (Fat soluble)	Margarine, nuts, leafy vegetables, vegetable oils, whole wheat	Used in cell respiration Protects red blood cells from destruction	Anemia in premature infants No known deficiency in adults
K (Fat soluble)	Synthesized by colon bacteria Green leafy vegetables, cereal	Essential for normal blood clotting	Slow blood clotting

for proper bowel function, reducing the symptoms of chronic constipation, diverticula disease, and hemorrhoids, and may lower the risk of heart diseases and some cancers. However, some of the health benefits associated with a high-fiber diet may come from other components present in these foods, not just from fiber itself. For this reason, fiber is best obtained from foods, rather than a supplement.

BIOCHEMICAL INDIVIDUALITY AND RECOMMENDED DAILY DIETARY ALLOWANCES

Developing universal "minimum daily requirements" that apply to everyone is an extremely difficult task. Nutritional requirements among individuals might vary for several reasons. Malabsorption disorders sometimes require that an individual needs greater than the average daily dosage of certain nutrients. Differences in the microbial environment of the intestine and genetic factors influencing biochemical reactions must also be considered. People experiencing psychological or physical stress often require a greater amount of certain nutrients to help the body maintain homeostasis, or a relatively constant internal environment.

In recognition of individual variations in nutritional requirements, a table of **Recommended Dietary Allowances (RDA)** has been approved by the Food and Nutrition Board of the National Academy of Sciences, Table 18-4. It contains the daily recommendations for protein, fat-soluble vitamins, water-soluble vitamins, and minerals. The allowances are intended to provide for individual variations among most normal persons as they live in the United States under usual environmental stresses.

DIETARY GUIDELINES FOR AMERICANS

In April 1992 the U.S. Department of Agriculture unveiled the "Food Guide Pyramid," made up of six food groups, Figure 18-1. This pyramid replaces the traditional pie chart with the basic four food groups. The recommended groups and amounts are as follows:

- Bread, cereal, and pasta—6 to 11 servings
- Vegetables—3 to 5 servings
- Fruit—2 to 4 servings
- Milk, yogurt, and cheese—2 to 3 servings
- Meat, poultry, fish, dry beans, eggs, and nuts—2 to 3 servings
- Fats, oils, and sweets—use sparingly

A scientific advisory committee was appointed by the U.S. government to develop dietary guidelines for the U.S. public. The importance of consuming a variety of foods to provide the essential nutrients at a caloric level

TABLE 18-4 *Recommended Dietary Allowances*

FOOD AND NUTRITION BOARD, NATIONAL ACADEMY OF SCIENCES–NATIONAL RESEARCH COUNCIL RECOMMENDED DIETARY ALLOWANCES.[a] REVISED 1989. DESIGNED FOR THE MAINTENANCE OF GOOD NUTRITION OF PRACTICALLY ALL HEALTHY PEOPLE IN THE UNITED STATES

Age (years) or Condition	Weight (kg)	Weight (lb)	Height[b] (cm)	Height (in)	Protein (g)	FAT-SOLUBLE VITAMINS Vitamin A (μg RE)[c]	Vitamin D (μg)[d]	Vitamin E (μg α-TE)[e]	Vitamin K (μg)	WATER-SOLUBLE VITAMINS Vitamin C (mg)	Thiamin (mg)	Riboflavin (mg)	Niacin (mg NE)[f]	Vitamin B6 (mg)	Folate (μg)	Vitamin B12 (μg)	MINERALS Calcium (mg)	Phosphorus (mg)	Magnesium (mg)	Iron (mg)	Zinc (mg)	Iodine (μg)	Selenium (μg)
Infants																							
0.0-0.5	6	13	60	24	13	375	7.5	3	5	30	0.3	0.4	5	0.3	25	0.3	400	300	40	6	5	40	10
0.5-1.0	9	20	71	28	14	375	10	4	10	35	0.4	0.5	6	0.6	35	0.5	600	500	60	10	5	50	15
Children																							
1-3	13	29	90	35	16	400	10	6	15	40	0.7	0.8	9	1.0	50	0.7	800	800	80	10	10	70	20
4-6	20	44	112	44	24	500	10	7	20	45	0.9	1.1	12	1.1	75	1.0	800	800	120	10	10	90	20
7-10	28	62	132	52	28	700	10	7	30	45	1.0	1.2	13	1.4	100	1.4	800	800	170	10	10	120	30
Males																							
11-14	45	99	157	62	45	1,000	10	10	45	50	1.3	1.5	17	1.7	150	2.0	1,200	1,200	270	12	15	150	40
15-18	66	145	176	69	59	1,000	10	10	65	60	1.5	1.8	20	2.0	200	2.0	1,200	1,200	400	12	15	150	50
19-24	72	160	177	70	58	1,000	10	10	70	60	1.5	1.7	19	2.0	200	2.0	1,200	1,200	350	10	15	150	70
25-50	79	174	176	70	63	1,000	5	10	80	60	1.5	1.7	19	2.0	200	2.0	800	800	350	10	15	150	70
51+	77	170	173	68	63	1,000	5	10	80	60	1.2	1.4	15	2.0	200	2.0	800	800	350	10	15	150	70
Females																							
11-14	46	101	157	62	46	800	10	8	45	50	1.1	1.3	15	1.4	150	2.0	1,200	1,200	280	15	12	150	45
15-18	55	120	163	64	44	800	10	8	55	60	1.1	1.3	15	1.5	180	2.0	1,200	1,200	300	15	12	150	50
19-24	58	128	164	65	46	800	10	8	60	60	1.1	1.3	15	1.6	180	2.0	1,200	1,200	280	15	12	150	55
25-50	63	138	163	64	50	800	5	8	65	60	1.1	1.3	15	1.6	180	2.0	800	800	280	15	12	150	55
51+	65	143	160	63	50	800	5	8	65	60	1.0	1.2	13	1.6	180	2.0	800	800	280	10	12	150	55
Pregnant					60	800	10	10	65	70	1.5	1.6	17	2.2	400	2.2	1,200	1,200	320	30	15	175	65
Lactating 1st 6 months					65	1,300	10	12	65	95	1.6	1.8	20	2.1	280	2.6	1,200	1,200	355	15	19	200	75
2nd 6 months					62	1,200	10	11	65	90	1.6	1.7	20	2.1	260	2.6	1,200	1,200	340	15	16	200	75

[a] The allowances, expressed as average daily intakes over time, are intended to provide for individual variations among most normal persons as they live in the United States under usual environmental stresses. Diets should be based on a variety of common foods to provide other nutrients for which human requirements have been less well defined. See text for detailed discussion of allowances and of nutrients not tabulated.

[b] Weights and heights of Reference Adults are actual medians for the U.S. population of the designated age, as reported by NHANES II. The median weights and heights of those under 19 years of age were taken from Hamill et al. (1979) (see page 337). The use of these figures does not imply that the height-to-weight ratios are ideal.

[c] Retinol equivalents. 1 retinol equivalent = 1 μg retinol or 6 μg β-carotene. See text for calculation of vitamin A activity of diets as retinol equivalents.

[d] As cholecalciferol. 10μg cholecalciferol = 400 IU of vitamin D.

[e] α-Tocopherol equivalents. 1 mg d-α tocopherol = 1 α-TE. See text variation in allowances and calculation of vitamin E activity of the diet as α-tocopherol equivalents.

[f] 1 NE (niacin equivalent) is equal to 1 mg of niacin or 60 mg of dietary tryptophan.

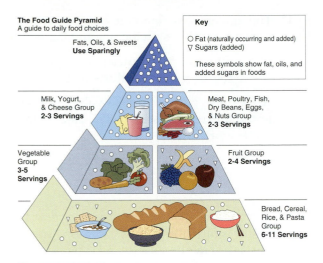

The Food Guide Pyramid
A guide to daily food choices

Key

○ Fat (naturally occurring and added)
▽ Sugars (added)

These symbols show fat, oils, and added sugars in foods

Fats, Oils, & Sweets
Use Sparingly

Milk, Yogurt, & Cheese Group
2-3 Servings

Meat, Poultry, Fish, Dry Beans, Eggs, & Nuts Group
2-3 Servings

Vegetable Group
3-5 Servings

Fruit Group
2-4 Servings

Bread, Cereal, Rice, & Pasta Group
6-11 Servings

● **FIGURE 18–1**   *Food guide pyramid.*

to maintain desirable body weight is emphasized. The following specific guidelines are advocated by the committee to help prevent the most prevalent and devastating diseases in our society: diabetes, cancer, hypertension, and heart disease.

1. Eat a variety of foods.

2. Maintain a desirable weight.

3. Avoid too much fat, saturated fat (mostly animal fat), and cholesterol.

4. Eat foods with adequate starch and fiber (roughage).

5. Avoid too much sugar.

6. Avoid too much sodium.

7. If you drink alcoholic beverages, do so in moderation.

● NUTRITION LABELING

Since May 1994 the Food and Drug Administration has required nutrition labeling for most foods offered for sale and regulated by the FDA, Figure 18-2. The nutrition label is required to include information on total calories and on amounts of calories from fat, cholesterol, sodium, total carbohydrates, dietary fiber,

STREET SMART

Stress is the body's response to physical, emotional, and behavioral stimuli. A certain amount of stress is good for a body, but only in moderation. Extreme stress can cause a breakdown in the body by pressuring certain organ systems to perform at a constantly high level.

To be prepared for the negative impacts of stress, the body needs proper nutrition. For EMS providers this may be easier said than done. Proper nutrition on the run is difficult to obtain.

Attention should be given to ensure that adequate hydration is obtained. Storing a liter of water in the front of an ambulance, for example, is an easy way to have fluids readily available.

Proper nutrition, in the form of vegetables and the like, should be included in every meal whenever possible. It is possible to eat on the run and still obtain proper nutrition. An EMS provider may want to consider eating a more Mediterranean-style diet.

Although EMS can be fast paced at times, encouraging EMS providers to eat high-calorie convenience foods, attention should be given to weight. Excess weight can itself become a stressor on the body.

These considerations must be weighed in light of the fact that fatigue and stress can affect appetite and that gastrointestinal problems such as nausea and diarrhea can adversely impact nutrition.

The body, like a machine, needs fluids and fuel to operate properly. Without proper hydration and nutrition, the machine fails. Cardiovascular disease, hypertension, and other debilitating stress-related disorders can be the result. ■

Nutrition Facts

Serving Size: 1/2 Cup
Servings Per Container: 4

Amount Per Serving

Calories 100   Calories from Fat 30

	% Daily Value*
Total Fat 3g	**5%**
Saturated Fat 0g	0%
Cholesterol 0mg	**0%**
Sodium 340mg	**14%**
Total Carbohydrate 15g	**5%**
Dietary Fiber 1g	4%
Sugars 0g	
Protein 2g	

Vitamin A 0%   •   Vitamin C 0%
Calcium   0%   •   Iron   2%

*Percent Daily Values are based on a 2,000 calorie diet. Your daily values may be higher or lower depending on your calorie needs:

	Calories	2,000	2,500
Total Fat	Less than	65g	80g
Sat Fat	Less than	20g	25g
Cholesterol	Less than	300mg	300mg
Sodium	Less than	2,400mg	2,400mg
Total Carbohydrate		300g	375g
Dietary Fiber		25g	30g

Calories per gram:
Fat 9 • Carbohydrate 4 • Protein 4

Ingredients: Flour, Water, Yeast Vegetable Oil, Salt, Artificial Flavor and Color.

● **FIGURE 18–2**   *A sample of nutrition labeling.*

sugars, protein, vitamin A, vitamin C, calcium, and iron, in that order. The information on the package should represent the packaged product before consumer preparation.

This final rule establishes a standard format for nutrition information on food labels consisting of the following:

1. The quantitative amount per serving of each nutrient, except vitamins and minerals

2. The amount of each nutrient as a percent of the RDA for a 2000-calorie diet

3. A footnote with reference values for selected nutrients based on 2000-calorie and 2500-calorie diets

4. Caloric conversion information

● **EATING DISORDERS**

Obesity is one of the most common "nutritional diseases" in our society and is the second leading cause of preventable death in the United States. This global health problem affects millions of people, leaving them at risk for diabetes, cardiovascular disease, and other weight-related disorders.

Of the many diseases associated with obesity, none is as dramatic as diabetes. The Centers for Disease Control and Prevention (CDC) reported that obesity-related diabetes has increased 57% since 1991 alone. Diabetes, even when well-controlled, can lead to hypertension, brain attacks (stroke), heart attacks (acute myocardial infarction), and blindness.

Because most cases of obesity are due to an excessive intake of calories in proportion to expenditure, a daily reduction of caloric intake and an increase in exercise are recommended for most overweight individuals.

Unfortunately, the desire to be thin has resulted in a complex disorder, mostly seen in young women, called **anorexia nervosa**. In true anorexia nervosa, there is no real loss of ap-

STREET SMART -

Anorexia is, by definition, a loss of appetite. Anorexia nervosa is a psychiatric condition, whereas anorexia itself may be a symptom of other potentially life-threatening medical conditions.

Anorexia, coupled with unexplained weight loss, may be signs of drug addiction, cancer, or tuberculosis, for example. Some medications may also induce anorexia. Any loss of appetite for a prolonged period should be reported to a health care professional. ■

MEDICAL HIGHLIGHTS

How many people have family recipes that cure colds, hay fever, asthma, and arthritis? Today scientists are looking at antioxidants, nutrients found in plant foods (such as vitamin C, carotenoids, vitamin E, and certain minerals), because of their potentially beneficial role in reducing the risk of cancer and certain other chronic diseases. Most of this research is in its earliest stages, but experts agree that certain food in moderation seem to boost healing.

Some foods believed to have healing power include the following:

- Barley—The soluble fiber in barley may be just as effective as oat bran in lowering cholesterol.*

- Carrots—Beta-carotene, a chemical found in carrots that offers an edge against cancer, may also protect against heart disease.

- Cheese—Identified in dental research as a food that fights, rather than creates, cavities. Tooth-friendly cheeses include cheddar, Monterey jack, edam, gouda, Roquefort, mozzarella, and Stilton.

- Chili peppers—Eating chili peppers helps clear a stuffed-up nose. The eye-watering, nose-running properties of peppers are good for people suffering from bronchitis, sinusitis, and colds.†

- Garlic—An all-around healing food; it lowers blood pressure and cholesterol levels and fights infection.

- Persimmons—A more powerful source of vitamin C than oranges, one persimmon is equal to 218 milligrams of vitamin C; one orange is equal to 70 milligrams of vitamin C.

- Prunes—Contain 60% of a fiber called pectin, which is known to reduce cholesterol. They are also high in iron, potassium, and beta-carotene.

- Dried beans—Help to lower cholesterol.

- Fish oil—Contains omega-3, a fatty acid currently being tested to help with inflammation from arthritis. Effective types of fish include mackerel, salmon, bluefish, oysters, mussels, crabs, and clams.

- Spinach and collard greens—Have two specific compounds that may be protective against the leading cause of irreversible blindness in older people, condition known as age-related macular degeneration.‡ ■

*Based on research conducted at Montana University.

†Based on research conducted by Dr. Irwin Zen at UCLA.

‡According to the November 9, 1994, edition of the *Journal of the American Medical Association*.

petite, but rather a refusal to eat because of a distorted body image and a fear of weight gain.

The criteria for diagnosis of anorexia nervosa are identified by the American Psychiatric Association as follows:

1. Intense fear of becoming obese that does not diminish as weight loss progresses

2. Disturbance of body image, such as claiming to feel fat even when emaciated

3. Weight loss of at least 25% of the original body weight

4. Refusal to maintain body weight over a minimum normal weight for age and height

5. No known physical illness that would account for the weight loss

6. Amenorrhea, or the cessation of menstruation

Another eating disorder associated with fear of weight gain is **bulimia**. It is characterized by episodic binge eating followed by purging behavior such as self-induced vomiting and laxative abuse. Bulimic patients are most often women somewhat older than those with anorexia nervosa. In some instances a young woman alternates between the two disorders.

The treatment of anorexia nervosa and bulimia is difficult and lengthy. The goals are restitution of normal nutrition and resolution of the underlying psychological problems. Early intervention is essential; the starvation associated with anorexia can cause irreversible tissue damage, and the purging associated with bulimia can cause homeostatic imbalances that lead to cardiac irregularities and, in extreme cases, death.

● REVIEW QUESTIONS

Select the letter of the choice that best completes the statement.

1. Materials needed by the individual cells for proper cell function are:
   a. proteases
   b. enzymes
   c. amylases
   d. nutrients

2. A gram of fat contains:
   a. 9 calories
   b. 4 calories
   c. 5 calories
   d. 7 calories

3. The main source of energy for the body is provided by:
   a. fats
   b. carbohydrates
   c. proteins
   d. water

4. To build and repair body tissue, you need:
   a. fats
   b. carbohydrates
   c. proteins
   d. water

5. The most common bone disease is:
   a. osteomyelitis
   b. fracture
   c. osteoporosis
   d. bone cancer

6. The minerals necessary to build bone and teeth are:
   a. iodine and calcium
   b. calcium and potassium
   c. calcium and phosphorus
   d. fluorine and calcium

7. Iodine is required for the formation of the:
   a. adrenal hormone
   b. thyroid hormone
   c. parathyroid hormone
   d. pituitary hormone

8. A vitamin needed to prevent night blindness is:
   a. vitamin A
   b. vitamin K
   c. vitamin C
   d. vitamin D

9. The vitamin essential for blood clotting is:
   a. vitamin A
   b. vitamin K
   c. vitamin C
   d. vitamin D

10. A food that has been identified to help lower cholesterol is:
    a. cheddar cheese
    b. garlic
    c. white bread
    d. broccoli

● APPLYING THEORY TO PRACTICE

1. In the spring of 1992 the U.S. Department of Agriculture (USDA) changed from the basic four food groups to the six-group pyramid plan, the model for Recommended Dietary Allowances. Compare your daily diet with the food pyramid plan. Should you consider changing your diet to meet these requirements?

2. Plan a 3-day meal plan, including between-meal snacks, that meets both recommended calorie intake and dietary allowances for yourself. Adjust this diet to meet the needs of a 12-year old male, height 62 inches. Adjust this diet to meet the needs of a 70-year old female, height 60 inches.

3. Nutritionists recommend 50% to 60% of carbohydrates daily in a 2000 calorie diet. What proportion of the diet would 60% be? How many calories would be in carbohydrates?

4. A 60-year-old woman informs you that she takes lots of calcium in foods such as milk, cheese, and ice cream to prevent osteoporosis. You know she has a high blood cholesterol level. How would you counsel her regarding her diet?

19 Urinary/Excretory System

Objectives

- Explain the function of the excretory organs
- Describe the structure and function of the organs in the urinary system
- Explain how the kidneys regulate water balance
- List and describe some common disorders of the urinary system
- Define the key words that relate to this chapter

Key Words

acid load
acute kidney failure
afferent arteriole
aldosterone
alkaline reserve
angiotensin
anuria
Bowman's capsule
buffering
calyces
catheterization
chronic renal failure
collecting tubule
cystitis
dialysis
dialyzer
distal convoluted tubule
dysuria
efferent arteriole
filtrate
fistula
glomerular filtration rate (GFR)
glomerulonephritis
glomerulus
glycosuria

hematuria
hemodialysis
hilum
hydronephrosis
kidney
kidney stones (renal calculi)
loop of Henle
nephron
neurogenic bladder
oliguria
osmoreceptor
peritoneal dialysis
pH value
proximal convoluted tubule
pyelonephritis
pyuria
renal column
renal fascia
renal papilla
renal pelvis
renal pyramid
renin
retroperitoneal
threshold

(continues)

⬤ URINARY SYSTEM

Food is utilized as energy through the processes of digestion, absorption, and metabolism. The blood and lymph transport products of digestion to the tissues. After the cells of the tissues have used the food and oxygen needed for growth and repair, waste products formed by the process are taken away and excreted from the body. The excretory organs eliminate the metabolic wastes and undigested food residue.

The excretory organs through which elimination takes place include the kidneys, the skin, the intestines, and the lungs. The lungs, generally considered part of the respiratory system, serve an excretory function in that they give off carbon dioxide and water vapor during exhalation. The urinary system functions largely as an excretory agent of nitrogenous wastes, salts, and water, whereas the skin excretes dissolved wastes present in perspiration, mostly dissolved salts. The indigestible residue, water, and bacteria are excreted by the intestines. The excretion of waste products is described and summarized in Table 19-1.

The urinary system performs the main part of the excretory function in the body, Figure 19-1. The most important excretory organs are the **kid-**

TABLE 19-1 *Elimination of Waste Products*

ORGAN	PRODUCT OF EXCRETION	PROCESS OF ELIMINATION
Lungs	Carbon dioxide and water vapor	Exhalation
Kidneys	Nitrogenous wastes and salts dissolved in water to form urine	Urination
Skin	Dissolved salts	Perspiration
Intestines	Solid wastes and water	Defecation

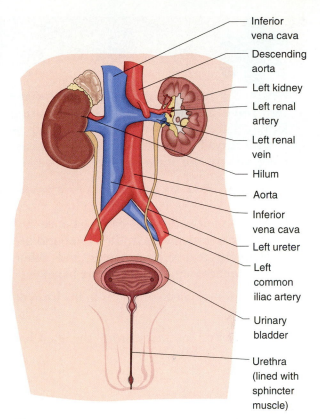

⬤ **FIGURE 19–1** *The structures of the urinary system.*

neys. Their primary excretory function is removal of the nitrogenous waste products. If the kidneys fail to function properly, toxic wastes start to accumulate in the body. Toxic wastes accumulating in the cells cause them to "suffocate" and literally poison themselves.

The urinary system consists of two kidneys (that form the urine), two ureters, a bladder, and a urethra. Each kidney has a long, tubular ureter that carries urine to the urinary bladder. This is a temporary storage sac for urine, from which urine is excreted through the urethra.

⬤ FUNCTIONS OF THE URINARY SYSTEM

Functions of the urinary system include the following:

1. Excretion, which is the process of removing nitrogenous waste material, certain salts, and excess water from the blood

2. Maintenance of acid-base balance by evaluating elements in the blood and selectively reabsorbing water and other substances to maintain the pH balance

3. Secretion of waste products in the form of urine

4. Elimination of urine from the bladder, where it is stored

KIDNEYS

The kidneys are bean-shaped organs resting high against the dorsal wall of the abdominal cavity; they lie on either side of the vertebral column, between the peritoneum and the back muscles. Because the kidneys are located behind the peritoneum, they are said to be retroperitoneal. They are positioned between the twelfth thoracic and third lumbar vertebrae. The right kidney is situated slightly lower than the left because of the large area occupied by the liver.

Each kidney and its blood vessels are enclosed within a mass of fat tissue called the adipose capsule. In turn, each kidney and adipose capsule is covered by a tough, fibrous tissue called the renal fascia.

There is an indentation along the concave medial border of the kidney called the hilum. The hilum is a passageway for the lymph vessels, nerves, renal artery and vein, and ureter. At the hilum the fibrous capsule continues downward, forming the outer layer of the ureter. Cutting the kidney in half lengthwise reveals its internal structure. The upper end of each ureter flares into a funnel-shaped structure known as the renal pelvis.

The kidneys have the potential to work harder than they actually do. Under ordinary circumstances, only a portion of the nephron is used. Should one kidney not function or have to be removed, more nephrons and tubules open up in the second kidney to assume the work of the nonfunctioning or missing kidney.

Medulla and Cortex

The kidney is divided into two layers: an outer, granular layer called the cortex and an inner, striated layer, the medulla. The medulla is red and consists of radially striated cones called the renal pyramids. The base of each renal pyramid faces the cortex, whereas its apex (renal papilla) empties into cuplike cavities called calyces. These in turn empty into the renal pelvis.

The reddish brown cortex is composed of millions of microscopic functional units of the kidney called nephrons. Cortical tissue is interspersed between renal pyramids, separating and supporting them. These interpyramidal cortical supports are the renal columns. The renal columns and the renal pyramids alternate with one another, Figure 19-2.

NEPHRON

The nephron is the basic structural and functional unit of the kidney. Most of the nephron is located within the cortex, with only a small, tubular portion in the medulla. Each kidney has more than 1 million nephrons, which together compose 140 miles of filters and tubes.

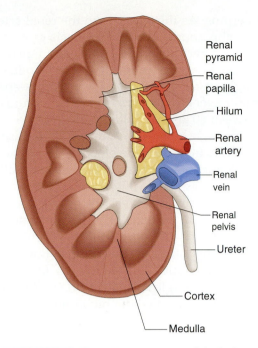

Renal
pyramid

Renal
papilla

Hilum

Renal
artery

Renal
vein

Renal
pelvis

Ureter

Cortex

Medulla

● **FIGURE 19–2**   *The structures of the kidney.*

A nephron begins with the **afferent arteriole**, which carries blood from the renal artery. The afferent arteriole enters the double-walled, hollow **Bowman's capsule**.* Within the capsule the afferent arteriole finely divides, forming a

*Named for Sir William Bowman (1816–1892), English anatomist and ophthalmologist.

knotty ball called the **glomerulus**, which contains some 50 separate capillaries. The combination of Bowman's capsule and the glomerulus is known as the renal corpuscle. Bowman's capsule sends off a highly twisted tubular branch referred to as the **proximal convoluted tubule**.

The proximal convoluted tubule descends into the medulla to form the **loop of Henle**. In Figure 19-3, observe that the loop of Henle has a straight descending limb, a loop, and a straight ascending limb. When the ascending limb of Henle's loop returns to the cortex, it turns into the **distal convoluted tubule**. Eventually this convoluted tubule opens into a larger, straight vessel known as the **collecting tubule**. Several distal convoluted tubules join to form this single straight collection tubule. The collecting tubule empties into the renal pelvis, then into the ureter.

As Figure 19-3 shows, the walls of the renal tubules are surrounded by capillaries. After the afferent arteriole branches out to form the glomerulus, it leaves Bowman's capsule as the **efferent arteriole**. The efferent arteriole branches to form the peritubular capillaries surrounding the renal tubules. All these capillaries eventually join together to form a small branch of the renal vein, which carries blood from the kidney.

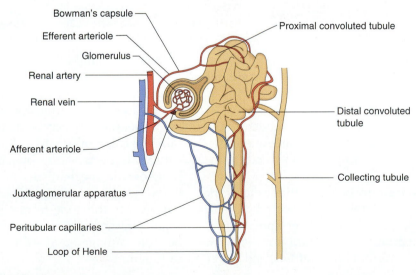

Bowman's capsule

Efferent arteriole

Glomerulus

Renal artery

Renal vein

Afferent arteriole

Juxtaglomerular apparatus

Peritubular capillaries

Loop of Henle

Proximal convoluted tubule

Distal convoluted tubule

Collecting tubule

● **FIGURE 19–3**   *Structure of the nephron.*

The Path of the Formation of Urine

Blood enters the afferent arteriole and passes through the glomerulus to Bowman's capsule. There it becomes filtrate (blood minus the red blood cells and plasma proteins) and continues through the proximal convoluted tubule to the loop of Henle; from there it progresses to the distal convoluted tubule and on to the collecting tubule (at this point about 99% of the filtrate has been reabsorbed). Approximately 1 milliliter of urine is formed per minute; this urine goes to the renal pelvis and then to the ureter; from there it moves to the bladder, the urethra, and finally to the urinary meatus.

URINE FORMATION IN THE NEPHRON

The kidney nephrons form urine through three processes: (1) filtration by the glomerulus, (2) reabsorption within the renal tubules, and (3) secretion by the tubular cells.

Filtration

The first step in urine formation is filtration. In this process, blood from the renal artery enters the smaller afferent arteriole, which in turn enters the even smaller capillaries of the glomerulus. As the blood from the renal artery travels this course, the blood vessels grow narrower and narrower. This results in an increase in blood pressure. In most of the capillaries throughout the body, blood pressure is about 25 millimeters of mercury; in the glomerulus, it is between 60 and 90 millimeters.

This high blood pressure forces a plasma-like fluid to filter from the blood in the glomerulus into Bowman's capsule. This fluid is called the filtrate. It consists of water, glucose, amino acids, some salts, and urea. The filtrate does not contain plasma proteins or red blood cells because they are too large to pass through the pores of the capillary membrane. Bowman's capsule filters out 125 milliliters of fluid from the blood in a single minute. In 1 hour, 7500 milliliters of filtrate leave the blood; this amounts to some 180 liters in a 24-hour period.

As the nephric filtrate continues along the tubules, 99% of this water is reabsorbed back into the bloodstream; therefore only 1 to 1.5 (1000 to 1500 milliliters) liters of urine is excreted per day.

Reabsorption

This process includes the reabsorption of useful substances from the filtrate within the renal tubules into the capillaries around the

STREET SMART

Chronic hypertension, generally defined as a persistent diastolic pressure greater than 90 millimeters of mercury (mm Hg), is common in the United States; it is present in about 15% of the population. Hypertension is twice as common among African-Americans, and the incidence of hypertension tends to increase with age.

Hypertension forces the kidneys to work harder. The result of this increased pressure to filtrate and then reabsorb water and sodium, an increased glomerular filtration rate (GFR), is higher than normal levels of salts and water in the blood. Higher levels of sodium and water lead to increased blood volume, which in turn affects the work of the heart.

Causes of hypertension can include kidney diseases, endocrine disorders, and certain vascular anomalies. Regardless of the cause, hypertension upsets the normal homeostatic mechanisms and causes many body systems to readjust to the higher pressure. Over the long-term, the more fragile organs in the body, such as the kidneys, may become damaged and start a gradual decline in function. ■

STREET SMART

Early physicians, including Galen, the father of medicine, were able to diagnosis diabetes mellitus because of the presence of two key symptoms that come from the kidneys.

The first symptom was the massive amounts of urine, called polyuria, that a person with diabetes would pass. In fact, *diabetes*, literally translated, means "to pass through."

The other symptom was due to the large amounts of glucose in the urine, called gly-cosuria. Flies were attracted to night pots of fresh urine left by persons with diabetes. A taste of the urine revealed sweetness. In fact, *mellitus*, literally translated, means "sweet."

Therefore diabetes mellitus, sweet urine, has been recognized as a human disease since antiquity. The recent marked increase in diabetes mellitus has been attributed to obesity, another human disorder that has been recognized since antiquity. ■

tubules (peritubular capillaries). These include water, glucose, amino acids, vitamins, bicarbonate ions (HCO_3^-), and the chloride salts of calcium, magnesium, sodium, and potassium. Reabsorption starts in the proximal convoluted tubules; it continues through the Henle's loop, the distal convoluted tubules, and the collecting tubules.

The proximal tubules reabsorb approximately 80% of the water filtered out of the blood in the glomerulus (180 liters). Water absorbed through the proximal tubules constitutes obligatory water absorption by osmosis. Simultaneously, glucose, amino acids, vitamins, and some sodium ions are actively transported back into the blood. However, when levels exceed normal limits, the selective cells lining the tubules no longer reabsorb substances such as glucose but allow it to remain in the tubule to be eliminated in the urine. The term used to describe the limit of reabsorption is threshold. Passing this level is referred to as "spilling over the threshold." For example, people who have diabetes spill sugar frequently; therefore sugar can be found in their urine (glycosuria). As another example, when a person is taking medications, the tubules only reabsorb a certain amount of the drug; therefore the medication may have to be taken every 4 to 6 hours to maintain a therapeutic dosage of the drug in the blood.

In the distal convoluted tubules, approximately 10% to 15% of water is reabsorbed into the bloodstream, depending on the needs of the body. This type of water absorption is called optional reabsorption. It is controlled by antidiuretic hormone (ADH) and aldosterone. ADH and aldosterone help maintain balance of body fluids, Figure 19-4.

Secretion

The process of secretion is the opposite of reabsorption. Some substances are actively secreted into the tubules. Secretion transports substances from the blood in the peritubular capillaries into the urine in the distal and collecting tubules. Substances secreted into the urine include ammonia creatinine, hydrogen ions (H^+), potassium ions (K^+), and some drugs. The electrolytes are selectively secreted to maintain the body's acid-base balance.

Acid-Base Balance

The reabsorption of bicarbonate ions (HCO_3^-) is a particularly important function of the kidneys. The enzymes and chemical reactions within the body operate in a narrow range of acidity (pH). When the body has too much acid in the blood, called an acid load, it must neutralize or eliminate that acid load to maintain proper cellular function and homeostasis.

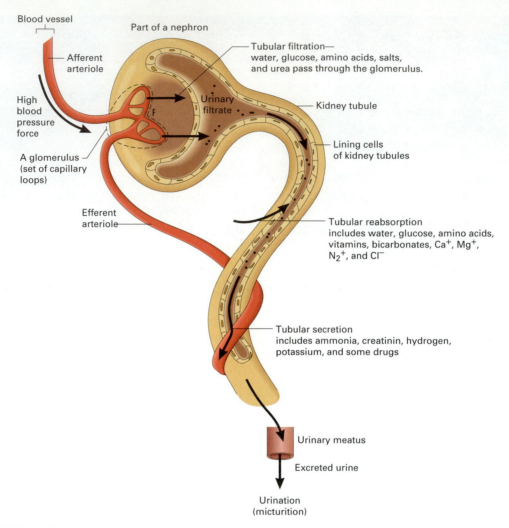

Blood vessel

Part of a nephron

Afferent arteriole

Tubular filtration—
water, glucose, amino acids, salts,
and urea pass through the glomerulus.

High blood pressure force

Urinary filtrate

F

Kidney tubule

A glomerulus (set of capillary loops)

Lining cells of kidney tubules

Efferent arteriole

Tubular reabsorption
includes water, glucose, amino acids,
vitamins, bicarbonates, Ca^+, Mg^+,
N_2^+, and Cl^-

Tubular secretion
includes ammonia, creatinin, hydrogen,
potassium, and some drugs

Urinary meatus

Excreted urine

Urination (micturition)

● **FIGURE 19–4**   *Processes and structures of the nephron.*

As a review, whenever an electrolyte separates—*ionizes*—in water and releases a hydrogen ion (H^+), it is called an acid. Common byproducts of cellular metabolism include carbonic acid, lactic acid, keto acids, and phosphoric acid. The concentration of hydrogen ions in those acids are measured as **pH value**.

The first means of neutralizing acid, a process called **buffering**, is by combining acid (H^+) with bicarbonate (HCO_3^-), an alkali, and creating the byproducts of water (H_2O) and carbon dioxide (CO_2).

$$HCO_3^- + H^+ = H_2O + CO_2$$

The water (H_2O) is then eliminated via the kidneys and the carbon dioxide (CO_2) is eliminated via the lungs.

The amount of bicarbonate buffer available, called the **alkaline reserve**, determines the blood's ability to neutralize acid.

The body's first defense against high acidity levels is the chemical buffering system in the blood, which is in large part the bicarbonate in the blood. These chemical reactions occur within seconds and maintain homeostasis until the alkaline reserves are depleted.

The secondary line of defense are the lungs and kidneys. The lungs will attempt to blow-off carbon dioxide, forcing more acid to convert to water and carbon dioxide and lowering the acid load as quickly as possible. It takes several minutes for lungs to effectively rid the body of excess acid.

Finally, if the buffering system and the lungs cannot compensate for the excessive acid load, as occurs in shock syndrome, then the kidneys start to conserve (reabsorb) more bicarbonate to add to the blood's alkaline reserve. This process of increased reabsorption can take up to 24 hours to begin.

Urinary Output

The amount of urinary output is 1000 to 2000 milliliters per 24 hours, with an average of 1500 milliliters per day. Volume varies with diet, fluid intake, temperature, and physical activity.

The kidneys are one of the first of the core organs to be affected by low blood pressure, hypotension, and loss of sufficient circulating blood, hypoperfusion.

When urinary output drops to below 40 milliliters per hour, it can be assumed that the kidneys are being hypoperfused and the patient's other core organs, including the heart, lungs, and brain, are also hypoperfused.

For this reason, when a patient comes into an emergency department with signs of hypoperfusion, or shock, the patient is quickly catheterized. Catheterization is a medical procedure in which a tube with a balloon, called an indwelling catheter, is placed through the urethra to drain the bladder and measure the urine amount. By carefully watching trends of urine amounts, and thus kidney function, the success or failure of resuscitation can be measured.

Another factor regulating secretion is the amount of solutes in the filtrate. Again consider the patient with diabetes, in whom there is an increase in the amount of glucose; it spills over into the urine, increasing the urine volume eliminated that day because more fluid is allowed to pass through to dilute the glucose content.

When large amounts of urine are produced by the kidneys, it is called polyuria. When small amounts of urine are produced by the kidneys, as a result of hypoperfusion, for example, it is called oliguria. When the kidneys stop making urine altogether, it is called anuria. Anuria is a sign of acute renal failure. Without urine production, large amounts of acids and electrolytes, especially potassium, collect and can poison the body. This accumulation of metabolic waste is called uremia.

Urinalysis, an examination of the urine, can determine the presence of blood cells, bacteria, acidity level, specific gravity (weight), and physical characteristics such as color, clarity, and odor. A urinalysis is the most common noninvasive diagnostic test done.

Normally urine does not contain glucose. As part of a routine urinalysis, the urine is frequently tested for the presence of glucose. If glucose is present, more tests for diabetes are in order. If the patient is diagnosed with diabetes, the urine may be tested for glucose using a "dipstick." If the patient is "spilling sugar," the insulin dose may be adjusted.

● URETERS

Urine passes from the kidneys out of the collecting tubules into the renal pelvis, down the ureter, into the urinary bladder. There are two ureters (one from each kidney) carrying urine from the kidneys to the urinary bladder. They are long, narrow tubes, less than a quarter inch wide and 10 to 12 inches long. Mucous membrane lines both renal pelves and the ureters. Beneath the mucous membrane lining of the ureters are smooth muscle fibers. When these muscles contract, peristalsis is initiated, pushing urine down the ureter into the urinary bladder.

● URINARY BLADDER

The urinary bladder, a hollow muscular organ made of elastic fibers and involuntary muscle, acts like a reservoir. It stores the urine until about 1 pint (500 milliliters) is accumulated. The bladder then becomes uncomfortable and must be emptied. Emptying the bladder, or voiding, takes place by muscular contractions of the bladder that are involuntary, although they can be controlled to some extent through the nervous system. Contraction of the bladder muscles forces the urine through a narrow canal, the urethra, which extends to the outside opening, the urinary meatus.

● CONTROL OF URINARY SECRETION

The secretion of urine is under both chemical and nervous control.

Chemical Control

The reabsorption of water in the distal convoluted kidney tubules and the collecting ducts is influenced by antidiuretic hormone. ADH helps to increase the size of the cell membrane pores in the epithelial cells of the distal tubule and collecting ducts by increasing their permeability to water. The secretion and regulation of the ADH is under the control of the hypothalamus. In the hypothalamus, highly sensitive receptor cells, called **osmoreceptors**, are sensitive to the osmotic pressure of blood plasma. An increase in the osmotic blood pressure resulting from salt retention causes an increase in ADH secretion. This inhibits normal urine formation, and water may also be held in the tissues. Figure 19-5 shows the effect of salt retention on human tissues.

There are other hormones involved in the reabsorption process. **Aldosterone** secreted by the adrenal cortex promotes the excretion of potassium and hydrogen ions and the reabsorption of sodium ions; chloride ions and water are also absorbed. As the blood passes through the glomerulus to Bowman's capsule, specialized cells are able to detect a drop in blood pressure. A hormone called **renin** is released by the kidneys into the bloodstream. Renin stimulates the release of aldosterone by the adrenal cortex. By interaction with a serum protein, or globulin, renin converts into **angiotensin** in the blood. Angiotensin is a powerful blood vessel constrictor (**vasopressor**) that increases blood pressure and stimulates aldosterone production. In the absence of aldosterone, sodium and water are excreted in large amounts and potassium is retained. Any dysfunction to the adrenal cortex produces pronounced changes in the salt and water content of body fluids.

Diuretics increase urinary output by inhibiting the reabsorption of water. Alcohol and caffeine are examples of common diuretics. Alcohol inhibits the secretion of ADH from the pituitary gland. This increases urinary output and may cause dehydration. (This explains why after drinking alcohol the night before, you may wake up feeling "parched" and dried out.) Caffeine increases the loss of sodium ion, thus increasing the loss of water.

Nervous Control

The nervous control of urine secretion is accomplished directly through the action of nerve impulses on the blood vessels leading to the kidney and on those within the kidney leading to the glomeruli. Indirect nerve control is achieved through the stimulation of certain endocrine glands, whose hormonal secretions control urinary secretion.

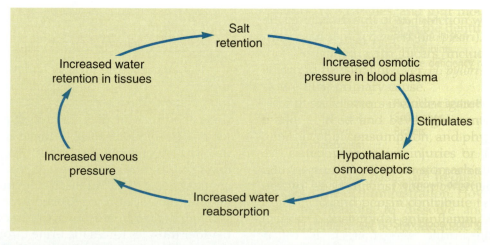

● **FIGURE 19–5**   *How salt retention influences water retention in tissues.*

STREET SMART

Antidiuretic hormone is also known by another name, vasopressin. Vasopressin has recently received international recognition for its use during cardiac arrest resuscitation. Advanced EMS providers can use vasopressin immediately following defibrillation, instead of epinephrine. Vasopressin (Pitressin) is a powerful smooth muscle stimulant that increases blood pressure. Vasopressin can be thought of as long-acting epinephrine. ■

DISORDERS OF THE URINARY SYSTEM

Acute kidney failure may be sudden in onset. Causes can be nephritis (inflammation of the nephron), shock, injury, bleeding, sudden heart failure, or poisoning. The symptoms of acute kidney failure include oliguria, which is scanty or diminished production of the urine, or anuria, which is absence of urine formation. Suppression of urine formation is dangerous; unless anuria is relieved, uremia will develop. Uremia is a toxic condition that occurs when the blood retains urinary waste products. Symptoms resulting from uremia are headaches, dyspnea, nausea, vomiting, and, in extreme cases, coma and death.

Chronic renal failure is a condition in which there is a gradual loss of function of the nephrons.

Glomerulonephritis is an inflammation of the glomerulus of the nephron. The filtration process is affected. Plasma proteins are filtered through and protein is found in the urine as albumin (albuminuria). In addition, red blood cells are present (**hematuria**).

Acute glomerulonephritis occurs in some children about 1 to 3 weeks after a bacterial infection, usually strep throat. The illness is treated with antibiotics and recovery takes place.

Chronic glomerulonephritis occurs when the filtration membrane is permanently affected. There is diminished function of the kidney, which may result in kidney failure.

Hydronephrosis occurs when the renal pelvis and calyces become distended because of an accumulation of fluid. The urine "backs up" because of a blockage in the ureter or pressure on the outside of the ureter, which may narrow the passageway. The blockage may be caused by a kidney stone. Other conditions that may cause hydronephrosis are pregnancy and an enlarged prostate gland, which causes pressure on the ureters or bladder. The treatment for this condition is the removal of the obstruction.

Pyelonephritis is the inflammation of the kidney tissue and the renal pelvis. This condition generally results from an infection that has spread from the ureters. One of the symptoms is **pyuria**, the presence of pus in the urine. The course of treatment includes the administration of antibiotics.

Kidney stones, or **renal calculi**, are stones formed in the kidney. Some materials contained in urine are only slightly soluble in water. Therefore when stagnation occurs, the microscopic crystals of calcium phosphate, along with uric acid and other substances, may clump together to form kidney stones. These kidney stones slowly grow in diameter. They eventually fill the renal pelvis and obstruct urine flow in the ureter. Usually the first symptom of a kidney stone is extreme pain, which occurs suddenly in the kidney area or lower abdomen and moves to the groin. Other symptoms include nausea and vomiting, burning, frequent urge to void, chills, fever, and weakness. There may also be hematuria. Diagnosis is made by symptoms, ultrasound, and x-ray studies such as intravenous pyelogram (IVP) and kidney, ureter, and bladder (KUB). Treatment includes an increase in fluids, which increases urinary output. This may help to flush out the stone. Medications are given to help dissolve the stone. If this is not successful, a urethroscopic examination, or lithotripsy, may be done.

Cystitis is the inflammation of the mucous membrane lining of the urinary bladder. The most common cause of cystitis is from the bacteria *Escherichia coli,* which is normally found in the rectum, or from urethritis; cystitis usually leads to painful urination (**dysuria**) or frequent urination (polyuria). This condition is more common in women. The length of the female urethra is about 1.25 to 2 inches. Organisms can easily enter the urethra from outside the body. The treatment of cystitis involves antibiotics and urinary antiseptics, along with increased fluid intake. The patient should be taught proper wiping techniques after urination. The patient with cystitis must be reminded to complete the prescribed amount of medication to prevent reinfection.

Incontinence is also known as involuntary micturition (urination). In this condition an individual loses voluntary control over urination. Incontinence occurs in babies prior to toilet training, because they lack control over the external sphincter muscle of the urethra. Thus urination occurs whenever the bladder fills. Similarly, a person who has suffered a stroke, or one whose spinal cord has been severed, may have no bladder control. In these latter conditions a patient may require an indwelling catheter.

Neurogenic bladder is a condition caused by damage to the nerves that control the urinary bladder. This results in dysuria, the inability to empty the bladder completely, and incontinence.

Dialysis

Dialysis is the type of treatment used for kidney failure. Dialysis involves the passage of blood through a device with a semipermeable membrane to rid the blood of harmful wastes,

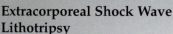

MEDICAL HIGHLIGHTS

Extracorporeal Shock Wave Lithotripsy

A surgical procedure called extracorporeal shock wave lithotripsy (ESWL) may be done to remove kidney stones located high in the ureters or the renal pelvis. ESWL uses shock waves created outside the body to travel through the skin and body tissues until the waves hit the dense stones. The stones become sandlike and are passed through the urinary tract. There are several devices used. The patient is positioned in the water bath while the shock waves are transmitted. Most devices use either x-ray or ultrasound to help the surgeon locate the stone during the treatment.

This procedure can be done on an outpatient basis. Recovery time is short, and most people resume normal activities in a few days. Some complications may occur, such as hematuria, bruising, and minor discomfort on the back or abdomen. In addition, the shattered stone fragments may cause discomfort as they pass through the urinary tract. Previous treatment for kidney stones involved nephrolithotomy, an opening into the kidney, with a week's hospital stay and 4 to 6 weeks of recovery.

Uteroscopic Stone Removal

Uteroscopic stone removal is done for mid-ureter and lower stones. A surgeon passes a small fiberoptic instrument called a urethroscope through the urethra and bladder into the ureter. The surgeon then locates the stone and either removes it with a cagelike device or shatters it with a special instrument that produces a form of shock wave. ■

extra salt, and water. Dialysis devices serve as a substitute kidney. The two forms of dialysis are hemodialysis and peritoneal dialysis.

Hemodialysis is a process for purifying blood by passing it through thin membranes and exposing it to a solution, called a dialysate, that continually circulates around the membrane. Substances in the blood pass through the membranes into the lesser concentrated dialysate in response to the laws of diffusion. The part of the unit that actually substitutes for the kidney is a glass tube called a **dialyzer**, which is filled with thousands of minute hollow fibers attached firmly at both ends, Figure 19-6. Blood from the patient flows through the fibers, which are surrounded by circulating dialysate. The dialysate is individualized for each patient to provide the appropriate levels of sodium, bicarbonate, and other substances. These cross the membrane and enter the blood. At the same time, extra water and waste products leave the blood to enter the dialysate.

The patient is connected to the dialysis unit by means of needles and tubing that take blood from the patient to the machine and return it to the patient. A **fistula** (an opening between an artery and a vein) or a graft (a vein inserted between the artery and a vein) is surgically constructed to provide a site for inserting the needles. Artificial veins may last from 3 to 5 years.

Most patients are assigned to a dialysis center for periodic treatment; however, treatment can also be done in the home if the patient and family are willing to assume responsibility. It is usually done two to three times a week and each treatment lasts from 2 to 4 hours. To avoid side effects, the patient is advised to follow special diet instructions and take medications as prescribed.

Peritoneal dialysis uses the patient's own peritoneal lining instead of a dialyzer to filter the blood. A cleansing solution called the dialysate travels through a catheter implanted into the abdomen. Fluid, wastes, electrolytes, and chemicals pass from tiny blood vessels in the peritoneal membrane into the dialysate. After several hours, the dialysate is drained from the abdomen, taking the wastes from the blood with it. The abdomen is filled with fresh dialysate and the cleaning procedure begins again. The most common types of peritoneal dialysis is continuous ambulatory peritoneal dialysis (CAPD). The dialysate stays in the abdomen for 4 to 6 hours. The process of draining the dialysate and replacing it with fresh solution takes about 30 minutes. Most people change the solution four times a day, Figure 19-7.

Automated peritoneal dialysis, a type of peritoneal dialysis that can be done at night while the patient is asleep, takes 6 to 8 hours.

The main complication of peritoneal dialysis is peritonitis, an inflammation of the peritoneal lining.

Kidney Transplants

Kidney transplants are done in cases of prolonged debilitating diseases and renal failure involving both kidneys. Usually the patient has been on dialysis for a long time waiting for a compatible organ. The transplant requires a donor organ from an individual who has a similar immune system to prevent rejection. Blood and other cellular material must match to ensure the greatest potential for success in a transplant. The patient is usually in a state of relatively poor physical condition as a result of the effects of the extended illness. This status, plus

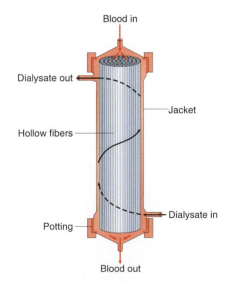

● **FIGURE 19–6**   *A dialyzer.*

Blood in

Dialysate out

Hollow fibers

Potting

Jacket

Dialysate in

Blood out

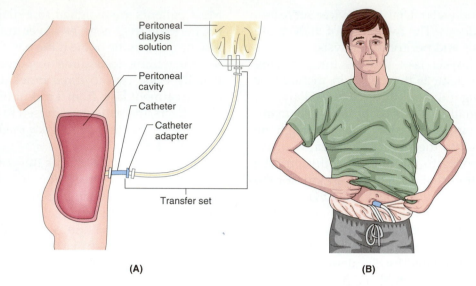

Peritoneal dialysis solution

Peritoneal cavity

Catheter

Catheter adapter

Transfer set

(A)

(B)

⬤ **FIGURE 19–7** *Peritoneal dialysis.*

the tendency of the body to reject a "substance" that is foreign and not of the same cellular structure, sometimes results in the organ's not surviving in the new host. The use of drugs to control the body's natural defensive mechanism of rejection increases the rate of success.

⬤ REVIEW QUESTIONS

Select the letter of choice that best completes the statement.

1. The kidneys are responsible for excreting:
   a. carbon dioxide and water
   b. solid wastes and water
   c. nitrogenous wastes and water
   d. perspiration

2. In addition to kidneys, the organ responsible for excretion of carbon dioxide and water is:
   a. lungs
   b. kidneys
   c. skin
   d. large intestine

3. The kidneys are located in which area?
   a. abdominal
   b. pelvic
   c. peritoneal
   d. retroperitoneal

4. A ball of capillaries is called the:
   a. Bowman's capsule
   b. cortex
   c. glomerulus
   d. medulla

5. The process of plasmalike fluid passing through the glomerulus to Bowman's capsule is called:
   a. filtration
   b. reabsorption
   c. secretion
   d. excretion

6. The hormone ADH affects reabsorption in the:
   a. glomerulus
   b. proximal convoluted tubule
   c. loop of Henle
   d. dismal convoluted tubule

7. The pathway of urine formation is:
   a. kidney, ureter, urethra, bladder
   b. ureter, pelvis, urethra, bladder
   c. kidney, urethra, bladder, ureter
   d. kidney, ureter, bladder, urethra

8. The average normal daily urinary output is:
   a. 600 milliliters
   b. 1200 milliliters
   c. 1800 milliliters
   d. 2400 milliliters

9. Inflammation of the urinary bladder is called:
   a. nephritis
   b. cystitis
   c. pyelitis
   d. urethritis

10. Involuntary urination is known as:
    a. polyuria
    b. anuria
    c. incontinence
    d. frequency

● COMPLETION

If laboratory facilities and supervision are available, obtain and examine several specimens of fresh normal urine.

1. What is the color of the specimen?

2. Is it clear or cloudy?

3. Is the urine acidic, alkaline, or neutral? To test, dip blue litmus paper into the urine. If acid is present, it will turn red. Dip red litmus paper in. If urine is alkaline, it will turn the paper blue. If neither paper changes color, the urine is neutral.

4. What is the specific gravity of a specimen? To test, use a urinometer.

5. Using Acetest reagent tablets, examine the urine for acetone. Have the results and your interpretation checked by the instructor.

Place the reagent tablet on a clean white sheet of paper. Place a drop of urine on the tablet. In 30 seconds, compare the resulting color with the color chart enclosed with the tablets. Record the result on the chart.

6. Using Clinitest tablets or Clinistix reagent strips, test for sugar. Have the results and your interpretation checked by the instructor.

Clinitest tablets: Place five drops of urine and ten drops of water in a test tube. Add the Clinitest tablet. Observe the reaction. Then shake the test tube and compare the color of the solution with the color scale enclosed with the tablets. Record the result.

Clinistix reagent strips: Dip the test end of the Clinistix in the urine and remove it. (Avoid contact with fingers or other objects because misleading results may occur.) If the moistened end turns blue, the result is positive. When sugar is present, the blue color appears in less than 1 minute. Record the result.

● MATCHING

Match each term in Column A with its description in Column B.

Column A	Column B
_____ 1. nephron	a. tubes that connect the kidneys with the bladder
_____ 2. glomerulus	b. mass of capillaries
_____ 3. bladder	c. structure that absorbs filtrate from the capillary mass
_____ 4. urethra	d. one of millions of tiny filtering units
_____ 5. ureter	e. returns blood to the inferior vena cava
_____ 6. ADH	f. hormone that regulates water reabsorption
_____ 7. collecting tubules	g. contraction of bladder muscles
_____ 8. Bowman's capsule	h. canal that opens to the outside of the body
_____ 9. kidney	i. primarily acts as a reservoir
_____ 10. renal vein	j. allow urine to drain into the renal pelvis
_____ 11. anuria	k. bean-shaped organ
_____ 12. dysuria	l. scanty urine
_____ 13. pyuria	m. blood in the urine
_____ 14. hematuria	n. no urine
_____ 15. oliguria	o. pus in the urine
_____ 16. carbon dioxide	p. painful urination
_____ 17. calculi	q. helps regulate body temperature
_____ 18. urine	r. blood retains urinary waste products
_____ 19. cystitis	s. stones in the kidneys
_____ 20. uremia	t. waste product eliminated through the lungs
	u. inflammation of the mucous membranes lining the bladder
	v. water and nitrogenous wastes

●APPLYING THEORY TO PRACTICE

1. The amount of daily water loss is approximately 1500 to 1800 milliliters through urinary output, 500 milliliters through the skin, and 500 milliliters through respiration. Keep a log for 24 hours. Measure your liquid intake and urinary output. Are you taking in enough fluid to maintain your body in good fluid balance?

2. You have just run a mile and sweated profusely. When you urinate you notice there is only a small amount and it is concentrated. Explain what has happened.

3. You have to take an antibiotic. The instructions say to take it every 6 hours. Why is it necessary to maintain this over 24 hours?

4. A patient is complaining of a severe back pain. After a patient examination and history, you suspect kidney stones. The patient inquires, "How did I get stones in my kidney?" Explain the cause and treatment.

5. In kidney failure, dialysis may be necessary. Define *dialysis*. What type do you think would be best for a vision-impaired 70-year-old? What type do you think would be best for a mother with children ages 2, 6, and 10?

20 Reproductive System

Objectives

- Compare somatic cell division (mitosis) with germ cell division (meiosis)
- Explain the process of fertilization
- Identify the organs of the female reproductive system and explain their functions
- Explain menopause and the changes that occur during this time
- Describe the stages and changes that occur during the menstrual cycle
- Identify the organs of the male reproductive system and explain their functions
- List some common disorders of the reproductive system
- Define the key words that relate to this chapter

Key Words

abortion
abruptio placentae
amenorrhea
areola
artificial insemination
bag of waters
Bartholin's glands
benign prostatic
    hypertrophy (BPH)
breast
breast cancer
breast tumor
bulbourethral gland
    (Cowper's gland)
cervical cancer
cervix
chlamydia
circumcision
clitoris
coitus
colostrum
corona radiata
corpus luteum
cryptorchidism
dilation

ductus deferens
dysmenorrhea
eclampsia
ectopic pregnancy
effacement
ejaculatory duct
embryo
endometrial cancer
endometriosis
endometrium
epididymis
epididymitis
episiotomy
fallopian tube (oviduct)
fertilization
fetal heart tones
fibroid tumors
fimbria
foreskin (prepuce)
fundus
gamete (germ cell)
genital warts
glans penis
gonorrhea
graafian follicle

(continues)

Key Words (continued)

human chorionic gonadotropin (HCG)	pelviscopy
hymen	penile shaft
hysterectomy	penis
impotence	perineum
in vitro fertilization	placenta
infertility	placenta previa
involution	preeclampsia
labia majora	pregnancy
labia minora	premenstrual syndrome (PMS)
labor	priapism
laparoscopy	progesterone
leukorrhea	prostatectomy
lumpectomy	prostate gland
mammogram	puberty
mastectomy	quickening
meiosis	salpingitis
menarche	scrotum
menopause	seminal vesicle
menstrual cycle	seminiferous tubule
menstruation	spermatogenesis
microsurgery	spermatozoa
miscarriage	spontaneous abortion
mittelschmerz	sterile
mons pubis	supine hypotensive syndrome
mucous plug	syphilis
myometrium	teratogenic abortion
oogenesis	testes
orchitis	toxic shock syndrome
os	trimester
ova	uterus
ovarian cancer	vagina
ovary	vas deferens
ovulation	vestibule
oxytocin	yeast infection
Pap smear	zygote
pelvic inflammatory disease (PID)	

All living organisms, whether unicellular or multicellular, small or large, must reproduce to continue their species. Humans and most multicellular animals reproduce new members of their species by sexual reproduction.

● FUNCTIONS OF THE REPRODUCTIVE SYSTEM

The reproductive system possesses the following characteristics:

1. Has the necessary organs capable of accomplishing reproduction, the creation of a new individual.

2. Manufactures the hormones necessary for the development of the reproductive organs and secondary sex characteristics.
   - Females—estrogen and progesterone
   - Male—testosterone

Specialized sex cells, or **gametes (germ cells)**, must be produced by the gonads of both male and female sex organs before sexual reproduction can take place. The female gonads, called the ovaries, produce egg cells (ova). The male gonads, the testes, produce sperm. Normal cell division is known as mitosis. In the formation of the germ cells, a special process of cell division occurs called **meiosis**. In the female the specific meiotic process is called **oogenesis**; in the male, it is called **spermatogenesis**.

In humans the somatic (body) cells, including skin, fat, muscle, nerve, bone cells, and so on, contain 46 chromosomes in the nucleus. Forty-four of these are autosomes (nonsex chromosomes). The remaining two are sex chromosomes. Each chromosome has a partner of the same size and shape so that they can be paired, Figure 20-1. In the female the somatic cells contain 22 pairs of autosomes and a single pair of sex chromosomes (both are X chromosomes). In the male the combination is also 22 autosomal pairs and a single pair of sex chromosomes. However, the male sex chromosomal pair consists of an X and Y chromosome.

Oogenesis and spermatogenesis reduce the chromosome number of 46 to 23 in the gametes or germ cells. All multicellular organisms start from the fusion of two gametes: the sperm (spermatozoon) from the male and the ovum from the female. Figure 20-2 shows the structure of a spermatozoon and an ovum.

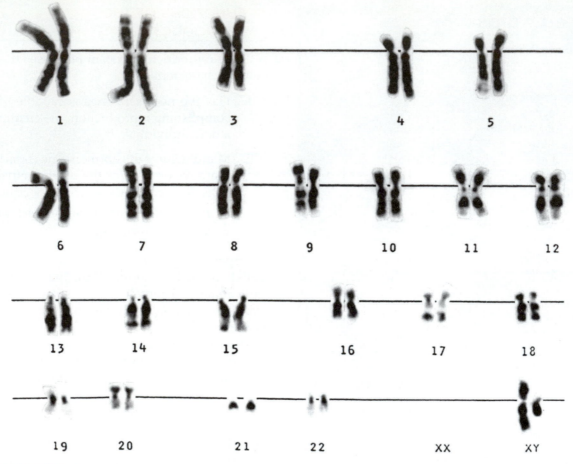

● **FIGURE 20–1**   *Karyotype of human from a male somatic cell. A karyotype is the arrangement of chromosome pairs according to size and shape.*

● FERTILIZATION

During sexual intercourse, or **coitus**, sperm from the testes is deposited into the female vagina, Figure 20-3. Spermatozoa entering the female reproductive tract live for only a day or two at the most, although they may remain in the tract up to 2 weeks before degenerating. Approximately 100 million spermatozoa are contained in 1 milliliter (1 cubic centimeter [cc]) of ejaculated seminal fluid. They are fairly uniform in shape and size. If the count is less than 20 million per milliliter, the male is considered to be **sterile**. These millions of sperm cells swim toward the ovum that has been released from the ovary. The large quantity of sperm is necessary because a great number are destroyed before they even approach the ovum. Many die from the acidity of the secretions in the male urethra or the vagina.

Some cannot withstand the high temperature of the female abdomen, and others lack the propulsion ability to progress from the vagina to the upper uterine (fallopian) tubes.

For a sperm to penetrate and fertilize an ovum, the **corona radiata** must first be penetrated. This is the layer of epithelial cells surrounding the zona pellucida, see Figure 20-2. Eventually, only one sperm cell penetrates and fertilizes an ovum. To accomplish this successfully, the sperm head produces an enzyme called hyaluronidase. Hyaluronidase acts upon hyaluronic acid, a chemical substance that holds together the epithelial cells of the corona radiata. As a result of the action of the hyaluronidase, the epithelial cells fall away from the ovum. This exposes an area of the plasma membrane for sperm penetration. Figure 20-3 illustrates the route of the ovum and the sperm.

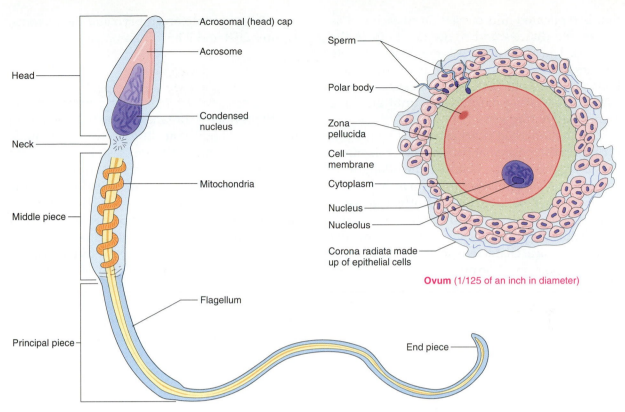

● FIGURE 20–2   *Structures of the human sperm and ovum.*

True **fertilization** occurs when the sperm nucleus combines with the egg nucleus to form a fertilized egg cell, or **zygote**. The type of fertilization that occurs in humans is referred to as internal fertilization; fertilization takes place within the female's body.

Fertilization restores the full complement of 46 chromosomes possessed by every human cell, each parent contributing one chromosome to each of the 23 pairs.

Deoxyribonucleic acid (DNA) is found in the chromosomes. It contains the genetic code

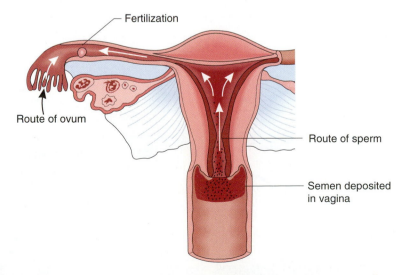

● FIGURE 20–3   *Route of the sperm and ovum.*

that is replicated and passed on to each cell as the zygote divides and re-divides to form the embryo. The early process whereby the zygote repeatedly divides to form an early embryo is known as cleavage. After early cleavage, actual embryonic development occurs until the fetus is completely formed.

All the inherited traits possessed by the offspring are established at the time of fertilization. This is a point to remember when working with parents. A young mother-to-be may hope that her baby will be a girl with curly hair, or a prospective father may insist that he wants a son. The health care provider can assure them that the sex and physical characteristics, such as eye color and curly hair, are determined at the time of fertilization. The sex chromosomes of the male parent determine the sex of the child, but other characteristics are a combination of both parents.

FETAL DEVELOPMENT

If fertilization occurs, the zygote travels down the fallopian tube and is implanted in the endometrial wall of the uterus. The zygote

rapidly grows into an embryo and then a fetus, Figures 20-4 and 20-5.

DIFFERENTIATION OF REPRODUCTIVE ORGANS

Reproductive organs are the only organs in the human body that differ between the male and female, and yet there is still a significant similarity. This likeness results from the fact that female and male organs develop from the same group of embryonic cells. For approximately 2 months, the embryo develops without a sexual identity. Then the influence of the X or Y chromosome begins to make a difference.

The gonads (sexual organs) of the female begin to evolve at about the tenth or eleventh week of pregnancy. The ovaries of the female embryo develop from the same type of tissue as the testes of the male embryo. However, the testes evolve from the medulla of the gonad, whereas the ovary develops from the cortex of the gonad. Figure 20-6 illustrates how the undifferentiated external genitalia develop into fully differentiated structures. In the male the

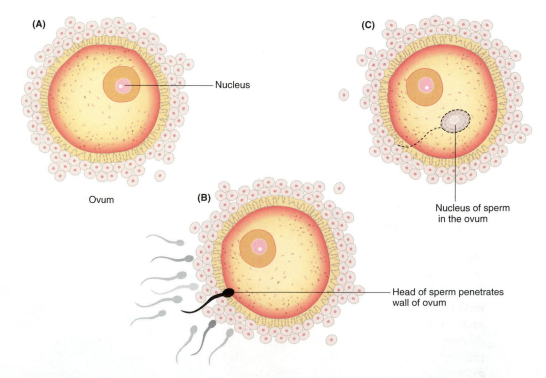

(A)

Nucleus

Ovum

(B)

(C)

Nucleus of sperm in the ovum

Head of sperm penetrates wall of ovum

● **FIGURE 20–4** *Fertilization.*

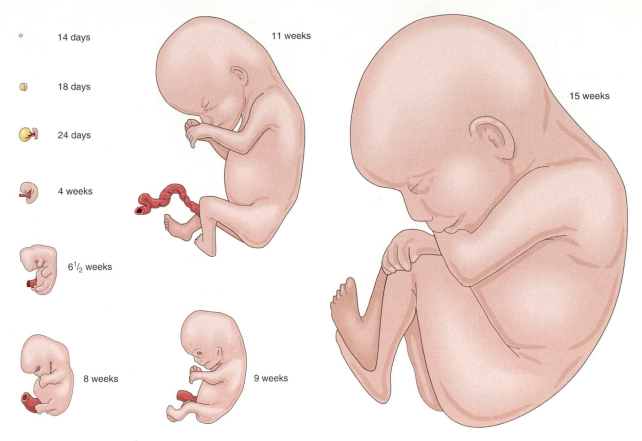

14 days

18 days

24 days

4 weeks

6½ weeks

8 weeks

9 weeks

11 weeks

15 weeks

● **FIGURE 20–5**   *Growth of an embryo into a fetus once fertilization has occurred.*

tubercle becomes the **glans penis**, the folds become the **penile shaft**, and the swelling develops into the scrotum. In the female the tubercle becomes the clitoris, the folds the labia minora, and the swelling the labia majora. Internally there is also a differentiation from initially similar structures. The embryonic müllerian ducts degenerate and the wolffian ducts become the epididymis, vas deferens, and the ejaculatory duct in the male. In the female the wolffian ducts degenerate and the müllerian ducts develop into the fallopian tubes, the uterus, and the upper portion of the vagina. It is believed that the presence of the testes in the male is the differentiating factor in the development. Without the androgens (male hormones) from the testes, a female develops. With the androgens, a male develops. Another substance, called the müllerian inhibitor, works in partnership with the androgen to produce the sex differentiation.

● ORGANS OF REPRODUCTION

The function of the reproductive system is to provide for continuity of the species. In humans the female reproductive system is composed of two ovaries, two fallopian tubes, the uterus, and the vagina. The male reproductive system is made up of two testes, seminal ducts, glands, and the penis. The principal male organs are located outside the body, in contrast to the female organs, which are largely located within the body.

● FEMALE REPRODUCTIVE SYSTEM

Placement of the female reproductive organs in the pelvic cavity are shown in Figure 20-7. As shown in Figure 20-8, the female reproductive system consists of two ovaries, two fallopian tubes, the uterus, and the vagina. Accessory organs are the breasts.

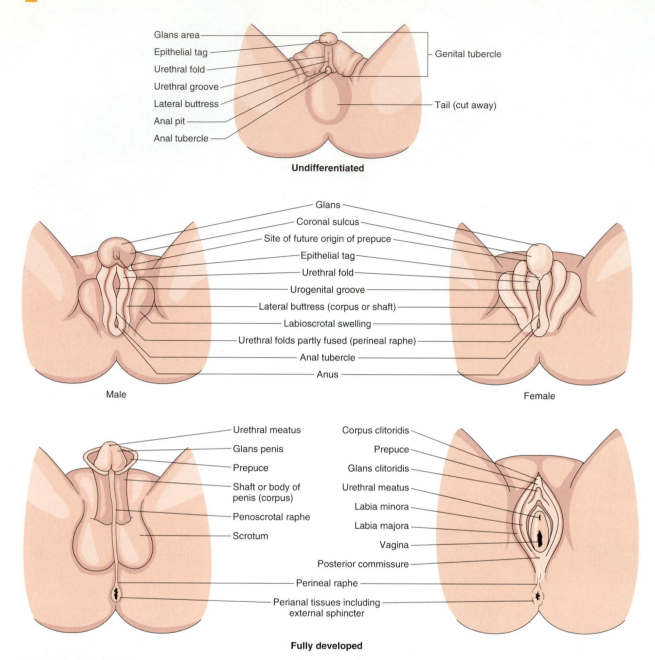

Glans area
Epithelial tag
Urethral fold
Urethral groove
Lateral buttress
Anal pit
Anal tubercle
Genital tubercle
Tail (cut away)

Undifferentiated

Glans
Coronal sulcus
Site of future origin of prepuce
Epithelial tag
Urethral fold
Urogenital groove
Lateral buttress (corpus or shaft)
Labioscrotal swelling
Urethral folds partly fused (perineal raphe)
Anal tubercle
Anus

Male   Female

Urethral meatus
Glans penis
Prepuce
Shaft or body of penis (corpus)
Penoscrotal raphe
Scrotum

Corpus clitoridis
Prepuce
Glans clitoridis
Urethral meatus
Labia minora
Labia majora
Vagina
Posterior commissure
Perineal raphe
Perianal tissues including external sphincter

Fully developed

● **FIGURE 20–6**   *Development of undifferentiated external genitalia into fully differentiated structures.*

Ovaries

The **ovaries** are the primary sex organs of the female. They are located on either side of the pelvis, lateral to the uterus, in the lower part of the abdominal cavity. Each ovary is about the shape and size of a large almond, measuring about 3 centimeters long and 1.5 to 3 centimeters wide. An ovarian ligament, a short fibrous cord within the broad ligament, attaches each ovary to the upper lateral part of the uterus.

Ovaries perform two functions. They produce the female germ cells, or **ova**, and the female sex hormones, estrogen and **progesterone**. Table 20-1 outlines the functions of the female sex hormones.

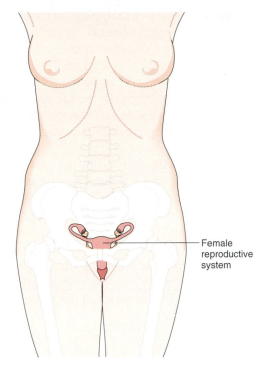

● **FIGURE 20–7** *Placement of the female reproductive system in the lower pelvic cavity.*

Each ovary contains thousands of microscopic hollow sacs, called **graafian follicles**, in varying stages of development. An ovum slowly develops inside each follicle. The process of development from an immature ovum to a func-

tional and mature ovum inside the graafian follicle is called maturation. In addition, the graafian follicle produces the hormone estrogen.

Usually a single follicle matures every 28 days throughout the reproductive years of a woman. The reproductive years begin at the time of **puberty** and **menarche** (the initial menstrual discharge of blood).

Occasionally two or more follicles may mature, releasing more than one ovum. As the follicle enlarges, it migrates to the outside surface of the ovary and breaks open, releasing the ovum from the ovary. This process is called **ovulation**; it occurs about 2 weeks before the menstrual period begins. The time of ovulation may vary, depending on emotional and physical health, state of mind, and age. During a woman's reproductive years, she produces about 400 ova.

The ovum consists of cytoplasm and some yolk. This yolk is the initial food source for the growth of the early embryo. After ovulation, the ovum travels down one of the fallopian tubes, or oviducts. Fertilization of the ovum takes place only in the upper third of the oviduct. The time of fertilization is limited to a day or two following ovulation. After fertilization, the zygote (fertilized egg) travels to the well-prepared uterus and implants itself in the wall of the endometrium (uterus lining).

The development of the follicle and release of the ovum occur under the influence of

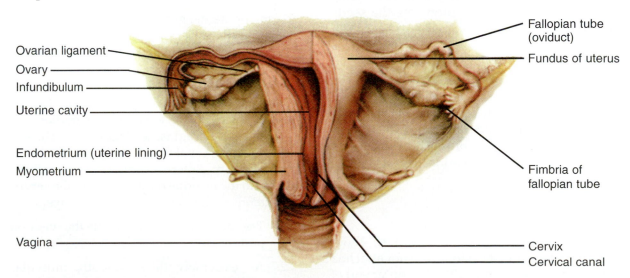

Ovarian ligament

Ovary

Infundibulum

Uterine cavity

Endometrium (uterine lining)

Myometrium

Vagina

Fallopian tube (oviduct)

Fundus of uterus

Fimbria of fallopian tube

Cervix

Cervical canal

● **FIGURE 20–8** *Structures of the female reproductive system.*

TABLE 20-1 *Functions of Estrogen and Progesterone*

HORMONE	FUNCTION
Estrogen	1. Affects the development of the fallopian tubes, ovaries, uterus, and vagina. 2. Produces secondary sex characteristics: • Broadening of the pelvis, making the outlet broad and oval to permit childbirth • Ceasing of growth and transformation of epiphysis (growth plate) to bone • Development of softer and smoother skin • Development of pubic and axillary hair • Depositing of fat in the breasts and development of the duct system • Depositing of fat in the buttocks and thighs • Development of sexual desire 3. Prepares the uterus for the fertilized egg.
Progesterone	1. Develops excretory portion of mammary glands. 2. Thickens the uterine lining so it can receive the developing embryo. 3. Decreases uterine contractions during pregnancy.

two hormones of the pituitary gland: follicle-stimulating hormone (FSH) and luteinizing hormone (LH). FSH also promotes the secretion of estrogen by the ovary.

After ovulation, the ruptured follicle enlarges, takes on a yellow fatty substance, and becomes the **corpus luteum** (yellow body). The corpus luteum secretes progesterone, which maintains the growth of the uterine lining. If the egg is not fertilized, the corpus luteum degenerates, progesterone production stops, and the thickened glandular endometrium sloughs off (see Menstrual Cycle).

Fallopian Tubes

The **fallopian tubes**, or **oviducts**, about 10 centimeters (4 inches) long, are not attached to the ovaries, see Figure 20-8. The outer end of each oviduct curves over the top edge of each ovary and opens into the abdominal cavity.

This portion of the oviduct, nearest the ovary, is the infundibulum. Because the infundibulum is not attached directly to the ovary, it is possible for an ovum to accidentally slip into the abdominal cavity and be fertilized there. If the fertilized egg implants in the fallopian tube instead of the uterus, it is called an **ectopic pregnancy**. An ectopic pregnancy can also occur outside the uterine cavity.

The area of the infundibulum over the ovary is surrounded by a number of fringelike folds called **fimbria**. Each oviduct is lined with mucous membrane, smooth muscle, and ciliated epithelium. The combined action of the peristaltic contractions of the smooth muscles and the beating of the cilia helps to propel the ova down the oviduct into the uterus. Conception (fertilization) takes place in the outer third of the fallopian tube.

Uterus

The **uterus** is a hollow, thick-walled, pear-shaped, and highly muscular organ. The nongravid (nonpregnant) uterus is approximately 7.5 centimeters long, 5 centimeters wide, and 2.75 centimeters thick. This is about 3 inches long, 2 inches wide, and 1 inch thick. The uterus lies behind the urinary bladder and in front of the rectum. The uterine cavity is extremely small and narrow. During pregnancy, however, the uterine cavity greatly expands to accommodate the growing embryo and a large amount of fluid.

The uterus is divided into three parts: (1) the **fundus**, the bulging, rounded upper part above the entrance of the two oviducts into the uterus; (2) the body, or middle portion; and (3) the **cervix**, the cylindrical, lower narrow portion that extends into the vagina, see Figure 20-8. There is a short cervical canal that extends from the lower uterine cavity (internal orifice, or os, of the uterus) to the external os at the end of the cervix. The uterine wall is composed of three layers:

1. The outer serous layer, or the visceral peritoneum

2. An extremely thick, smooth, muscular middle layer, the **myometrium**

3. An inner mucous layer, the **endometrium**

The endometrium, which lines the oviducts and the vagina, is also lined with ciliated epithelial cells, numerous uterine glands, and many capillaries.

During development of the embryo/fetus, the uterus gradually rises until the top part is high in the abdominal cavity, pushing on the diaphragm. This may cause the expectant mother some difficulty in breathing during the late stages of pregnancy.

Vagina

The **vagina** is the short canal that extends from the cervix of the uterus to the vulva. The vagina is composed of smooth muscle with a mucous membrane lining. This type of muscle tissue allows the vaginal canal to accommodate the penis during sexual intercourse; it also permits a baby to pass through the vaginal canal during the birthing process. A membrane called the **hymen** may be found at or near the entrance to the vagina. The hymen does have some openings that allow for the flow of blood during menstruation. During the first act of sexual intercourse, the openings in the hymen are enlarged and there may be slight bleeding, Figures 20-9 and 20-10.

External Female Genitalia

The external female genitalia, or **vulva**, contains the external organs of the reproductive area, see Figure 20-10. The large pad of fat that is covered with coarse hair on the mature female and overlies the symphysis pubis is known as **mons pubis**. The area surrounding the openings of the urethra and vagina is called the **vestibule**. The urethra opening is superior to the vagina. Above the urethral opening is a small structure called the **clitoris**, which contains many nerve endings. These receptors are stimulated during sexual intercourse.

The vagina is surrounded by folds of skin called the **labia minora** and the **labia majora**. At the entrance to the vagina are the **Bartholin's glands**, which contain mucus.

The **perineum** is the area between the vaginal opening and the rectum. The perineal area is composed of muscles that form a sphincter

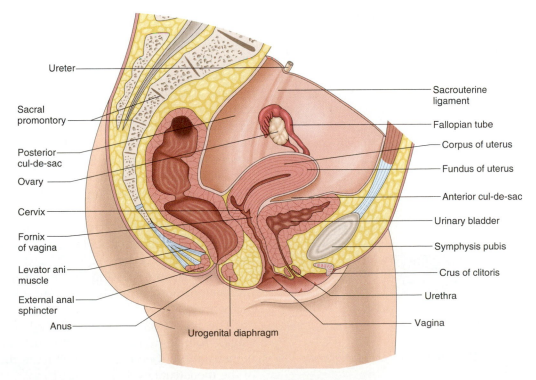

● **FIGURE 20–9**   *Structures of the female reproductive system.*

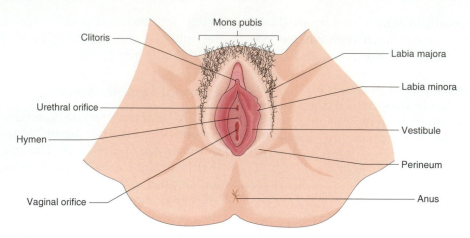

● **FIGURE 20–10** *External female genitalia.*

for the vestibule. In childbirth an incision called an **episiotomy** may be made from the vagina into the perineal area to facilitate childbirth.

Breasts

The **breasts** are accessory organs to the female reproductive system, Figure 20-11. They are composed of numerous lobes arranged in a circular formation. Clusters of secreting cells surround tiny ducts. A single duct extends from each lobe to an opening in the nipple. The **areola**, the darker area that surrounds the nipple, changes to a brownish

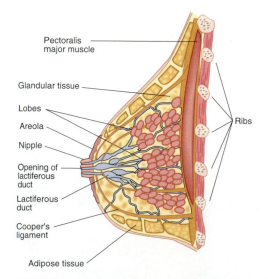

● **FIGURE 20–11** *Sagittal section of the female breast.*

color during pregnancy. Prolactin from the anterior lobe of the pituitary gland stimulates the mammary glands to secrete milk after childbirth.

● **MENSTRUAL CYCLE**

In females a mature egg develops and is ovulated from one of the two ovaries about once every 28 days, through a complex series of action between the pituitary and the ovary. Before the mature egg is released from the ovary, a series of events occurs to thicken the uterine lining (endometrium). This is necessary to receive and hold a fertilized egg for embryonic development. If the egg is not fertilized, the endometrium starts to break down. Eventually the old unfertilized egg and the degenerated endometrium are discharged out of the female reproductive tract (**menstruation**). The cycle then starts all over again with the development of another ovum and the buildup of the endometrium.

The **menstrual cycle** starts at puberty, as early as 9 years of age to as late as 17. Generally the age range is between 12 and 15. The changes that occur during the menstrual cycle involve hormones from the pituitary gland and the ovaries.

The menstrual cycle is divided into four stages: follicle, ovulation, corpus luteum, and menstruation. (See Figure 20-12 for a diagram of the menstrual cycle.)

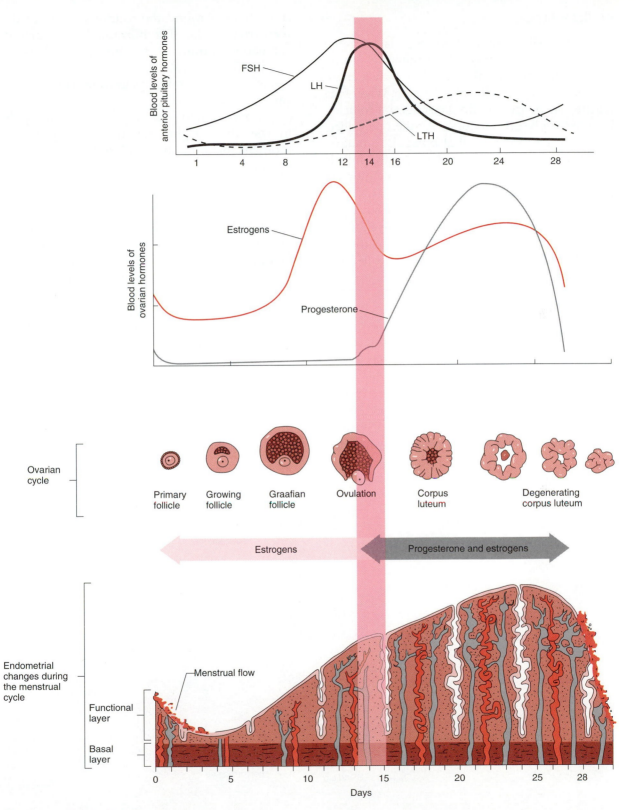

● FIGURE 20–12 *The menstrual cycle.*

Follicle Stage

Follicle-stimulating hormone is secreted from the anterior lobe of the pituitary gland on day 5 of the menstrual cycle. FSH is then circulated to an ovary via the bloodstream. When FSH reaches an ovary, it stimulates several follicles; however, only one matures. As the one follicle grows in size, an egg cell also begins to mature inside the follicle, Figure 20-13. As the follicle grows in size, it fills with a fluid containing estrogen. The estrogen stimulates the endometrium to thicken with mucus and a rich supply of blood vessels. These changes to the endometrium prepare the uterus for the implantation of an embryo. The follicle stage lasts about 10 days.

Ovulation Stage

When the concentration of estrogen in the female bloodstream reaches a high level, it causes the pituitary gland to stop FSH secretion. As this occurs, luteinizing hormone is secreted by the pituitary gland. At this point, there are three different hormones circulating in the female bloodstream—estrogen, FSH, and LH. Each hormone is present in different concentrations. Around the fourteenth day of the menstrual cycle, this hormonal combination somehow stimulates the mature follicle to break. When the follicle ruptures, a mature egg cell is released into fallopian tube. This event is called ovulation.

Some women experience abdominal pain in the area of the ovulating ovary at the moment of ovulation. This pain is called **mittelschmerz**.

Corpus Luteum Stage (Luteal Phase)

After ovulation, LH stimulates the cells of the ruptured follicle to divide quickly. This mass of reddish-yellow cells is called the corpus luteum. The corpus luteum, in turn, secrets a hormone called progesterone. Progesterone helps to maintain the continued growth and thickening of the endometrium, so if an embryo happens to be implanted into the uterine lining, the pregnancy can be maintained. That is why progesterone is often called the "pregnancy hormone." Progesterone also prevents the formation of new ovarian follicles by inhibiting the release of FSH. The corpus luteum stage lasts about 14 days.

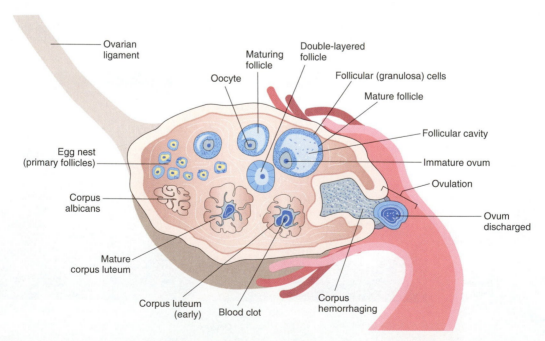

Ovarian ligament

Maturing follicle

Double-layered follicle

Oocyte

Follicular (granulosa) cells

Mature follicle

Follicular cavity

Egg nest (primary follicles)

Immature ovum

Ovulation

Corpus albicans

Ovum discharged

Mature corpus luteum

Corpus luteum (early)

Blood clot

Corpus hemorrhaging

● **FIGURE 20–13**   *An ovary showing the development of an ovum in a graafian follicle.*

Menstruation Stage

If fertilization does not occur and an embryo is not implanted in the uterus, the progesterone reaches a level in the bloodstream that inhibits further LH secretion. With decreased LH secretion, the corpus luteum breaks down, causing a decrease in progesterone secretion as well. As the progesterone level decreases, the lining of the endometrium becomes progressively thinner and eventually breaks down. The extra layers of the endometrium, the unfertilized egg, and a small quantity of blood that comes from the ruptured capillaries as the endometrium peels away from the uterus are discharged from the body through the vagina. This causes the characteristic menstrual blood flow; the menstruation stage starts around the twenty-eighth day of the cycle. The menstruation stage lasts about 4 days. While menstruation is occurring, the estrogen level in the bloodstream is decreasing. The anterior lobe of the pituitary gland is now stimulated to secrete FSH; consequently a new follicle starts to grow and the menstrual cycle starts again.

The relationship between the pituitary gland hormones and the ovarian hormones is one of feedback. That means that pituitary hormones control the functioning of the ovaries; in turn, the ovaries secrete hormones that control pituitary functioning. This is another example of the automatic regulation of many of the body's processes.

● MENOPAUSE

Menopause, or "change in life," is the time in a female's life when the monthly menstrual cycle comes to an end. It frequently occurs between ages 45 and 55. Menopause signals the end of follicle growth and ovulation; consequently, it means the end of childbearing. However, a normal libido usually remains.

The woman undergoing menopause experiences the following anatomical changes:

1. Atrophy of the internal reproductive structures:
   - Uterus
   - Fallopian tubes
   - Ovaries

2. Atrophy of the external genitalia

3. Change in the shape of the vagina to conical

4. Atrophy of the vaginal mucous membranes

5. Reduction of the secretory activity of the glands associated with the reproductive organs

These changes do not occur overnight; they happen gradually over a period of years. Pronounced physiological changes also occur. These include "hot flashes," dizziness, headaches, rheumatic pains in joints, sweating, and susceptibility to fatigue. Sometimes these physiological changes are accompanied by psychological changes, including abnormal fears, depression, excessive irritability, and a tendency to worry. Many of these physiological and psychological symptoms can be alleviated by the careful administration of female hormones.

Menopause can be induced prematurely (artificial menopause) by either deactivation or removal of ovarian tissue.

STREET SMART

During her adult life, a woman's heart is protected from some of the abnormal fat buildup that occurs in the heart, atherosclerosis, because of hormones. As a woman undergoes menopause, she loses the cardioprotective effects of hormones and her risk of heart attack rises dramatically. ■

● MALE REPRODUCTIVE SYSTEM

The male reproductive organs, Figure 20-14, consist of the following structures:

1. The two testes produce the male gametes, **spermatozoa**, and the male sex hormone testosterone. They are suspended from the body wall by a spermatic cord and encased in a pouch called the scrotum.

2. A system of ducts carries the sperm cells out of the testes through the epididymis, two seminal ducts (ductus deferens, or vas deferens), two ejaculatory ducts, and the urethra.

3. Accessory glands include the two seminal vesicles, two bulbourethral glands, and a prostate gland. These glands add a viscous fluid to the sperm cells to form seminal fluid.

4. The penis is a copulatory structure that transfers sperm cells to the female reproductive system.

Testes and Epididymis

The two **testes** are the primary male reproductive organs, Figure 20-15. They are found in a pouch lying outside the male body, called the scrotum. Each testis is about the size and shape of a small egg, approximately 4 centimeters long, 2.5 centimeters wide, and 2 centimeters thick. The testes are attached to an overlying structure called the **epididymis**. A fibrous tissue called the tunica albuginea covers the testes and sends incomplete partitions into the body of each testis. Each one of these partitions is called a lobule, and each testis contains 250 lobules.

Each testicular lobule contains one to four minute and highly convoluted (twisted) **seminiferous tubules**. FSH stimulates the production of sperm in the cells that line the tubules. As the sperm develop, they are released into the tubules. In males, mature sperm formation requires about 74 days. This function begins at about age 12, and the first mature sperm are ejaculated at about age 14. All the seminiferous tubules intertwine and join together to form a small meshlike network of

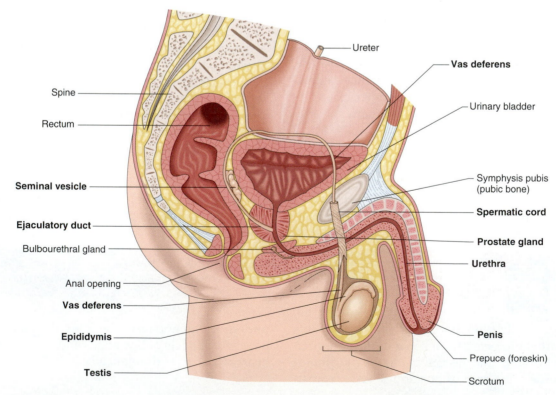

● **FIGURE 20–14**   *Structures of the male reproductive system.*

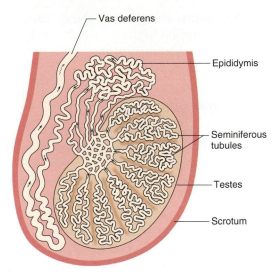

Vas deferens

Epididymis

Seminiferous tubules

Testes

Scrotum

● **FIGURE 20–15**   *Structures of the testes.*

tubules called the rete testis. The rete testis unite to form the epididymis. The seminiferous tubules are supported by a type of tissue called interstitial tissue. The interstitial cells lining the interstitial tissue produce the male hormone testosterone. Testosterone is secreted in relatively steady amounts during the adult life of the male. Testosterone stimulates the growth and development of the male reproductive organs, underlies the sex drive, and is responsible for the secondary sex characteristics. These include deepening of the voice, growth of hair (beard and body hair, especially in the axillary and pubic area), increase in muscle mass, and thickening of the bones of the skeletal system.

The epididymides connect the testes with the ductus deferens and help in the final development of the sperm cells.

Descent of the Testes

At the embryonic stage, testes are formed and developed in the abdominal wall slightly below the kidneys. During the last 3 months of fetal development, the testes migrate downward through the ventral abdominal wall into the scrotum. In its descent, each testis carries with it the ductus deferens, blood and lymphatic vessels, and autonomic nerve fibers. These structures and their fibrous tissue covering form the spermatic cord.

Occasionally, as in premature babies, the testes do not descend; this condition is known as **cryptorchidism**. (If one testis does not descend, it is called unilateral cryptorchidism. When neither testis descends, the condition is called bilateral cryptorchidism.) If the testes stay inside the abdomen after puberty, spermatogenesis is affected. The increased body temperature destroys any sperm cells. A simple surgical procedure done before puberty can correct this condition.

Scrotum

The **scrotum** is an external sac that contains the testes.

Ductus Deferens, Seminal Vesicles, and Ejaculatory Ducts

The right and left **ductus deferens (vas deferens)** are continuations of the epididymides. The ductus deferens has a dual function. It serves as a storage site for sperm cells and as the excretory duct of the testis. Each ductus runs from the epididymis up through the inguinal canal. It then runs downward and backward to the side of the urinary bladder. It curves around the ureter and goes down to meet with the seminal vesicle duct on the posterior side of the bladder.

The **seminal vesicles** are two highly convoluted membranous tubes. A duct leads away from a seminal vesicle that joins to the ductus deferens to form the ejaculatory duct on either side. The seminal vesicles produce secretions that help to nourish and protect the sperm on its journey up the female reproductive system. At the precise moment of ejaculation, the seminal fluid is added to the sperm cells as they leave the ejaculatory ducts.

The **ejaculatory ducts** are short and very narrow. They begin where the ductus deferens and the seminal vesicle duct join, then descend into the prostate gland to join with the urethra, into which they discharge their contents, see Figure 20-14.

Penis

The external organs are the scrotum and the penis. Internally the scrotum is divided into two sacs, each containing a testis, epididymis, and lower part of the vas deferens. The **penis** contains erectile tissue that becomes enlarged and rigid during intercourse. Loose-fitting skin, called the **foreskin**, or **prepuce**, cover the end of the penis. The foreskin can be removed in a simple operation known as **circumcision**.

Prostate Gland

The **prostate gland** is located in front of the rectum and just under the urinary bladder, and it surrounds the opening of the bladder leading into the urethra. It surrounds the beginning portion of the urethra that is called the prostatic urethra. The prostate gland is about the shape and size of a chestnut. It is covered by a dense, fibrous capsule and contains glandular tissue surrounded by fibromuscular tissue that contracts during ejaculation. The contraction of the prostate gland closes off the prostatic urethra during ejaculation, preventing the passage of urine through the urethra. This contraction of the muscular tissue also aids in the expulsion of semen during an ejaculation. The prostate gland secretes a thin, milky alkaline fluid that enhances sperm motility. It also gives semen its characteristic musky odor. Fluid in the ductus deferens is highly acidic, as are female vaginal secretions. Therefore the alkaline prostatic fluid probably neutralizes the acidic semen and vaginal secretions. This enhances the viability and motility of the sperm cells.

Bulbourethral Glands

The **bulbourethral glands**, also known as **Cowper's glands**, are located on either side of the urethra below the prostate gland. They add an alkaline secretion to the semen that helps the sperm to live longer within the acidic medium of the female reproductive tract.

Erection and Ejaculation

The urethra extends down the length of the penis, opening at the urinary meatus of the glans. The urethra serves two purposes: to empty urine from the bladder and to expel semen. Sexual intercourse becomes possible because of the columns of erectile tissue in the penis. When a male is sexually aroused, nerve impulses cause the erectile tissue to engorge with blood, increasing in size and becoming firm. Blood entering the dilated arteries squeezes the veins against the penile structures, prohibiting venous return.

Once stimulation of the glans results in maximum stimulation of the seminal vesicles, impulses are sent to the ejaculatory center and orgasm occurs. Orgasm is the result of muscular contractions from the vas deferens, ejaculatory ducts, and prostate glands. Secretions stored in these structures along with the sperm are forcibly expelled through the urethra, after which the engorgement gradually subsides.

Impotence

Impotence is the inability to have or sustain an erection during intercourse. *Primary* impotence refers to the patient who has never had an erection. *Secondary* impotence refers to the patient who is currently impotent but has had intercourse in the past. Transient periods of impotence are not considered a dysfunction and

STREET SMART

Erection and ejaculation are both controlled by the autonomic nervous system. Erections are sustained, or aborted, by competition of the two divisions of the autonomic nervous system. If the patient sustains a spinal cord injury above the lumbar region, he suffers an abnormal, painful erection called **priapism**. Priapism occurs without sexual desire and is indicative of disease or injury. ■

probably occur in half the adult male population between the ages of 40 and 70; the incidence increases with age.

Impotence was thought to be 80% psychogenic until the mid-1980s. Doctors now know that the vast majority of cases involve organic causes, often multiple ones. Psychological factors such as anxiety and stress can also be causes of impotence.

The type of therapy chosen depends on the specific cause of the dysfunction. Treatment may be sexual therapy if the cause is thought to be related to psychological factors. At the present time, penile implants and injection therapy are being used to treat impotence. A new medication, called sildenafil (Viagra), is often useful in the treatment of erectile dysfunction. Viagra must be taken with caution when the patient is taking other medications such as nitroglycerin.

CONCEPTION

When a sperm unites with an egg, or ovum, it becomes one cell, called a zygote; the chromosomes of each are combined and fertilization is complete. The zygote continues to divide, forming a ball in the process, and travels from the fallopian tube to the uterus, where it implants itself in the uterine wall. This is the start of **pregnancy**.

The outer cells of the zygote become the **placenta**, while the rest of the cells becomes the **embryo**. This process of fertilization and implantation takes about 7 to 10 days.

The placenta is vital to the embryo's survival. The placenta creates a hormone called **human chorionic gonadotropin (HCG)**. The presence of HCG in the urine confirms pregnancy. HCG prevents the sloughing off of the uterine lining, as occurs during menstruation, and stimulates the ovaries to continue to excrete high levels of estrogen and progesterone. Placental hormones also stimulate the development of the breasts.

PREGNANCY

A typical pregnancy lasts about 37 to 40 weeks, which are divided into three **trimesters**. In the first trimester the mother may not be aware she is pregnant. The developing embryo is safe within the protective confines of the uterus and the pelvis. It is during this first trimester that many of the effects of alcohol, drugs, and the like can have a negative impact on the developing fetus, potentially causing birth defects. If the fetus is not viable (capable of living outside the uterus [womb]), the mother's body may expel it. This process is called a **miscarriage** by lay people; health care professionals refer to it as a **spontaneous abortion**.

On average, about 30% to 40% of woman have bleeding during the first 20 weeks of pregnancy and about 20% actually lose the pregnancy. Because the lack of a menstrual period is the basis for the belief that a woman is pregnant, this bleeding can create some confusion about a woman's pregnancy.

During the second trimester, the fetus is developing his or her organs and becoming more "humanlike." The mother may have experienced morning sickness, a period of nausea with or without vomiting, as a result of elevated hormone levels.

During the last trimester, the fetus is growing and the swollen uterus is very visible. The uterus containing the growing fetus is too large to remain inside the confines of the pelvis and is now vulnerable to external trauma. The mother, whose center of balance is changed, is more ungainly and unstable on her feet as well.

Changes of Pregnancy

There are changes throughout the body during pregnancy. The mother's blood volume increases by as much as a third. In fact, urine output, cardiac output, and respiratory rate all increase as a result of the pregnancy.

At about the twentieth week, the mother may feel the baby's movement, called **quickening**; this signals that the infant may be viable if delivered. For EMS providers, the quickening represents the first opportunity that they may have to hear the **fetal heart tones**. Each successive day in the uterus improves the infant's chance of survival. Table 20-2 summarizes the physical changes that occur during pregnancy.

TABLE 20-2 *Physiological Changes during Pregnancy*

	FIRST TRIMESTER	SECOND TRIMESTER	THIRD TRIMESTER
Genital Tract			
Cervix	Softening of cervix Mucous plug formation		
Uterus	Growth of muscle fibers		Enlargement of chamber
Fundal height	Suprapubic	Umbilicus	Subdiaphragmatic
Breasts	Enlargement		Colostrum production
Cardiovascular System			
Heart rate		Increase 10 BPM	
Blood pressure		Decrease	Increase by 15 mm Hg
Cardiac output	Increase	Increase by > 1/3	Decline to 20%
Blood volume	Increase by 20%	Increase by 40%	
Respiratory System			
Oxygen consumption		Increase by 15%	
Respiratory rate		Slight increase	
Gastrointestinal System			
Esophagus	Salivation Vomiting (morning sickness)	Acid reflux	
Intestines			Constipation
General Changes			
Weight gain	3–4 pounds	12–14 pounds	8–10 pounds

BPM, *Beats per minute.*

CHILDBIRTH

As in pregnancy, childbirth is divided into three stages. During the first stage of labor, the infant starts to descend down into the birth canal. In front of the infant's head, blocking progress, is the cervical opening called the **os**.

The infant must pass through the cervix to reach the birth canal, or vagina. By repeated rhythmic contractions the cervix is flattened (**effacement**) and the opening enlarged (**dilation**). This process is called **labor** and may take as much as 20 hours or longer to complete. The onset of labor is often announced when the **mucous plug** is expelled from the os of the cervix or the **bag of waters** (amniotic sac) ruptures. The hormone **oxytocin**, released from the posterior pituitary gland, stimulates labor.

During the second stage of childbirth, the infant is forced out of the vaginal canal and into the world. Health care professionals, including nurse-midwives and EMS providers, quickly place the infant to the mother's breast. The stimulation of the nipple causes the release of more oxytocin, which in turn pushes the placenta (afterbirth) out the uterus. As the uterus expels first the infant and then the placenta, it shrinks, becoming smaller and smaller, in a process called **involution**, until it returns to its normal size, about the size of a pear. Delivery of the placenta signals the end of pregnancy and the start of motherhood.

BREASTFEEDING

Breastfeeding is a natural act that fulfills many needs. With a new infant demanding time and energy from the mother, another pregnancy is ill advised. For a short time, while oxytocin is being excreted, the mother's menstrual cycle does not return. Oxytocin is released every time the nipple is stimulated during breastfeeding.

Mother's first milk is called **colostrum**. Colostrum lacks fats but has many of the nutrients that the growing infant needs. This early milk also contains antibodies that help protect the infant from disease for a time. This naturally acquired passive immunity is important to an infant's survival. However, the main purpose of mother's milk is to provide nutrition and fluid to the newborn infant.

● COMPLICATIONS OF PREGNANCY

Not all pregnancies result in childbirth. In fact, one in five pregnancies is lost before childbirth. This is often the result of an identifiable problem that makes the pregnancy high risk. A high-risk pregnancy exists when there is a substantial risk of serious illness to or death of either the mother or the infant.

Add to the number of pregnancies lost before childbirth the number of infants who die during the first 6 weeks after birth (the neonatal period), and it is easy to understand why perinatal death exceeds all other causes of death combined until age 65. Because of complications of pregnancy, the most dangerous period in most people's lives is from the moment of conception until the end of the neonatal period. Therefore EMS providers should understand high-risk pregnancy.

Occasionally the cause of the high-risk pregnancy lies in the mother's age. Very young mothers have a higher rate of prenatal complications and therefore experience high-risk pregnancies. These teenage mothers have a higher rate of anemia and pregnancy-induced hypertension. The infants born of these mothers are more likely to be premature and suffer from low birth weight. These infants are also predisposed to mental retardation and injury at birth. As a general rule, the younger the mother, the greater the chances of complications for both mother and child.

Teenage pregnancy, especially new mothers less than 16, is a rapidly growing percentage of pregnancies. In fact, approximately 1500 teenagers give birth every day in the United States and another 1500 terminate their pregnancy.

Conversely, pregnancy later in life also carries with it a greater risk of complications. Complications of pregnancy for women in their 40s include pregnancy-related diabetes (gesta-tional diabetes) and Down syndrome. Down syndrome is a genetic, or chromosomal, disorder that affects 1 in every 370 children born to women over the age of 35. The babies of these older woman are also more likely to be premature or underweight.

Some complications of pregnancy are the result of illness during the pregnancy. For example, if a woman contracts measles during her pregnancy, she is at higher risk of delivering a child with a birth defect. In fact, any infection or toxin that causes abnormal development of the embryo, resulting in a birth defect, is called a teratogen.

Potentially life-threatening obstetric complications can be divided into two general classifications. The first concerns maternal bleeding during the pregnancy, called a hemorrhagic disorder, and the second classification revolves around higher than normal blood pressures during pregnancy, or hypertensive disorders.

Hemorrhagic Disorders

The first hemorrhagic disorder naturally occurs during the first trimester. During conception, the egg and the sperm unite to form an ovum and the ovum normally implants itself in the uterus. Occasionally, about once in every 200 pregnancies, the ovum implants itself outside the uterus. This is called an ectopic pregnancy; the ovum can implant in the abdomen or in the ovary, but most commonly it implants itself in the fallopian tube and is called a tubal pregnancy.

Many women may be unaware that they have a tubal pregnancy. The only sign that anything is different is a missed or abnormal period. If the ovum continues to mature and enlarge, it can rupture the fallopian tube, resulting in severe life-threatening hemorrhage. An ectopic pregnancy is a medical emergency and is so serious that, as a rule, any female of child-bearing age with lower abdominal pain is assumed to have an ectopic pregnancy until proven otherwise.

For a number of reasons, a pregnancy may not be viable and the products of conception, including the ovum, are expelled from the body. When this occurs before the twentieth week of pregnancy, it is called an **abortion**. The majority of abortions occur naturally, called spontaneous abortions within the first 8 weeks of pregnancy. If the abortion is performed for medical reasons—for example, the pregnancy risks the life of the mother—it is called a therapeutic abortion. If the abortion is performed for other than medical reasons, it is called an induced abortion. If only part of the products of conception are passed, it is called an incomplete abortion. Complications of an incomplete abortion include severe bleeding (hemorrhage) and infection (sepsis).

In some cases the placenta implants itself low in the uterus over the opening of the uterus to the vaginal birth canal, called the os. This condition is called **placenta previa**. The impact of a placenta previa is twofold. One, the exit from the uterus to the birth canal is obstructed. In some cases the infant must be delivered by cesarean section. Two, the underside of the placenta, now exposed to the opening of the uterus, tends to bleed painlessly. This bleeding can be severe and life-threatening, resulting in loss of life to either mother or child. Placenta previa occurs in about 1 in 200 pregnancies.

Another complication of pregnancy that can lead to severe, life-threatening hemorrhage is **abruptio placentae**. Abruptio placentae occurs when the placenta detaches from the uterine wall prematurely. This placental detachment can be minor, usually along the margins, or severe, resulting in bleeding into the uterus, as well as deprivation of the life-giving blood to the fetus.

Trauma, either accidental or intentional, can cause abruptio placentae. Any pregnant woman with severe vaginal bleeding (external hemorrhage) or signs of hypoperfusion (concealed hemorrhage) should be evaluated for abruptio placentae.

Hypertensive Disorders

The other classification of potentially life-threatening complications of pregnancy are the hypertensive disorders. Formerly called toxemia of pregnancy, which literally means the poisoned pregnancy, the most grave of these hypertensive disorders is **eclampsia**.

Eclampsia is divided into two stages. The first is called **preeclampsia**. Preeclampsia typically occurs between the twentieth week of pregnancy and the first week after delivery (postpartum). Signs of preeclampsia include water retention, as evidenced by excessive edema of the extremities, unexpected weight gain, protein spilled into the urine, and hypertension. Hypertension is one of the classic signs of preeclampsia; blood pressure is elevated more than 15 mm Hg diastolic above normal for the patient.

STREET SMART

Gravida, another term for a pregnant woman, literally means "heavy with child." The additional weight of a full-term pregnancy is usually about 28 to 29 pounds; 11 to 12 pounds of that is the products of conception (fetus and amniotic fluid).

When a pregnant woman lies flat on her back, such as what might occur if her spine is being immobilized to a backboard, the weight of the enlarged uterus compresses the inferior vena cava. This effectively reduces the amount of blood returning from the lower extremities to the heart. The result is that the patient's blood pressure drops, she becomes hypotensive, and she may complain of feeling dizzy or lightheaded.

This set of symptoms is called the **supine hypotensive syndrome**; it is also known as vena caval syndrome. Supine hypotensive syndrome is easily preventable. The EMS provider need only turn the patient on her side in the left lateral recumbent position, elevate her right hip about 15 degrees, or manually shift the woman's abdomen to the left. ■

The transition between preeclampsia and eclampsia is often frightening. The hallmark between the two stages is usually a convulsion that leads to coma. One in fifteen woman who have an eclamptic convulsion die secondary to either intracranial hemorrhage or cardiopulmonary failure, and 20% of the infants die in the mother's uterus (in utero) as a result of hypoxia.

Diabetes and Pregnancy

A discussion about the complications of pregnancy is not complete without addressing diabetes. As mentioned earlier, some women develop diabetes during their pregnancy, called gestational diabetes, and the diabetes resolves after childbirth.

It is generally thought the diabetes is the result of the inability of the pancreas to produce sufficient amounts of insulin for both mother and child, a form of type II diabetes.

Pregnant women who develop diabetes during pregnancy usually have large infants that sometimes have difficulty passing through the birth canal. The degree of diabetes can range from mild, requiring no additional insulin, to severe, resulting in renal disease. Even with diligent control of blood sugar levels, there still is a 15% perinatal fetal mortality rate.

● CONTRACEPTION

Some religious and ethnic groups oppose birth control, and this text does not ignore that issue. This subject matter is presented factually, from a clinical viewpoint, as information required for practice as a health care worker. As the word implies, contraception is literally "against" conception. One choice in contraception is abstinence. Abstinence is the voluntary restraint of sexual intercourse and is a positive, healthy choice many people make.

Several reasons may be given to avoid pregnancy:

- To avoid health risks to the woman. A woman in poor health may not survive a pregnancy.

- To space pregnancies. Some women are very fertile and could conceive every year. The in-

fant death rate is reported to be 50% higher at 1-year intervals than at 2 or more years.

- To avoid having babies with birth defects. Some women have chromosome defects or are genetic disease carriers (or married to carriers) and choose not to risk pregnancy.

- To delay pregnancy early in marriage to allow a time for adjustment to avoid additional stress in the new relationship and establish a strong marriage.

- To limit family size. It is sometimes a personal decision and other times a reality of limited resources.

- To avoid pregnancy among unmarried couples. Single parenthood is difficult.

- To curb population growth. The concern over worldwide food supply and supportive environment prompts some to promote contraception.

Several methods to prevent conception and their relative percentage of effectiveness are listed in Table 20-3. Selection is usually made by the woman in consultation with her doctor. The cost, ease of use, degree of effectiveness, and likelihood of side effects must be taken into consideration when selecting a method.

● INFERTILITY

Infertility is when conception cannot occur. Some causes of infertility may be damage to fallopian tubes, a low sperm count, hormonal imbalance, and other disorders. Medical advances have led to a variety of different methods to increase fertility, including the following:

> **Artificial insemination**—a procedure in which the semen is placed into the vaginal canal by means of canula and syringe, usually around the time of ovulation.

> **In vitro fertilization**—a procedure in which the female is given ovulation-inducing drugs that stimulate the development of multiple ovarian follicles. A laparoscopy is done at a precise time to remove the ovarian follicles and extract the ova. The ova are then cultured in vitro

TABLE 20-3 *Different Methods of Preventing Conception*

% EFFECTIVE	METHOD	DESCRIPTION/COMMENTS
100%	Abstinence	Refraining from sexual intercourse; always effective.
100%	Sterilization	Tubal/ligation (cutting of the fallopian tubes) in the female. The cut ends can be sewn back in opposite directions or cauterized. The surgical procedure is done through a laparoscope inserted into the abdomen. The procedure is considered permanent. A vasectomy in the male, with the ends being sewn in opposite directions. The surgery is performed through a small incision at the base of the scrotum. Vasectomies are usually not reversible; however, in some instances, reconstructive surgery has been successful, especially in cases in which the sterilization was performed recently.
95%–99%	Birth control pills	Many different kinds are available. They are a combination of hormones that prevent ovulation; no ovum, therefore no pregnancy. Failure occurs when pills are not taken as prescribed. Side effects can be prohibitive for some women. Available only by prescription and requires regular visits to a physician. Cost is a factor to consider.
93%–99%	IUD	The intrauterine device is a small piece of plastic or coiled material inserted into the uterus to prevent implantation of a fertilized egg, presumably by providing irritation to the endometrium. Failure can occur if the device is expelled during the first few months after being inserted. Initial insertion costs involved, and cost of removal. Side effects bother some women.
90%–99%	Diaphragm	A thin piece of dome-shaped rubber with a firm ring that is inserted into the vagina to cover the cervix and provide a barrier to sperm. It is most effective when used in combination with a contraceptive cream placed into the dome before inserting. Failure usually results from improper insertion; a defect in the rubber, such as a hole; failure to insert before any penile penetration; or failure to maintain in place at least 6 hours after intercourse. Initial cost for examination, fit, and purchase. No side effects. Requires cleaning and inspection after each use.
85%–97%	Condom	A thin sheath of rubber or latex that fits over an erect penis to catch the semen. A properly used condom is very effective. It must be unrolled onto an erect penis *before* any penetration occurs. It is important to leave about half an inch of free air space at the tip (unless the condom is constructed with a tip) to catch the semen; otherwise, the force of the ejaculation may burst the condom. It must also remain in place throughout intercourse. After ejaculation has occurred, care must be taken to withdraw with the condom in place. It may require grasping with the fingers. This is the only contraceptive that also provides a level of protection against sexually transmitted diseases. It is relatively inexpensive, easy to use, and readily available. Only a latex condom is also effective against the AIDS virus.
70%–75%	Spermicides	Contraceptive foams, jellies, and creams with sperm-killing ingredients, inserted by applicator, deep into the vagina before intercourse. It must remain in place for a least 6 to 8 hours afterward. Each application is good for only one act of intercourse. They should not be relied on alone as an effective contraceptive. Combined with a diaphragm or condom, they are effective. Few side effects (some report allergic reactions), easily used, and readily available. Must not be confused with lubricants such as K-Y or Lubafax, which contain *no* spermicide.
?	Douching	Absolutely not reliable. It only takes a couple of minutes for sperm to enter the cervix. In reality, douching cannot be accomplished quickly enough. In fact, it may even assist sperm in moving toward the cervix.
70%–80%	Withdrawal	This method has been practiced since ancient times. It simply requires that the penis be withdrawn and ejaculation occur outside the vagina. It is not very effective because some sperm are deposited in the vagina before ejaculation occurs. In addition, the man may not be able to withdraw in time. It requires a lot of concentration to control. It is also not advised because it may lead to a sexual dysfunction if practiced for a prolonged period.
65%–85%	Rhythm	The practice of abstinence during an 8-day period from day 10 to 17 of the menstrual cycle, when conception is theoretically possible. The method works fairly well for women who are extremely regular in their cycles and couples who can practice strong self-control. However, it requires a careful assessment of at least 6 months of cycles to establish ovulation days. If cycles vary in length, the period of abstinence must be increased to cover the longest possible time.

with the male's spermatozoa under careful laboratory conditions. If fertilization is successful, and when the zygote is at the four- to eight-cell stage, it is transferred to the uterus of the female.

ADVANCES IN MICROSURGERY FOR FEMALE INFERTILITY

Microsurgery is performed with the aid of magnification. The use of the operating microscope has produced better surgical results because it allows magnification from two- to thirtyfold. This procedure also allows the use of fine suture material and delicate handling.

Pelviscopy is a special type of operative laparoscopy in which extensive procedures are performed. This involves the use of magnification through lenses and frequently the use of a video camera, which allows a surgical assistant to work with the surgeon. This procedure is used in the treatment of ectopic pregnancy, fibroids, ovarian cysts, tumors, endometriosis, and pelvic adhesions.

Gamete Intrafallopian Tube Transfer (GIFT)

In gamete intrafallopian transfer, a laparoscope is used to recover the eggs from the ovary and to transfer the sperm and eggs back into the ends of the fallopian tube after fertilization. This tubal embryo transfer is one of the newer areas of in vitro fertilization; using the laparoscope to place the embryos in the ends of the tubes has resulted in excellent pregnancy rates.

DISORDERS OF THE REPRODUCTIVE SYSTEM

Female Reproductive Disorders

Amenorrhea is a term used to define the absence of the menstrual cycle. This is normal if the female is pregnant. Psychological factors, anorexia, and hormonal imbalance are other causes of this condition.

Premenstrual syndrome (PMS) is a group of symptoms exhibited just prior to the menstrual cycle, caused by water retention in the body tissue. Irritability, nervousness, mood swings, and weight gain are some of the most common symptoms. PMS is no longer considered a myth and is treated with medication and diet to reduce water retention.

Dysmenorrhea is a term used to describe painful menstruation. Dysmenorrhea is characterized by cramps, which may be caused by excessive production of an inflammatory substance such as prostaglandin. Aspirin-like substances that block the action of prostaglandin are helpful.

Endometriosis, a word that comes from *endometrium,* is a disease that affects women during their reproductive years. In this condition, endometrial tissue is found outside the uterus, around the ovaries and other organs in the abdominopelvic cavity.

Every month, like the lining of the uterus, the tissue responds to hormonal changes. The tissue gets bigger, breaks down, and causes bleeding. Endometrial tissue outside the uterus has no way to leave the body. The result is internal bleeding, inflammation of the surrounding areas, and formation of scar tissue. This condition causes infertility, heavy or irregular bleeding, and pain before and during menstruation and during or after sexual activity. The cause is unknown, but different theories exist. One theory is that during menstruation some of the tissue backs up through the fallopian tubes, implants in the abdomen, and grows. Some experts feel it is related to an autoimmune problem. Others suggest that endometrial tissue is distributed from the uterus to other parts of the body through the lymph system.

Diagnosis is made by **laparoscopy**, a minor surgical procedure done under anesthesia in which the patient's abdomen is distended with carbon dioxide gas to make the organs easier to see. A laparoscope (a tube with a light on it) is inserted through a tiny incision in the abdomen. By moving the instrument around the abdomen, the surgeon can check the condition of the organs and see the endometrial implants, if they are present. The surgeon can also remove endometrial tissue with this method. In addition to laparoscopic surgery, another treatment is the use of hormonal drugs to stop ovulation and force endometriosis into remission during the time of treatment. Menopause generally ends the activity of mild or moderate endometriosis.

Fibroid tumors are usually benign growths that occur in the uterine wall. Fibroids may enlarge to cause pressure on other organs or may cause excessive bleeding. To treat fibroids, a **hysterectomy** (removal of the uterus) may be done.

Breast tumors are either benign or malignant. Benign tumors are usually fluid-filled cysts that enlarge during the premenstrual cycle. Women are taught to do periodic breast self-examinations to detect any developing lumps. Breast examinations are done by palpating the breasts in a circular fashion. Any suspected lump should be reported to a doctor immediately.

Breast cancer, or malignant tumor, is the most common cancer in women. Early detection and treatment is vital to survival. Surgical treatment consists of a **lumpectomy** (removal of tumor only) or **mastectomy** (removal of the breast). Other types of treatments include radiation and chemotherapy (anticancer drugs). Benefits are associated with all types of treatment; the patient and physician select the most appropriate treatment. **Mammogram** is a special type of x-ray that can detect tumors of the breast before they can be palpated. This test is recommended on an annual basis for all women over the age of 40.

Endometrial cancer is the most common type of uterine cancer. It usually affects women after menopause. Women are instructed to immediately report to their physician any vaginal bleeding that occurs after menopause. Hysterectomy and irradiation are the usual types of treatment.

Ovarian cancer is a leading cause of cancer death in women. It usually occurs between the ages of 40 and 65. Early diagnosis is difficult and treatment is aggressive surgery to remove all reproductive organs.

Cervical cancer is frequently seen in women between the ages of 30 and 50. The test to detect cancer of the cervix is called the **Pap smear**, in which a sample of cell scrapings is taken from the cervix and cervical canal for microscopic study. When a woman becomes sexually active, this test should be done on an annual basis. Early detection and treatment are vital to the prognosis of the disease.

Infections of Female Reproductive Organs

Pelvic inflammatory disease (PID) may be caused by infections that occur in the reproductive organs and spread to the fallopian tubes and peritoneal cavity. This disease may also be secondary to another infection such as gonorrhea. The inflammation causes pain, high temperature, and possible scarring of the fallopian tubes. Treatment consists of medications such as antibiotics and analgesics.

Salpingitis is an inflammation of the fallopian tubes that may result in permanent damage.

Toxic shock syndrome is a bacterial infection caused by a staphylococcal organism. Symptoms are fever, rash, and hypotension, which may result in shock. The patient is treated with antibiotics.

Vaginal **yeast infections** are generally caused by the organism *candida albicans*. This fungus is part of the body's natural organisms. A problem arises when the environment of the vagina is altered. A yeast infection develops when the vagina becomes less acidic. This change results in an overgrowth of *candida* organisms, causing an infection.

Symptoms include itching, burning, and redness in the vagina and vulva. There may also be an odorless, thick, white discharge (leukorrhea) resembling cottage cheese. Treatment with an antibiotic (for another illness) that alters the normal bacteria of the vagina may cause a yeast infection to occur. Yeast infections are more common in people with diabetes, pregnant women, and those with other causes of hormonal changes. Treatment is the use of a fungicidal agent that destroys the organism. This may be used as a vaginal cream or vaginal insert.

Male Reproductive Disorders

Epididymitis is a painful swelling in the groin and scrotum caused by infection of the epididymis. This is treated with antibiotic therapy.

Orchitis is an inflammation of the testes. It may be a complication of mumps, flu, or another infection. Symptoms are swelling of the scrotum, fever, and pain. This disease is treated with antibiotic therapy, pain relievers, and cold compresses.

Prostatitis is an infection of the prostate gland. The prostate gland lies below the urinary bladder, and the prostatic urethra passes through the gland. Urinary symptoms are often the first indication there is a prostatic problem. The patient complains of difficulty in urination. Treatment with antibiotics is effective.

Benign prostatic hypertrophy (BPH) indicates an enlarged prostate. The prostate gland continues to grow during most of a man's life; the enlargement usually does not cause problems until late in life. More than half of men in their 60s and as many as 90% in their 70s have some symptoms of BPH. The prostate enlarges but the capsule around the prostate does not, which causes the prostate to press up against the urethra like a clamp around a tube. The bladder becomes thick and irritable. Then the bladder begins to contract even when it contains only small amounts of urine, causing frequent urination. As the bladder weakens, it loses the ability to empty itself and urine remains in the bladder. The narrowing of the urethra may cause retention of urine and an infection may occur.

Diagnosis is made by rectal exam, ultrasound, and cystoscopy. A cystoscope is a flexible tube with a lens and a light system that is inserted into the urethra. This enables the physician to see the inside of the urethra and the bladder.

Treatment may depend on the extent of the symptoms. At the present time a prostatectomy is the usual treatment.

Prostate cancer is the most common cancer in males over the age of 50. Males over the age of 40 should have annual rectal examinations, which can detect enlargement of the prostate. A prostate-specific antigen (PSA) blood screening test detects an abnormal substance released by cancer cells. Symptoms include frequency of urination, dysuria (painful urination), urgency, nocturia (night voiding), and in some cases hematuria (blood in the urine). The most com-

mon treatment is a **prostatectomy** (removal of the prostate gland). This procedure is called a transurethral resection of the prostate (TURP). An instrument is inserted into the penis and resects, or cuts away, the prostate gland, which is then removed through the penis. There is no abdominal incision and recovery time is short.

SEXUALLY TRANSMITTED DISEASE

Sexually transmitted diseases (STDs), also known as venereal diseases, are transmitted through the exchange of body fluids such as semen, vaginal fluid, and blood. STDs can be serious, painful, and cause long-term complications, including sterility, chronic infection, scarring of the fallopian tubes, ectopic pregnancy, cancer, and death. The most common STDs are chlamydia, genital herpes, and genital warts.

Some of these diseases have no symptoms. Several of the more common symptoms include the following:

- In females, an unusual discharge from the vagina, pain in the pelvic area, burning or itching around the vagina, unusual bleeding, and vaginal pain during intercourse.

- In males, a discharge from the penis.

- In both females and males, sores or blisters near the mouth or genitalia, burning and pain during urination or bowel movements, flulike symptoms, and swelling in the groin area.

The patient who is at a physician's office or a health care center to be checked for an STD may feel some embarrassment. It is critical that the health care worker treat the person in a nonjudgmental manner because every day that the disease is untreated leads to more severe health problems. Some STDs are diagnosed by physical examination, whereas others require blood or other laboratory tests. For bacterial diseases such as gonorrhea, chlamydia, and syphilis, treatment is with antibiotics. Viral infections usually cannot be cured, but the symptoms can be relieved.

Protection from STDs includes abstinence and practicing safe sexual behavior. Abstinence is the voluntary refraining from sexual activity, a positive, healthy choice many people make. Safe sex means using condoms and looking for any signs of venereal disease *before* sexual activity occurs. Once a person is aware of the disease, he or she must notify any sexual partners so they can also be checked for the disease. It is often necessary for previous sexual partners to also be notified. All sexually transmitted diseases need to be treated. A high incidence of STD is leading to an increase in sterility in young females.

Chlamydia is caused by the *chlamydia trachomatis* organism and is the most common curable sexually transmitted disease in the United States. It is the major cause of non-gonococcal urethritis, bacterial vaginitis, and pelvic inflammatory disease. Up to 80% women and 25% of men have no symptoms. If symptoms do occur they are the usual symptoms of STDs. A screening test called a DNA probe assay may be done for this disease. The test examines secretion from the cervix, urethra, or rectum. Treatment is with antibiotics; however, immunity does not develop after being infected.

Genital warts, or human papillomavirus, is another common sexually transmitted disease. Warts can appear on the shaft of the penis or on the vagina. It is usually asymptomatic. In many cases the warts are not visible to the naked eye. In other cases they look like small, hard, round spots resembling a cauliflower. Although genital warts are usually painless, they become sore, itchy, and may burn if hit, rubbed, irritated, or ignored for a long period. Diagnosis is made primarily by examination. To find very small warts, the genital area may be examined with a magnifying instrument. Treatment involves the use of an acid to destroy wart tissue, or cryosurgery. Cryosurgery uses liquid nitrogen, which is placed on the wart and a small area of the surrounding skin. The liquid nitrogen freezes the skin, causing ice crystals, which results in the sloughing off of the wart.

Gonorrhea is an STD resulting from a bacterial infection caused by *Neisseria gonorrhoeae*. The symptoms in the male may be painful urination and the discharge of pus from the penis. In the female the early stages

of the disease may be asymptomatic (no symptoms). This disease is treated with antibiotic therapy. There is a problem with some strains of the organism that have become resistant to the usual treatment.

Complications may occur if the inflammation spreads to the epididymis of the male or the fallopian tube of the female. The tubes may become scarred and blocked, which results in sterility. In addition, if a pregnant woman contracts the disease and it is untreated, her baby may be born with gonorrheal eye infection.

Genital herpes is a sexually transmitted viral infection. The herpes lesions may cause a burning sensation, and small, blisterlike areas may appear in the genitalia. Other symptoms may be painful irritation and discomfort while sitting or standing. Herpes symptoms may simply disappear after 2 weeks; however, the symptoms continue to reappear throughout the lifetime of the individual. Females who are diagnosed with herpes must consult with their physicians on whether or not to have a cesarean section to prevent herpes from infecting their newborns during childbirth.

Syphilis is a bacterial sexually transmitted disease. This disease, prevalent at one time, is once again on the increase in association with the AIDS epidemic.

Syphilis has four stages. In the first stage, a sore (chancre) appears at the site of infection. A chancre heals whether or not a person gets treatment. The second stage occurs 6 to 12 weeks after the initial infection. Symptoms include discolored spots or patches on the hands and the soles of the feet; moist, raised, or elevated skin lesions; mucous patches in the mouth, throat, and cervix in women; a rash over the body; and flulike symptoms. The discolored spots disappear with or without treatment. In the early stage, there are no symptoms. In the tertiary stage, or final stage, which occurs 10 to 40 years after the first stage, tissue and liver damage occur; this may cause heart disease, brain damage, paralysis, and death. Syphilis is diagnosed by recognition of the signs and symptoms, examination of the lesion under a microscope, and a blood test. Syphilis is treated with penicillin or another antibiotic.

● REVIEW QUESTIONS

Select the letter of choice that best completes the statement.

1. One of the male hormones is:
   a. progesterone
   b. luteinizing hormone
   c. follicle-stimulating hormone
   d. testosterone

2. Ovulation usually occurs:
   a. the day before the menstrual period begins
   b. 1 week before the menstrual period begins
   c. 3 weeks before the menstrual period begins
   d. 2 weeks before the menstrual period begins

3. The ovaries contain:
   a. 30 graafian follicles
   b. thousands of graafian follicles
   c. hundreds of graafian follicles
   d. 6 graafian follicles

4. The development of the follicle and release of the ovum are under the influence of:
   a. follicle-stimulating hormone and luteinizing hormone
   b. estrogen and corpus luteum
   c. progesterone and follicle-stimulating hormone
   d. estrogen and luteinizing hormone

5. Which one of the following statements is *not* correct?
   a. The fallopian tubes are about 4 inches long.
   b. The fallopian tubes serve as ducts for the ovum on its way to the uterus.
   c. The fallopian tubes are also called oviducts.
   d. The fallopian tubes are attached to the ovaries.

● MATCHING

Match each term in Column A with its correct description in Column B.

Column A	Column B
_____ 1. scrotum	a. secondary sex characteristics
_____ 2. testosterone	b. external sac that holds the testes
_____ 3. facial and pubic hair	c. excreted from the pituitary gland
_____ 4. epididymis and penis	d. formed in the seminiferous tubules
_____ 5. spermatozoa	e. male gamete
	f. secondary reproductive organs
	g. male hormone produced in the testes

● COMPLETION

Fill in the blanks.

1. Painful or difficult in menstruation is known as _____.

2. Amenorrhea is normal when a person is _____.

3. Gonorrhea is a sexually transmitted disease. The male complains of _____ and the female complains of _____.

4. The test done to detect breast tumors is called _____.

5. Sterility in women results from inflammation of the fallopian tube, which can be caused by _____ and _____.

6. A group of symptoms that occur before the menstrual cycle is called _____.

7. The onset of ovulation is known as _____, and the cessation of ovulation is known as _____.

8. A sexually transmitted disease that results in small blisterlike areas is known as _____.

9. An enlarged prostate may cause problems with _____.

10. The best methods of preventing sexually transmitted diseases are _____ and _____.

●APPLYING THEORY TO PRACTICE

1. A young pregnant woman comes into the doctor's office and states, "I told my husband I will give him a son, because in my family I was the only girl and I have four brothers." Is this a valid statement? Explain to the expectant mother how the sex of the newborn is determined.

2. If a person has a sperm count of 16 million, he is considered sterile. Fertilization only requires the union of one egg and one sperm; why then are so many sperm necessary for fertilization to occur?

3. You are asked to describe the fertilization process. Explain how the sperm travels from the testes and arrives at the fallopian tube in time to meet the ovum.

4. You are invited to a middle school to address 11- to 14-year-olds and discuss puberty. Plan a program to describe how females are affected by estrogen and progesterone and how males are affected by testosterone.

5. A 50-year-old female patient tells you it has gotten very hot in the ambulance and requests that you put on the air conditioner. The temperature outdoors is 30° F. She further states that the doctor told her about changes that usually occur at midlife. Explain to the patient the physiological and psychological changes attributed to menopause.

● LABELING

Label the structures of the male reproductive system on the following diagram.

1. _____
2. _____
3. _____
4. _____
5. _____
6. _____
7. _____
8. _____
9. _____
10. _____
11. _____
12. _____
13. _____
14. _____
15. _____
16. _____
17. _____
18. _____
19. _____
20. _____
21. _____
22. _____

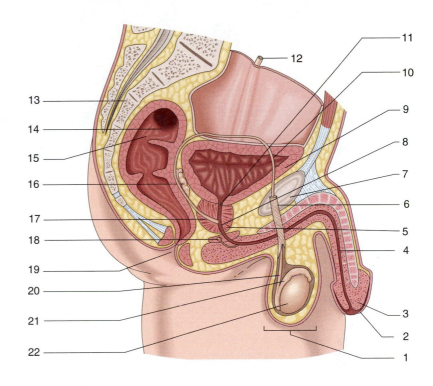

21

Genetics and Genetically Linked Diseases

Objectives

- Define *mutation*
- Differentiate between the two basic types of mutations
- Name three human genetic disorders and describe the cause and symptoms of each
- Explain genetic counseling
- Define the key words that relate to this chapter

Key Words

amniocentesis
black biology
chorionic villi sampling
chromosomal mutation
chromosome
congenital disorder
cystic fibrosis
Duchenne's muscular dystrophy
gene
gene mutation
genetic counseling
genetic disorder
genetics
hemophilia
Huntington's disease
interferon
lethal gene
mutagenic agent
mutation
phenylketonuria (PKU)
recombinant DNA
sickle cell anemia
somatic cell mutation
Tay-Sachs disease
thalassemia (Cooley's anemia)
trisomy 21 or Down syndrome (mongoloidism)

GENETICS

In sexual reproduction a new individual is created from the union of the sperm cell and the egg cell. This process is called fertilization. Contained in the nucleus of each gamete are structures called **chromosomes**. The chromosomes contain deoxyribonucleic acid (DNA), the hereditary material referred to in Chapter 2. The DNA is packaged in small functional units found along the length of a chromosome, called **genes**. A gene is an area of DNA that carries information for the cellular synthesis of a specific protein. These genes are transmitted to the zygote and then control the development and characteristics of the embryo as it grows and matures. Eventually, as a result of the combined influence of all the genes on all the chromosomes, a new individual is formed. The new individual possesses all the necessary characteristics or traits needed for survival. In addition, because the genes come from two parents, the offspring resemble both parents in some ways. However, it is also different from each parent in some ways. The mixture of the genes from both parents results in the production of a unique individual.

Genetics is the branch of biology that studies how the genes are transmitted from parents to offspring. Occasionally a gene or chromosome is changed, or mutated, in a gamete, and this mutated gene or chromosome is inherited by the offspring. The inheritance of such a mutated gene or chromosome causes the appearance of a new and different trait, called a **mutation**. Sometimes the mutation is beneficial or harmless to an organism. Unfortunately, most inherited mutations are not beneficial. Still, it must be emphasized that mutations in the genetic material are responsible for biological evolution on this planet.

TYPES OF MUTATIONS

There are two types of mutations. One is called a **gene mutation**. When this mutation occurs, a new or altered gene is produced to replace a normal preexisting gene. The other type is a **chromosomal mutation**. This mutation involves a change in the number of chromosomes found in the nucleus or a change in the structure of a whole chromosome.

Somatic Cell Mutation

Gene mutations occur occasionally at random in all cells of the human body. For instance, skin cells often undergo mutation as an individual ages. Mutations that occur in individual body (somatic) cells are not transmitted to the offspring. This specific type of mutation is called a **somatic cell mutation**. A somatic cell mutation is not likely to affect other cells or the function of the organism as a whole. As an example, a single cell may lose the ability to make a certain protein and die without having an impact on the total organism.

Gametic Cell Mutation

Mutations that occur in the nucleus of the gametes (sperm and egg cell) are passed on to the next generation. If either a gene or chromosomal mutation is present in a gamete at the moment of fertilization, all the cells of the embryo and the developed organism will have the mutation in at least half their DNA.

STREET SMART

Some mutations are not compatible with life. If the mutation involves a developing embryo, the pregnancy may not be sustained. In that case the body rids itself of the unwanted pregnancy by a process called spontaneous abortion, also referred to as a miscarriage. ■

LETHAL GENES

On the whole, inherited mutations are generally negative. At times they might even result in the formation of lethal genes. A lethal gene is a gene that results in death.

The time at which lethal genes exert their deadly influence varies. Some genes interfere with mitosis of the zygote and life ends before the zygote divides. Some lethal genes interfere with implantation of the fertilized egg in the uterus. Death occurs so early that a woman never knows that conception has occurred. A lethal gene that prevents normal formation of the heart or normal blood production causes death at about 3 weeks after fertilization because this is the time when circulating blood becomes vital for continued existence. Others may kill at various times during development, depending on the time their products become vital for survival. Some lethal genes causing neonatal deaths involve abnormalities of the lungs and shifts in the circulatory system that must channel blood from the heart to the lungs instead of to the umbilical cord.

Certain lethal genes do not exert their effects until later in life. Tay-Sachs disease causes death several years after birth. Duchenne's muscular dystrophy causes death in the teens and early childhood. Huntington's disease usually results in death at 40 to 50 years of age.

It is estimated that each person carries two or three different recessive lethal genes. Two similar recessive genes must be present in an individual for the gene to be expressed. Because there are so many kinds of lethal genes, one's chance of marrying someone with even one matching lethal gene is small. Statistically,

should this happen, the lethal gene would be expressed in only one fourth of the offspring.

When close relatives marry, the chance of the offspring's inheriting two similar lethal genes increases. Persons with a common ancestry are more likely than nonrelatives to share many genes. As a result, spontaneous abortions, stillbirths, neonatal deaths, and congenital deformities are higher among progeny of people sharing similar gene pools.

HUMAN GENETIC DISORDERS

Some diseases caused by gene mutations in humans are phenylketonuria, sickle cell anemia, Tay-Sachs disease, Duchenne's muscular dystrophy, Huntington's disease, and cystic fibrosis.

It is important to note that there is a difference between genetic disorders and congenital disorders. A hereditary, or genetic, disorder is caused by a variation in the genetic pattern; a congenital disorder is something that evolves during fetal development and is not related to genetic malfunction.

Phenylketonuria

Phenylketonuria (PKU) is a human metabolic disorder caused by an enzyme deficiency. The individual with the trait cannot break down the amino acid phenylalanine and consequently there is a buildup of this substance in the body. Excess phenylalanine disrupts the normal development of the brain. If a person born with the defect eats proteins containing phenylalanine during childhood, mental retardation results. A newborn infant is tested for this defect, and if

STREET SMART

When a woman over the age of 35 becomes pregnant, her unborn child has a higher risk of having a genetic disorder. For example, a 40-year old woman who is pregnant has a 1 in 42 chance of delivering a baby with Down syndrome. The infant with Down syndrome has an extra chromosome, usually 21. A special test called an amniocentesis can diagnose many genetic disorders before birth. Parents should be counseled regarding options. More discussion about genetic counseling can be found at the end of the chapter. ■

the test is positive, a phenylalanine-restricted diet is prescribed. In most cases this diet can be liberalized as the child grows older and brain development and maturation are completed.

Sickle Cell Anemia

Sickle cell anemia is a blood disorder common in individuals of African descent. It is caused by a gene mutation resulting in an abnormal hemoglobin molecule in a red blood cell, Figure 21-1. Especially in times of low oxygen availability, the shape of a red blood cell changes from that of a biconcave disk to a crescent shape. This is referred to as sickling. The sickle shape causes the cells to clump together, thus clogging small blood vessels and capillaries. Because a sickle cell has an abnormal hemoglobin (the pigment that combines with oxygen), it also carries less oxygen to the tissues, resulting in fatigue and listlessness. Breakage of these cells is also common because their membranes are excessively fragile. See Figure 21-2 for a description of the tissue damage and physiological effects caused by sickle cell anemia.

Tay-Sachs Disease

Tay-Sachs disease is a genetic disorder caused by a mutation resulting in a deficiency of a lysosomal enzyme. The enzyme's function is to break down lipid molecules in the brain.

Without the enzyme, lipids accumulate in the brain cells and destroy them. This results in severe mental and motor deterioration leading to death several years after birth. This disorder is found most frequently among Jewish people of central European ancestry.

Huntington's Disease

Huntington's disease is characterized by the degeneration of the central nervous system, which ultimately results in abnormal movements and mental deterioration. In this disorder the product of an abnormal gene interferes with normal metabolism in nerve tissue.

Duchenne's Muscular Dystrophy

In **Duchenne's muscular dystrophy** the muscles suffer a loss of protein and the contractile fibers are eventually replaced by fat and connective tissue, rendering skeletal muscle useless. As the weakening process of the disease continues, the teen or young adult is confined to a wheelchair. In many cases the person with Duchenne's muscular dystrophy dies before the age of 20 from respiratory or heart failure.

Cystic Fibrosis

Cystic fibrosis is a disease of the exocrine gland. The lining of the digestive tract, the

Concavity, or dents

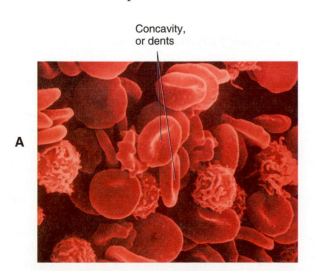

Normal red blood cell   Sickle-shaped red blood cell

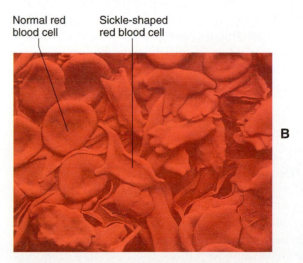

A   B

● **FIGURE 21–1**   *(A) Normal red blood cells (RBCs); seen from the sire, normal RBCs have a concavity (or dent) on the two sides. (B) Sickle-shaped (crescent-shaped) red blood cells.*

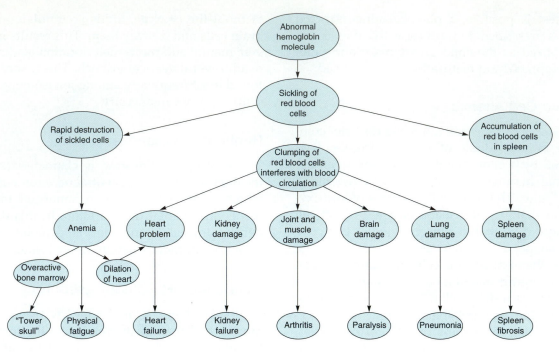

● **FIGURE 21-2** *Damage caused by sickle cell anemia.*

ducts of the pancreas, and the respiratory tract produce thick mucus that blocks the passageways. The blockage of the respiratory passages causes chronic bronchitis and pneumonia. Pulmonary therapy consists of a procedure called "cupping and clapping," which helps to dislodge the thick mucus from the respiratory tract. These treatments have helped to prolong the life span of patients with cystic fibrosis; however, only half the patients live to the age of 25. Science has discovered the gene that transmits this disease and may soon be able to treat and prevent this illness. The involvement of the lungs makes this one of the most fatal hereditary disorders.

Thalassemia

Thalassemia (Cooley's anemia) is a blood disease found among people of Mediterranean descent. Symptoms are the same as those associated with any anemia; there is also enlargement of the spleen and possible congestive heart disease. This disease is treated with blood transfusions to replace the defective hemoglobin molecules.

Hemophilia

Hemophilia is a sex-linked genetic disorder; that is, it is only transmitted on the X chromosome. In this disease the person is unable to produce the factor VIII, which is necessary for blood clotting. Persistent bleeding may occur as a result of an injury or spontaneously. Treatment consists of giving the person factor VIII intravenously.

Chromosomal Aberrations

Some mutations are caused by chromosomal aberrations. Some involve entire chromosomes and others involve parts of chromosomes. During meiosis (the cell division occurring when gametes are formed), a pair of chromosomes may adhere to each other and not pull apart at metaphase. As a result of this nondisjunction, duplicate chromosomes go to one daughter cell and none of this type of chromosome to the other. Nondisjunction of certain chromosomes referred to as sex chromosomes causes various abnormalities of sexual development such as Turner's syndrome in females and Klinefelter's syndrome in males.

One of the most common chromosomal abnormalities involves an extra chromosome designated as chromosome 21. This disorder is referred to as trisomy 21 or Down syndrome (mongoloidism). The risk of bearing a child with Down syndrome significantly increases with the age of the mother. Many physicians therefore recommend amniocentesis for all women who become pregnant after age 35. Cells from the amniotic fluid show trisomy 21 (as well as other chromosomal defects) if it is present. If a serious defect is detected, prospective parents have the option of therapeutic abortion.

Mutagenic Agents

Although most gene or chromosomal mutations occur spontaneously, the rate or speed of mutations can be increased. This happens when a cell, a group of cells, or an entire organism is exposed to certain chemicals or radiations. Agents that speed up the occurrence of mutations are called mutagenic agents. Mutagenic agents can be radiations like cosmic rays, ultraviolet rays from the sun, x-rays, and radiation from radioactive elements. Some mutagenic chemicals are benzene, formaldehyde, phenol, and nitrous acid.

In recent times the accelerated use of various chemical and physical agents with mutagenic properties has caused concern among some geneticists who fear possible significant alterations to genes and chromosomes that will be passed on to future generations. The increased use of ionizing radiation in medical diagnosis and the problem of the disposal of nuclear waste from reactors are examples. Certain chemical pollutants in the environment, such as herbicides and insecticides, are also suspected of causing genetic defects.

Because people are being exposed to more and more new substances, and because changes in genes are irreversible, caution should be the rule with regard to any unnecessary exposure to those suspected of being mutagens.

● GENETIC COUNSELING

Genetic counseling involves talking to parents or prospective parents about the possibility of genetic disorders. The counseling team usually is made up of members of the health care team, a genealogist, a nurse, laboratory personnel, and social service professionals. In genetic counseling a family history, called a pedigree, is obtained. Any and all facts that pertain to the parents or prospective parents and family members are considered. After careful analysis a genotype is determined; this analysis will be able to predict the possibility of a genetic disorder.

The prospective parents are made aware of what diagnostic tests are available during pregnancy. Chorionic villi sampling is a test that may be done as early as 8 to 10 weeks into the pregnancy. A sample of fetal cells is removed from the fetal side of the placenta and examined. Amniocentesis is withdrawal of amniotic

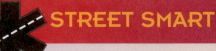

STREET SMART

Although genetic engineering could have potentially useful purposes, it could also be used for destructive purposes.

Although biological terrorism, the use of infectious agents as bio-weapons, has increasingly alarmed public safety officials, more alarming is the thought of genetically engineered bio-weapons.

There are treatments for many of the currently available biological warfare agents. However, it could take years to develop an antibiotic or a vaccination against a new biological agent.

The creation of these new biological weapons by gene splicing, for example, called black biology, is a growing concern. ■

fluid during the sixteenth week of pregnancy. An examination of the fluid is able to pick up as many as 200 possible genetic disorders. Prior to performing an amniocentesis, a sonogram is done to determine where the fetal structures are located so as to prevent any problems.

Genetic counseling helps prospective parents make informed decisions regarding having children.

● GENETIC ENGINEERING

Recent advances in the methods of gene transfer from the cell of one species to another offer exciting possibilities for the treatment of genetic deficiencies. Human insulin, human growth hormone, and human interferons (proteins that interfere with virus replication) are now being produced using the sophisticated technology of recombinant DNA. We can isolate a desired gene (to correct for a defective one) and grow millions of copies of it in the cells of bacteria and yeast, which in turn produce the gene product on a commercial scale.

Some scientists even envision a time when we will have the ability to introduce copies of normal genes into humans whose genes are defective, thus alleviating much human suffering.

● REVIEW QUESTIONS

Select the letter of the choice that best completes the statement.

1. The branch of science that deals with how human traits are passed down is called:
   a. genetic engineering
   b. biology
   c. genetics
   d. genetic counseling

2. When a change takes place in a gene, what has occurred?
   a. mutation
   b. lethal gene
   c. congenital defect
   d. mutant

3. A deficiency in breaking down fat molecules is characteristic of:
    a. sickle cell
    b. Tay-Sachs
    c. PKU
    d. Down syndrome

4. An extra chromosome can cause a defect known as trisomy 21 or:
    a. Cooley's anemia
    b. Huntington's disease
    c. Down syndrome
    d. PKU

5. A disease that produces thick mucus is called:
    a. PKU
    b. sickle cell
    c. Huntington's disease
    d. cystic fibrosis

●APPLYING THEORY TO PRACTICE

1. A young couple comes to the doctor's office and state that they have heard about genetic counseling. There is a family history of Tay-Sachs disease. Explain to them about genetic counseling and the probability of having a child with Tay-Sachs disease.

2. A friend tells you she has been advised to have an amniocentesis; she is 16 weeks pregnant. The thought of having someone stick a needle in her belly and what may happen to her baby is frightening. Explain the test to her.

3. PKU is a genetic disorder that can be detected while the infant is still in the hospital nursery. Explain the disease and the special dietary restrictions.

4. Sickle cell anemia trait can be diagnosed with a simple blood test. People are afraid to have this test done. List some of the factors that influence people's opinions regarding this test.

5. You are going to participate in a debate on the issue of genetic engineering. One side must present legal, scientific, and moral issues for the limited use of this science, whereas the other side will support unrestricted use of the technology.

Glossary

abdomen (ab'-do-mun): portion of body lying between the thorax and pelvis

abdominal cavity (ab-dom'-i-nul ka'-vih-tee): area containing the stomach, liver, gallbladder, a portion of the pancreas, spleen, small intestine, appendix, and part of the large intestine

abdominal hernia (ab-dom'-i-nul hur'-nee-uh): abnormal protrusion of an organ, or part of an organ, through the abdominal wall

abdominopelvic cavity (ab-do'-man-o pel'-vic ka'-vih-tee): area below diaphragm, with no separation between the abdomen and pelvis

abduction (ab-duck'-shun): movement away from midline or axis of the body

abortion (a-bor'-shun): expulsion of a pregnancy

abrasion (a-bray'-shun): damage to the uppermost layer of the skin

abruptio placentae (ab-rup'-tee-oh pla-sin-tay): premature placental detachment from the uterine wall

absence seizure (ab'-since see'-zure): loss of consciousness without loss of muscle tone

abscess (ab'-sess): pus-filled cavity

absolute zero (ab'-suh-lewt zee'-row): complete absence of heat, or about –273.2° C (–459.8° F)

absorption (ub-sorp'-shun): passing of a substance into body fluids and tissues

acetabulum (as"-e-tab'-you-lum): cup-shaped cavity in the innominate bone receiving the head of the femur

acetylcholine (as'-e-til-ko-len): chemical released when a nerve impulse is transmitted; a neurotransmitter

Achilles tendon (ack-i'-leez ten'-dun): cord at the rear of the heel

acid (as'-id): chemical compound that ionizes to form hydrogen ions (H^+) in aqueous solution

acid load (as'-id lode): condition in which the body has too much organic acid in the blood

acidosis (as"-i-do'-sis): disturbance in the acid-base balance from excess acid, or excessive loss of bicarbonate; depletion of alkaline reserve

acne vulgaris (ak'-ne vul-gayr'-us): common and chronic disorder of the sebaceous gland

acquired immunity (a-kwir'-ed im-yu'-net-e): immunity as a result of exposure to a disease

acquired immunodeficiency syndrome (a-kwir'-ed im-yu'-no-de-fish'-en-ce sin'-drom): *see* AIDS

acromegaly (ak'-ro-meg"-a-le): excess of growth hormone in adults; overdevelopment of bones of hand, face, or feet

action potential (ak'-shan po-ten'-shal): stimulation of a neuron that causes ions to move across the cell membrane, briefly changing the charge of the cell

active acquired immunity (ack'-tiv a-kwir'-ed im-yu'-net-e): two types—natural and artificial acquired immunity

active transport (ack'-tiv tranz'-port): process by which solute molecules are transported across a membrane against a concentration gradient, from an area of low concentration to one of high concentration

acute coronary syndrome (ACD) (ah-kut' kor'-i-nair-ee sin'-drome): group of symptoms indicating myocardial muscle damage that results from coronary artery disease

acute kidney failure (ah-kut' kid'-nee fayl'-ur): disorder of the urinary system caused by inflammation of the nephron, shock, injury, bleeding, sudden heart failure, or poisoning

acute myocardial infarction (AMI) (ah-kut' migh"-o-kahr'-de-al in-fark-shun): disorder resulting from loss of blood flow to the myocardium

Addison's disease (Ad'-e-sen di-zeez'): hypofunction of adrenal gland

adduction (a-duck'-shun): movement of part of body or limb toward the midline of body; opposite of abduction

adenitis (ad'-n-i'-tis): inflammation of a lymph gland

adenoids (ad'-e-noydz): pair of glands composed of lymphoid tissue, found in nasopharynx; also called pharyngeal tonsils

adenosine triphosphate (ATP) (a-den'-o-seen try-fos'-fate): chemical compound consisting of one molecule of adenine, one of ribose, three of phosphoric acid

adhesion (add-he'-shun): growth of extra tissue; typically occurs after abdominal surgery

adipose (ad'-i-pose): fatty or fatlike

adipose tissue (ad'-i-pose tish'-ew): body fat

adrenal crisis (a-dre'-nal kry'-sis): sudden loss of hormones produced by the adrenal gland

adrenal gland (a-dre'-nal gland): endocrine gland that sits on top of kidney; consists of cortex and medulla

Adrenalin (epinephrine) (ah-drin'-ah-lin [ep'-i-neff'-rin]): hormone that stimulates the sympathetic portion of the autonomic nervous system

adrenergic receptors (alpha and beta) (a'-dre-nair"-jic re-sep'-terz): type of nerve receptors found in the sympathetic portion of the autonomic nervous system

adrenocorticotropic hormone (ACTH) (a-dren"-o-kor-tih-co-trah'-pik hor'-moan): hormone of the pituitary gland that stimulates the growth and secretion of adrenal cortex

afferent arteriole (af'-ur-unt ahr-teer'-ee-ole): takes blood from the renal artery to Bowman's capsule of the kidney

afferent nerve (af'-ur-unt nerv): a nerve that carries nerve impulses from the periphery to the central nervous system; also known as sensory nerve

agglutinin (a-gloo'-ti-nin): antibody found in normal or immune serum, causing antigen and cellular clumping

agglutinogen (a-gloo'-tin-o-jen): chemical substance (antigen) that stimulates the formation of a specific agglutinin

agonal respiration (ag'-ah-nal res'-pa-ray'-shun): slow, gasping breathing associated with near-death

agranulocyte (ay-gran'-yoo-lo-site): nongranular white blood cell; also known as agranular leukocyte

AIDS (aydz): acquired immunodeficiency syndrome; a disease that suppresses the natural immune system

albinism (al'-bi-nizm): partial or total absence of melanin pigment from eyes, hair, and skin

albumin (al-bew'-min): plasma protein, maintains osmotic pressure

albuminuria (al-bew'-mi-new'-ree-uh): excess of albumin protein in urine

aldosterone (al-dos'-ta-ron'): hormone secreted by the adrenal cortex; regulates salt and water balance in the kidney

alimentary canal (al"-i-men'-tuh-ree ka-nal'): entire digestive tube from mouth (ingestion) to anus (excretion)

alkali (al'-kuh-li'): substance that, when dissolved in water, ionizes into negatively charged hydroxide (OH) ions and positively charged ions of a metal

alkaline reserve (al'-ka-lyn re-serv'): amount of chemical buffers available in the blood

alkalosis (al"-kuh-lo'-sis): excessive alkali; disturbance in acid-base balance from excess loss of acid

allergen (al'-er-jen'): substance that causes an allergic reaction

alopecia (al'-e-pe'-she): loss of hair; baldness

alveoli (al-vee'-o-li): alveolar sacs; air cells found in the lung

Alzheimer's disease (alts'-hi'-merz di-zeez'): progressive and irreversible neurological disease with degeneration of nerve endings in the cortex of the brain

American Sign Language (ah-mer'-i-kan sine lane'-guag): method of communication using standard hand gestures

amblyopia (am'-ble-o'-pe-a): dimness of vision

amenorrhea (a-men"-o-ree'-uh): absence of menstruation

amino acid (a-me'-no as'-id): small molecular units that make up protein molecules

amniocentesis (am'ne-osen-te'-sis): withdrawal of amniotic fluid for testing

amphiarthrosis (am-phi-är-thro'-sis): partially moveable joint (e.g., symphysis pubis)

ampulla of Vater (am-pul'-uh of vah-ter): a junction or common passageway formed from the common bile duct of the liver and the pancreatic duct; helps to empty bile into the duodenum

amylase (am'-e-layz): enzyme that converts starch or glycogen to glucose

amylopsin (am'-e-lop'-sin): pancreatic amylase

anabolism (anab'-o-lizm): building up of complex materials in metabolism

analgesic (an'-el-je'-zik): drug that reduces pain

anal sphincter (ay'-nul sfink'-tur): muscles surrounding anal opening

anaphylactic shock (an'-a-fa-lac"-tic shok): or anaphylaxis; severe and sometimes fatal allergic reaction

anaphylaxis (an'-a-fa-lax"-is): *see* anaphylactic shock

anastomose (an-as'-tah-moz): natural or surgical connection of two blood vessels

anatomical position (an-a-tom'-i-kel pa-zi'-shun): body standing erect, face forward, arms at side and palms forward

anatomy (a-nat'-a-me): study of structure of an organism

androgen (an'-dro-jen): male hormones

anemia (uh-nee'-mee-uh): blood disorder characterized by reduction in red blood cells or hemoglobin

aneurysm (an'-you-rism): widening, or sac, formed by dilation of a blood vessel

angina pectoris (anji'-nuh peck'-to-ris): severe chest pain caused by lack of blood supply to heart

angioplasty (an'-je-o-plas-te): balloon surgery to open blocked blood vessels

angiotensin (an'-je-o-ten"-sin): blood vessel constrictor that increases blood pressure and stimulates aldosterone production

anisocoria (an'-e-so-core-e-a): unequal pupils; may be naturally occurring

ankylosis (ank"-i-lo'-sis): abnormal immobility and consolidation of a joint

anorexia (an"-o-rek'-see-uh): loss of appetite

anorexia nervosa (an"-o-rek'-see-uh nur-vo'-suh): illness in which a person refuses to eat

antagonist (an-tag'-a-nist): muscle whose action opposes the action of another muscle

anterior (an-teer'-ee-ur): front or ventral

anterior nares (an-teer'-ee-ur nair'-ays): nostrils

anterior chamber (an-teer'-ee-ur chame'-bur): space between the cornea and iris

anterior pituitary lobe (an-teer'-ee-ur pih-tu'-ih-ta-ree lowb): part of the pituitary gland that secretes hormones

anterior wall (an-teer'-ee-ur wahl): front portion of the left ventricle

antibody (an'-tih-bod"-ee): substance produced by the body that inactivates a specific foreign substance that has entered the body

anticoagulant (an'-tih-ko-ag"-yoo-lunt): chemical substance that prevents or slows blood clotting (e.g., heparin)

anticonvulsant (an"-tih-kun-vul'-sunt): therapeutic agent that stops or prevents convulsions

antidiuretic hormone (an"-tih-dye-yoo-ret'-ik hor'-moan): hormone secreted by the posterior pituitary gland that prevents or suppresses urine excretion

antigen (an'-tih-jin): substance stimulating formation of antibodies against itself

antiprothrombin (an"-tih-pro-throm'-bin): chemical substance that directly or indirectly reduces or retards action of prothrombin (such as heparin)

antithromboplastin (an"-tih-throm-bo-plas'-tin): chemical substance inhibiting clot-accelerating effect of thromboplastins

anuria (a-noor'-e-a): absence of urine

anus (ay'-nus): outlet from rectum

anvil (an'-vil): middle ear bone, or ossicle, in a chain of three ossicles of the middle ear

aorta (ay-or'-tuh): largest artery in body, rising from left ventricle of the heart

aortic dissection (ay-or'-tik di-sek'-shun): tear or rupture of the aorta; often at the insertion of the ligamentum arteriosus during sudden deceleration

aortic-semilunar valve (ay-or'-tik-sem"-ee-loo-nur valv): made up of three half-moon–shaped cups, located between junction of aorta and left ventricle of heart

apex (ay'-peks): top of object; point or extremity of a cone

apex of the lung (ay'-pecks of the lung): upper extremity of lung, behind border of the first rib

aphasia (a-fay'-zhuh): loss of ability to speak; may be accompanied by loss of verbal comprehension

aplastic anemia (a-plas'-tik uh-nee'-mee-uh): anemia caused by a suppression of the bone marrow

apnea (ap'-nee-uh): temporary stoppage of breathing movements

aponeurosis (ap"-o-new-ro'-sis): flattened sheet of white, fibrous connective tissue; serves as attachment for flat muscles or as sheet enclosing/binding muscle groups

appendicitis (a-pen"-di-si'-tis): inflammation of the appendix

appendicular skeleton (ap"-en-dik'-yoo-lur skel'-uh-tun): part of skeleton consisting of pectoral and pelvic girdles and limbs

aqueous humor (a'-kwe-as hyoo'-mar): watery fluid found in anterior chamber of the eye

arachnoid (mater) (uh-rak'-noyd [may'-tur]): weblike middle membrane of meninges

areola (a-ree-o'-luh): pigmented ring around nipple; any small space in tissue

arrector pili muscle (ar-rek'-tor pi'-lee mus'-ul): smooth muscle attached to the side of each hair follicle

arrhythmia (a-rith'-mee-uh): absence of a normal rhythm in heartbeat

arteriole (ahr-teer'-ee-ole): small branch of artery

arteriosclerosis (ahr-teer"-ee-o-skleh-ro'-sis): hardening of arteries, resulting in thickening of walls and loss of elasticity

artery (ar'-ter-ee): blood vessel that carries blood away from heart

arthritis (ahr-thry'-tis): inflammation of a joint

articular cartilage (ar-tik'-ye-lar kar'-ta-lij): thin layer of cartilage over the ends of long bones

artificial acquired immunity (ar'-ta-fish'-el a-kwir-ed im-yu-net-e): immunity from injection of vaccine, antigen, or toxoid

artificial insemination (ar'-ta-fish'-el in-sem'-a-na'-shun): procedure in which semen is placed in vagina by means of cannula or syringe

ascending colon (ah-send'-ing ko'-luhn): portion of the colon located along the right side of the abdominal cavity

ascending tract (ah-send'-ing trakt): portion of the spinal cord that carries sensations from the extremities to the brain

ascites (a-si'-teez): accumulation of fluid in the peritoneal cavity

asphyxia (as-fik'-see-ah): lack of oxygen intake; often the result of a complete blockage of the airway

aspiration (as'-pur-ay"-shun): breathing in foreign bodies such as liquid or vomitus into the lungs

assimilation (a-sim"-i-lay'-shun): process of changing food into a form suitable for absorption by the circulatory system

associative neuron (a-so'-she-a'-tiv noor'-on): carries messages from sensory neuron to motor neuron

asthma (az'-ma): airways obstructed because of inflammatory reaction to a stimulus

astigmatism (a-stig'-ma-tiz'-em): irregular curvature of cornea or lens

ataxia (ah-tak'-see-uh): muscle incoordination, particularly of muscle groups involved in walking or reaching for objects

atelectasis (a-te-lec'-ta-sis): lungs fail to expand normally

atherosclerosis (ath"-er-o-scle-ro'-sis): gradual deposit of fats along an arterial wall that eventually block blood flow

athlete's foot (ath'-leets foot): fungal infection of the foot

atlas (at'-lus): first cervical vertebra; articulates with axis and occipital skull bone

atom (at-om): smallest piece of an element

atrial fibrillation (ay'-tree-ul fib"-ri-lay'-shun): cardiac arrhythmia, characterized by rapid, irregular atrial impulses and ineffective atrial contractions

atrial kick (ay'-tree-ul kik): contraction of the atria that augments cardiac output

atrial-septal defect (ay'-tree-ul-sep-tal de'-fekt): disorder in which there is a hole between the right and left portions of the heart

atrioventricular (AV) node (ay"-tree-o-ven-trik'-yoo-lur nod): or bundle; small mass of interwoven conducting tissue in the heart, where the upper portion of the heart's electrical system communicates with the lower portion of the heart's electrical system

atrioventricular valves (ay"-tree-o-ven-trik'-yoo-lur valvz): tricuspid and mitral (bicuspid) valves of heart

atrium (ay'-tree-um): upper chamber of heart

atrophy (a'-truh-fee): wasting away of tissue

aura (aw'-rah): sensation that occurs before a convulsion

auricle (aw'-ri-kul): (1) pinna, or ear flap of external ear; (2) atrium of the heart

auscultation (aw'-skul-tay"-shun): listening

autoimmune disorder (aw"-to-im-yune dis-or'-der): a condition in which a misdirected immune response from the body's immune system attacks normal cells

autoimmunity (aw"-to-im-yu'-net-e): action of antibodies against one's own body

autonomic (aw"-tuh-nom'-ik): independent; self-regulating

autonomic nervous system (aw"-tuh-nom'-ik nur'-vus sis'-tum): collection of nerves, ganglia, and plexuses through which visceral organs, heart, blood vessels, glands, and smooth (involuntary) muscles receive their innervation

autonomic sniff box (aw"-tuh-nom'-ik sniff boks): hollow space behind the thumb proximal to the radial pulse

autosome (aw'-to-sohm): non–sex-determining chromosome

axial muscle group (ack'see-ul mus'-ul groop): muscles of the head, face, neck, and trunk

axial skeleton (ack'see-ul skel'-e-tun): skeleton of head and trunk

axilla (ak-sil'-uh): armpit

axillary node (ak'-sil-ahr-e nod): lymph nodes under the arms

axis (ack'-sis): (1) imaginary line passing through center of the body; (2) second cervical vertebra

axon (acks'-on): nerve cell structure that carries impulses away from cell body to dendrites

avascular (a-vas'-ku-lar): without blood vessels

AV block (ay-vee blok): disturbance in conduction within the AV node of the heart

backward failure (bak'-word fail'-yur): condition in which the blood begins to back up from the heart; also called congestive heart failure

bactericidal (bak-teer"-i-sigh'-dul): bacterial destruction

ball-and-socket joint (bol and sok'-it joynt): diarthroses joint; allows the greatest freedom of movement

bag of waters (bag of wa'-terz): the membrane that encloses the infant and placenta within the uterus or womb

bag-valve-mask (BVM) device (bag-valv-mask di-vis'): equipment used to assist in providing respirations for a nonbreathing patient

barrier devices (bare'-ee-er di-vi'-sez): equipment that creates an impenetrable barrier against disease transmission

Bartholin's gland (Bar-thol'-inz gland): mucous glands at the opening of the vagina

base (bays): (1) lowest part of a body; (2) main ingredient of a substance; (3) chemical compound yielding hydroxyl ions (OH–) in an aqueous solution that reacts with acid to form a salt and water

basilar skull fracture (bays'-i-lar skull frak'-shure): break in the bones that makeup the floor of the cranium

basophil (bay'-suh-fil): leukocyte cell, substance, or tissue that shows an attraction for basic dyes

Bell's palsy (Belz pol'-zee): disorder that affects the facial nerve

belly (bel'-ee): central part of a muscle

benign (beh-nin'): nonmalignant

benign prostatic hypertrophy (BPH) (beh-nin' pro-sta'-tik hi'-per-tro-fee): enlarged prostate

bicarbonate ion (by-kahr'-buh-nate eye'-on): salt of carbonic acid characterized by ion HCO_3^-

biceps (bye'-seps): muscle on front part of upper arm

bicuspid (bye-kus'-pid): having two cusps

bicuspid (mitral) valve (bye-kus'-pid [my'-trul] valv): atrioventricular valve of the left side of the heart

bifurcation (bye"-fur-kay'-shun): division into two branches

bilateral symmetry (bye-lat'-ur-ul sim'-e-tree): relating to both sides of body

bile (biyl): substance produced by liver; emulsifies fat

bilirubin (bil"-ee-roo'-bin): one of two pigments that determines the color of bile; reddish in color

biochemistry (bye-o-kem'-is-tree): study of chemical reactions of living things

biology (bye-ol'-ah-jee): study of all forms of life

biopsy (bye'-op-see): excision of a piece of tissue from a living body for diagnostic study

bio-weapons (bye'-oh-wep'-ahns): terrorist weapon designed to spread lethal infectious microorganisms

bipedal (bye-ped'-ul): having two feet

black biology (blak bye-ol'-oh-gee): creation of new biological weapons by gene splicing

blood-brain barrier (blud brayn bar'-ee-ur): substance cannot penetrate the brain tissue

blood volume expander (blud vol'-yoom x-pan'-der): substance that remains in the blood for an extended period

blowout fracture (blo'-owt frak'-shure): break of the zygomatic bone that helps to house the eyeball

blown pupil (blown pew'-pil): extreme pupil dilation

B-lymphocyte (be-limf'-o-site): type of white blood cell synthesized in the bone marrow

body mass index (BMI) (bah'-de mass in'-dex): calculation to determine normal body weight using height and weight

boil (boyl): bacterial infection of the sebaceous gland

bolus (boh'-lus): rounded mass; food prepared by mouth for swallowing

bowel (bow'-ul): intestine

Bowman's capsule (boh-manz kap'-sel): double-walled capsule around the glomerulus of nephron

brachial (bray'-kee-al): pertaining to the upper arm

brachial artery (bray'-kee-al ar'-ter-ee): artery of the elbow, used to measure blood pressure

brachial pulse (bray'-kee-al puls): pulse point that can be felt under the humerus along the brachial artery

brachiocephalic artery (bray'-kee-o-se-fal'-ik ar'-ter-ee): artery rising from the right side of the aortic arch; it divides into right subclavian and right common carotid arteries

bradycardia (brad"-ee-cahr'-dee-uh): abnormally slow heartbeat, less than 60 beats per minute

brainstem (brayn'-stem): portion of the brain other than cerebral hemispheres and cerebellum

brain tumor (brayn too'-mer): abnormal growth cells within the brain

breast (brest): mammary gland in front of the chest; secretes milk after childbirth

breast cancer (brest kan'-ser): malignant growth of cells within the breast

breast tumor (brest too'-mer): abnormal growth of cells within the breast

Broca's area (bro'-cahz air'-ee-ah): inferior portion of the frontal lobe of the brain

bronchiectasis (bran"-kee-ek'-tah-sis): chronic dilation of the bronchial tubes

bronchitis (bran-kiy'-tis): inflammation of the bronchial tubes

bronchoscopy (bran-kas'-koh-pee): tubular, lighted instrument used to inspect the interior of the bronchial tubes

buccal (buk'-ul): pertaining to the cheek or mouth

buccal cavity (buk'-ul ka'-vih-tee): mouth cavity bounded by the inner surface of the cheek

buffer (buf'-er): compound that maintains the acid-base balance in a living organism

buffering (buf'-er-ing): means of neutralizing an acid or base to preserve neutrality

bulbourethral gland (bul"-bo-yoo-re'-thral gland): located on either side of urethra in male; adds alkaline substance to semen

bulimia (bul-ee'-mee-a): episodic binge eating

bundle (bun'-dal): pairs working as one unit

bunion (bun'-yun): swelling of bursa of foot

burn (burn): result of destruction of the skin by fire, boiling water, steam, sun, chemicals, or electricity; classified as follows: superficial (first degree)—only the epidermal layer is affected; partial thickness (second degree)—the epidermis and some dermis are affected; full thickness (third degree)—complete destruction of the epidermis, dermis, and subcutaneous layers

bursa (bur'-suh): small sac interposed between parts that move on one another

bursitis (bur-sigh'-tis): inflammation of a bursa

calcaneus (kal-kay'-nee-us): heel bone

calciferol (kal"-sif'ur-ol): vitamin D_2

calcify (kal'-si-fiy): to deposit mineral salts

calcitonin (kal-si-to'-nin): hormone secreted by thyroid gland that controls calcium ion concentration in body

calcium (Ca+) (kal'-si-um): most abundant electrolyte in the whole body; stored within the bones; essential for acid-base balance, nervous system function, blood pressure, and muscular activity

calculus (kal'-kew-lus): stonelike formation in any part of the body, usually composed of mineral salts

callus (kal'-us): area of hardened and thickened skin

calorie (kal'-or-ee): unit that measures the amount of energy

calyx (kay'-liks): or calyces; cup-shaped part of the renal pelvis

cancer (kan'-ser): malignant growth of cells

cancer of the larynx (kan'-ser of the lar-inx): malignant growth of cells within the throat

cancer of the lungs (kan'-ser of the lungs): condition caused by an oat cell that spreads rapidly

canine (kay'-nine): sharp teeth of mammals, between incisors and premolars

capillary (kap'-i-lair-ee): microscopic blood vessel that connects arterioles with venules

caput medusa (kap'-et me-du'-sa): distended abdominal veins that become visible under the skin as a result of liver disease, often secondary to alcoholism

carbohydrate (kar"-boh-high'-drayt): organic compound composed of carbon, hydrogen, and oxygen as sugar or starch

carboxyhemoglobin (kahr-bock"-see-hee'-moh-gloh-bin): compound of carbon monoxide and hemoglobin formed when carbon monoxide is present in blood

carcinoma (kahr"-si-noh'-muh): malignant tumor

cardiac (kahr'-dee-ak): relating to the heart

cardiac arrest (kahr'-dee-ak uh-rest'): syndrome resulting from failure of heart as a pump

cardiac arrhythmia (kahr'-dee-ak a-rith'-mee-uh): any change or abnormality in normal heart rhythm or beat

cardiac muscle (kahr'-dee-ak mus'-ul): muscle of the heart

cardiac sphincter (kahr'-dee-ak sfink'-tur): circular muscle fibers around the cardiac end of the esophagus

cardiac output (kahr'-dee-ak out'-put): amount of blood the heart can pump, calculated by multiplying stroke volume by heart rate

cardiopulmonary resuscitation (CPR) (kahr"-dee-oh-puhl'-mun-nair-ee ree-sus"-i-tay'-shun): prevention of asphyxial death by artificial respiration

cardiotonic (kar"-dee-oh-ton'-ic): drug to slow and strengthen the heart

caries (kair'-eez): decay of tooth or bone

carotid artery (kah-ro'-tid ar'-ter-ee): artery that supplies blood to the neck and head

carpal (kahr'-pul): bones of the wrist

carpal tunnel syndrome (kahr'-pul tuh'-nel sin'-drom): condition caused by repetitive wrist movements; characterized by swelling around the carpal tunnel, pain, muscle weakness, and tingling sensation in the hand

carpopedal spasm (kahr'-po-ped"-el spaz'-em): cramping of the hands and feet

cartilage (kar'-ta-lij): white, semi-opaque, nonvascular connective tissue

casein (kay'-see-in): protein obtained from milk

catabolism (ca-tab'-oh-lizm): breaking down and changing of complex materials with the release of energy; process in metabolism

catalyst (kat'-uh-list): chemical substance that alters a chemical process but does not enter into the process

cataract (kat'-uh-rakt): condition in which the eye lens becomes opaque

catheterization (kath"-e-ter-i-za'-shen): medical procedure in which a tube is placed through an orifice for drainage

caudal (kod'-el): indicates direction, near the tail end of the body

cauda equina (kod'-el e-kwi'-na): the tail-like appendage below the second lumbar vertebra consisting of nerve roots from the upper spinal cord

cautery (kaw'-ter-e): destroying tissue by heat, cold, chemicals or electricity, often to stop bleeding

cecum (see'-kum): pouch at the proximal end of the large intestine

cell (sel): basic unit of structure and function of all living things

cell membrane (sel mem'-brayn): structure that encloses the cell

cellular respiration (sel'-yu-lar res'-pa-ray"-shun): or oxidation; use of oxygen to release energy from the cell

central canal (sen'-tral ka-nal'): thin channel in the middle of the spinal cord that contains cerebrospinal fluid

central nervous system (sen'-tral ner'-vus sis'-tem): one division of the nervous system that consists of the brain and spinal cord

centrioles (sen'-tree-olz): two cylindrical organelles found near muscles in a tiny body called the centrosome; perpendicular to each other

centrosome (sen'-tro-sohm): tiny area near the nucleus of an animal cell; contains two cylindrical structures called centrioles

cerebellum (ser-eh-bel'-um): section of the brain located behind the pons and below the cerebrum, consisting of white matter on the inside and gray matter on the outside

cerebral aqueduct (ser-ee'-bral ak'-kweh-dukt): narrow tunnel connecting the third and fourth ventricles of the brain

cerebral cortex (ser-ee'-bral kor'-teks): gray matter covering upper and lower surfaces of the cerebrum

cerebral edema (ser-ee'-bral e-de'-ma): swelling of the brain tissue

cerebral hemorrhage (ser-ee'-bral hem'-ar-ij): bleeding from blood vessels in the brain

cerebral palsy (ser-ee'-bral pahl'-see): disturbance in voluntary muscular action resulting from brain damage; characterized by spastic paralysis of all four limbs

cerebrovascular accident (CVA) (ser'-ee-broh-vas'-cular ak'-su-dent): or stroke; sudden interruption of blood flow to the brain

cerebral ventricles (ser-ee'-bral ven'-tri-klz): four fluid-filled cavities within the brain

cerebrospinal fluid (ser-ee'-bro-spi"-nal flu'-id): substance that forms inside the four brain ventricles that protects the brain and the spinal cord

cerebrum (ser-ee'-brum): largest and highest part of the brain

cerumen (see-roo'-men): ear wax

cervical cancer (sur'-vi-kul kan'-ser): malignant growth of cells within the cervix

cervical vertebrae (sur'-vi-kul vur'-tuh-bray): first seven bones of the spinal column

cervix (sur'-viks): opening at the base of the uterus

chemistry (kem'-is-tree): study of structure of matter, composition of substances, their properties, and their chemical reactions

chemotaxis (kem"-o-tack'-sis): response of an organism or a cell to a chemical stimulus by either moving toward or away from the chemical stimulus

Cheyne-Stokes (chain-stoks): respiratory pattern that exhibits as a waxing and waning of depth and rate

chlamydia (klah-mihd'-ee-yah): sexually transmitted disease caused by *chlamydia trachomatis* bacterium

cholecystectomy (kol"-ah-sis-tek'-tuh-mee): removal of the gallbladder

cholecystitis (kol"-ah-sis-ti'-tis): inflammation of the gallbladder

cholecystokinin (kol"-ah-sis"-tih-kigh'-nen): hormone secreted by the duodenum and jejunum that stimulates pancreatic juice secretion

cholesterol (koh-les'-tur-ol): steroid normally synthesized in the liver and also ingested in egg yolks, animal fats, and tissues

cholinergic receptors (koh"-lin-er'-jik ree-sep'-turz): chemical messengers of the parasympathetic portion of the autonomic nervous system

chorionic villi sampling (koh"-ree-on'-ik vee'-lie samp'-el-ing): test done as early as 8 weeks into a pregnancy to help identify genetic disorders

choroid coat (koh'-royd cot): middle layer of the eye

choroid plexus (koh'-royd plek'-sus): network of blood vessels of the pia mater that helps to form cerebrospinal fluid

chromatin (kroh'-mah-ten): DNA and protein material in a loose and diffuse state; during mitosis, chromatin condenses to form the chromosomes

chromosomal mutation (kroh"-muh-soh"-mul mewtay'-shun): mutation that involves a change in the number of chromosomes in the organism's nucleus or a change in the structure of a whole chromosome

chromosome (kroh'-muh-sohm): nuclear material that determines hereditary characteristics

chronic obstructive pulmonary disease (COPD) (kron'-ik ub-struk'-tiv pul'-mun-ar-ee di-zeez'): chronic lung condition such as emphysema or bronchitis

chronic renal failure (kron'-ik re'-nal fayl'-ur): gradual loss of function of the nephrons

chyme (kime): food that has undergone gastric digestion

chymotrypsin (kigh"-mo-trip'-sen): enzyme that digests proteins or incompletely digested proteins, turning them into peptides, proteases, polypeptides, peptides, and finally into amino acids

cicatrix (sik'-a-triks): scar tissue

cilia (sil'-ee-uh): tiny lashlike processes of protoplasm

ciliary body (sil'-e-ar"-e bo'-dee): thick ring of smooth muscle that surrounds the lens of the eye; the iris attaches to the ciliary body

ciliary gland (sil'-e-ar"-e gland): a gland with ducts that open into the eyelashes

circumcision (sur"-kum-si'-shun): removal of the foreskin of the penis

circumduction (sur"-kum-duk'-shun): circular movement at a joint

cirrhosis (sa-ro'-sis): chronic, progressive inflammatory disease of the liver characterized by the formation of fibrous connective tissue

claudication (klo"-di-kay'-shun): pain in legs or buttocks when walking

clavicle (kla'-vi-kul): collarbone

clean wound (kleen woond): wound in which infection is not present

clitoris (kli-tor'-is): small structure located above the female urethra; has many nerve endings

clonic phase (klon'-ik fase): repetitive tightening and relaxing of the muscles of the body

clotting time (klot'-ing tym): time it takes for blood to clot

coagulation (ko-ag"-yu-lay'-shun): process of blood clotting

coagulation cascade (ko-ag"-yu-lay'-shun kas'-kade): the series of events that leads to blood clotting

coccyx (kok'-siks): tailbone

cochlea (kock'-lee-uh): spiral cavity of the internal ear containing the organ of Corti

cochlear duct (kock'-lee-ur dukt): endolymph-filled triangular canal containing the spiral organ of Corti

coenzyme (ko-ehn'-zim): nonprotein part of a specialized protein molecule

coitus (ko-oi'-tus): act of intercourse

colitis (ko-liy'-tis): inflammation of the colon

collagen (kol'-uh-jen): fibrous protein occurring in bone and cartilage

collecting tubule (ko-lek'-ting too'-byool): structure in nephron that collects urine from distal convoluted tubule

colon (ko'-luhn): known as the large intestine; about 5 feet in length and 2 inches in diameter; divided into ascending, transverse, descending, and sigmoid colon

colostomy (ko-los'-tah-mee): artificial opening from the colon onto the surface of the skin

colostrum (ko-los'-trum): mother's first milk, rich in antibodies

common bile duct (kah'-mun biyl dukt): formed by the union of the hepatic duct and cystic duct, which brings bile to the duodenum

common carotid artery (kah'-mun kah-ro'-tid ar'-ter-ee): principle blood supply to the brain and neck

comparative anatomy (kum-par'-ah-tiv a-nat'-a-me): study of similarities and differences of humans to other animals

compartment syndrome (kum-part'-ment sin'-drome): condition characterized by paresthesia, paralysis, and pulselessness as a result of compression of muscle tissues for an extended time

complete proteins (kum-pleet' pro'-teenz): proteins that contain all the essential amino acids; enable an animal to grow and carry on fundamental life activities

complex partial seizure (kom'-plecks par'-shel see'-zure): chaotic nervous activity involving an entire lobe of the brain

compound (kom'-pownd): elements combined together in definite proportion by weight to form a new substance

conduction defect (kon-duk'-shun de'-fekt): a defect in the electrical impulse system of the heart muscle

cones (konz): pigment in the retina responsible for colors and bright lights

congenital (kun-jen'-i-tul): present at birth

congestive heart failure (kon-jes'-tive hart fayl'-yer): condition in which the blood begins to back up from the heart into the lungs or venous circulation; also called backward failure

conjunctivitis (kon-junk"-tih-vi'-tis): inflammation of the membranes in front of the eye (pink eye)

connective tissue (ka-nek'-tiv tish'-yu): cells whose intercellular secretions (matrix) support and connect the organs and tissues of the body

constipation (kon"-stih-pa'-shun): difficulty in or lack of bowel movement over time

contractibility (kon-trak"-tih-bil'-ih-tee): ability of a muscle to reduce the distance between the parts of its contents or the space it surrounds

Cooley's anemia (koo'-leez uh-nee'-mee-uh): or Thalassemia minor; anemia caused by defect in hemoglobin formation

Core organs (kore or'-ganz): organs essential to sustain life: the heart, lungs, and brain

cornea (kor'-ne-ah): circular transparent area of the sclerotic coat; located in the front center of the eye

coronal plane (kor'-en-l playn): frontal plane at a right angle to the sagittal plane, divides the body into anterior and posterior

corona radiata (kor-oh'-nah ra-dee-ay'-tah): layer of epithelial cells around ova

coronary (kor'-o-nair"-ee): referring to the blood vessels of the heart

coronary artery bypass graft (CABG) (kor'-o-nair"-ee ar'-ter-ee biy'-pas graft): use of a surgically implanted vein to move blood around a block in an artery

coronary bypass (kor'-o-nair"-ee bye'-pas): shunt to go around an area of blockage in the coronary arteries, to provide blood supply to myocardium

coronary sinus (kor'-o-nair"-ee siy'-nus): pocket in posterior of right atrium into which the coronary vein empties

corpus (kor'-pus): body

corpus callosum (kor'-pus kal'-oh-sum): wide band of axonal fibers holding together two hemispheres of the cerebrum

corpus luteum (kor'-pus lut'-ee-um): yellow body formed from ruptured graafian follicle; produces progesterone

cortex (kor'-teks): outer part of an internal organ

costal (kos'-tul): pertaining to the ribs

coughing (kof'-ing): deep breath followed by forceful exhalation from the mouth

cranial (kray'-nee-al): refers to the brain or direction toward the head of the body

cranial cavity (kray'-nee-al ka'-vih-tee): portion of the dorsal cavity housing the brain

cranial nerves (kray'-nee-al nervz): twelve pairs of nerves in the peripheral nervous system that begin in different areas of the brain

cranium (kray'-nee-um): flat bones that make up the skull

cretinism (kree'-tin-izm): congenital and chronic condition resulting from the lack of thyroid hormone

cricoid cartilage (kri'-koid kar'-ta-lij): O-shaped ring of cartilage located inferior to the larynx

cricoid pressure (kri'-koid preh'-shur): manual pressure on the cricoid cartilage to occlude the trachea

cricothyrotomy (kri"-ko-thi-rot'-e-me): a surgical division of the cricoid and thyroid cartilage for the purpose of creating an airway

crown (krown): pertains to part of tooth that is visible

cryptorchidism (krip-tor-kih'-dizm): failure of testes to descend into the scrotal sac

Cushing's syndrome (koosh'-ings sin'-drome): disorder of hyperfunction of adrenal cortex

Cushing's triad (koosh'-ings try'-ad): symptoms of irregular breathing, bradycardia, and profound hypertension that are indicative of increased intracranial pressure

cutaneous (kew-tay'-nee-us): pertaining to the skin

cyanotic (si"-uh-noh'-tic): a bluish-gray tint of skin resulting from insufficient blood oxygen

cystic duct (sis'-tik dukt): duct from gallbladder to common bile duct

cystic fibrosis (sis'-tik fi-bro'-sis): disease of the exocrine gland causing chronic bronchitis and pneumonia

cystitis (sis-ti'-tis): inflammation of the mucous membrane of the urinary bladder

cytology (siy-tol'-uh-jee): study of cells

cytoplasm (sigh'-toh-plazm): protoplasm of the cell body, excluding the nucleus

cytoskeleton (si"-to-skel'-ah-tin): internal framework of the cell; made up of microtubule, intermediate filaments, and microfilaments

dead space (ded spase): space from the opening of the mouth to the bronchioles in which no gas exchange takes place

deciduous teeth (de-sid'-yoo-us teeth): temporary teeth, usually lost by 6 years of age

decompensated shock (de-kom"-pen-sa'-ted shok): failure of organs caused by shock and hypoperfusion

deep (deep): injury involving damage to an internal organ such as a stomach

deep vein thrombosis (DVT) (deep vayn throm-boh'-sis): blood clot typically originating in the lower legs

defecation (def"-eh-kay'-shun): elimination of waste material from the rectum

defibrillator (de-fib'-rul-ay-tor): electrical device used to discharge an electrical current to shock the pacemaker of the heart back to a normal rhythm

defibrillation (de-fib"-ri-la'-shun): application of an electrical charge across the heart to return the heart to asystole (flatline) so that natural pacemakers may resume activity

deglutition (dee"-gloo-ti'-shun): the act of swallowing

dehydration (de"-hi-dra'-shun): excessive fluid loss

delirium (de-leer'-e-um): state of mental confusion associated with excitement or frenzy

deltoid (del'-toyd): triangular-shaped muscle that covers the shoulder prominence; used for intramuscular injections in adults dementia (de-men'-shah): loss in at least two areas of complex behavior, such as language, memory, or visual and spatial abilities

dendrite (den'-drite): nerve cell process that carries nervous impulses toward the cell body

dental caries (den'-tal car'-ees): cavities

dentin (den'-tin): main part of the tooth located under the enamel

dentition (den-tish'-un): number, shape, and arrangement of teeth

deoxygenate (dee-ock'-si-jen-ate): process of removing oxygen from a compound

deoxyribonucleic acid (DNA) (dee-ok"-see-ri-boh-nu-klay'-ik as'-id): nucleic acid containing the elements of carbon, hydrogen, oxygen, nitrogen, and phosphorous; genetic material

deoxyribose sugar (dee-ock-see-ri'-bos shuh'-gar): sugar that has one less oxygen atom than the ribose sugar

dermatitis (dur"-muh-tiy'-tus): inflammation of the skin

dermatology (dur"-mah-tol'-ah-jee): study of the physiology and pathology of the skin

dermis (dur'-mis): true skin; lying immediately beneath the epidermis

descending colon (de-send'-ing ko'-luhn): portion of the colon that is located on the left side of the abdominal cavity

descending tract (de-send'-ing trakt): portion of the spinal cord that carries nerve impulses from the brain to the extremities

detached retina (de-tachd' reh'-tih-nah): vitreous fluid of the eye; contracts as it ages and pulls on the retina, causing a tear

developmental anatomy (de-vel-op-men'-tul a-nat'-a-me): studies the growth and development of an organism during its lifetime

deviated nasal septum (de'-ve-a-ted na'-sl sep'-tum): condition in which there is a bend in the cartilage structure of the septum

dextrose (deks'-trose): glucose, monosaccharide

5% dextrose in sterile water (D₅W) (five per'-sent deks'-trose in ster'-el wa'-ter): hypotonic solution used to combat dehydration

diabetes insipidus (dye'-a-be'-tees in-sip'-ah-dus): decrease of ADH of pituitary causing excessive loss of water

diabetes mellitus (dye"-a-be'-tees ma-liy'-tus): pancreas is unable to produce insulin or is unable to produce enough insulin for the cells to use glucose

dialysis (dye-al'-i-sis): separation of smaller molecules from larger molecules in a solution by selective diffusion through a semipermeable membrane

dialyzer (dye'-al-i-zer): device to perform dialysis; a kidney machine

diapedesis (dye"-ih-peh'-dee'-sis): passage of cells through unruptured vessel wall into tissues

diaphragm (dye'-uh-fram): muscular partition between the thorax and the abdomen

diaphysis (dye-af'-i-sis): shaft of long bone

diarrhea (dye"-ah-ree'-uh): excessive elimination of watery feces

diarthroses (dye-ar-throh'-ses): moveable joints (e.g., elbow, knee)

diastole (dye-as'-tuh-lee): resting period of the heart

diastolic pressure (dye-as-stol'-ik preh'-shur): lessened force of the blood, measured when the ventricles are relaxed

diencephalon (dye"-en-sef'-ah-lon): posterior part of the brain; contains the thalamus, hypothalamus, and pituitary gland

diffusion (dif-yu'-szen): molecules move from higher concentration to lower

digestion (dye-jes'-chun): complex process of the breaking down of food to be utilized by the body

dilation (dye-la'-shun): expansion of an orifice (opening)

dilator (dye'-la-tor): muscle that opens or closes an orifice

diphtheria (dip-theer'-i-uh): infectious disease of respiratory system; because of DPT vaccine it is uncommon today

diploë (dip'-lo-e): spongy tissue in between the two bones of the cranium

diplopia (di-ploh'-pee-uh): double vision

direct contact (dye'-rekt con'-takt): person-to-person exposure to an infectious disease

disaccharide (dye-sak'-a-ride): double sugar

dislocation (dis"-loh-kay'-shun): displacement of one or more bones of a joint or organ from original position

disseminated intravascular coagulation (DIC) (di-sem"-i-nat'-ed in"-tra-vas'-ku-lar ko-ag"-yu-lay'-shun): disorder in which the blood clots inappropriately in some places while failing to clot correctly in others

distal (dis'-tul): farthest from point of origin of a structure; opposite of proximal

distal convoluted tubule (dis'-tul kon"-vo-lu'-ted tu'-bul): the farthest portion of the ascending limb of the loop of Henle

diuretic (dye-yoo-re'-tik): drug that reduces the amount of fluid in the body

diverticulitis (dye-vur-tik"-yul-i-tis): numerous diverticula in the colon

dorsal (dor'-sul): pertaining to the back

dorsal cavity (dor'-sul ka'-vih-tee): posterior cavity of the body that houses the brain and spinal column

dorsalis pedis artery (dor-sal'-is pe'-dis ar'-ter-ee): pulse point on the anterior surface of the foot, below the ankle joint

Duchenne's muscular dystrophy (du-shenz' mus'-kew-ler dis'-tro-fee): disorder that weakens skeletal muscle, leading to fatal respiratory or heart failure ductus deferens (vas deferens) (duk'-tus def'-uh-renz [vas def'-uh-renz]): part of the excretory duct system of the testes that runs from the epididymis to the ejaculatory duct

duodenum (dew"-o-dee'-num): first part of small intestine, beginning at the pylorus

dura mater (dew'-ruh may'-tur): fibrous membrane forming the outermost covering of the brain and spinal cord

dwarfism (dworf'-izm): caused by hypofunction of growth hormone; growth of long bone is decreased

dysmenorrhea (dis-men"-o-ree'-uh): difficult or painful menstruation

dyspareunia (dis"-puh-roo'-nee-uh): difficult or painful sexual intercourse

dysphasia (dis-fa'-zya): impairment of speech and verbal comprehension

dyspnea (disp-nee'-uh): labored breathing or difficult breathing

dysrhythmia (dis-rith'-me-a): irregularity in heart rhythm

dysuria (dis-yoor'-ee-a): painful urination

eclampsia (e-klamp'-se-a): toxemia of pregnancy; literally, "poisoned pregnancy"

ectopic pregnancy (ek-top'-ik preg'-nan-se): pregnancy that develops outside of the uterus

eczema (ek'-se-mah): acute or chronic noncontagious inflammation of the skin

edema (e-de'-ma): excessive fluid in tissues

effacement (eh-fas'-ment): thinning of the cervical opening (os) in preparation for childbirth

effector (e-fek'-tor): muscle or organ that responds to a stimulus

efferent arteriole (ef'-er-ant ar-teer'-ee-ul): carries blood from glomerulus

efferent neuron (ef'-er-ant neur'-on) see motor nerve

ejaculatory ducts (e-jak'-yoo-luh-tor"-ee duktz): short and narrow ducts that begin where the ductus deferens and the seminal duct join

ejection fraction (e-jek'-shun): percentage of blood pumped out of the left ventricle in a single beat; portion of the total left ventricular volume

elastic (e-las'-tik): capable of returning to original form after being compressed or stretched

elasticity (e-las-tih'-sih-tee): ability of a muscle to return to its original length when relaxing

elastin (e-las'-tin): single elastic fibers

electrocardiogram (ECG) (e-lek"-tro-kar'-dee-u-gram): device used to measure the electric conduction system of the heart

electrolytes (e-lek'-tro-lights): electrically charged particles that help determine fluid and acid-base balance

electromyograph (e-lek"-troh-miy'-oh-graf): device used to measure electrical muscle activity

element (el'-e-ment): made up of like atoms; substance that can neither be created nor destroyed

embolism (em'-bo-lizm): obstruction of a blood vessel by a circulating blood clot, fat globule, air bubble, or piece of tissue

embolitic stroke (em'-bo-li-tic strok): blockage of a cerebral blood vessel by an embolus

embryo (em'-bree-oh): human young up to the first 3 months after conception; the young of any organism in early development stage

embryology (em-bree-ol'-u-jee): study of the formation of an organism from fertilized egg to birth

emesis (em'-eh-sis): vomitus

emphysema (em-fi-see'-muh): lung disorder in which inspired air becomes trapped and is difficult to expire

empyema (em-pye-ee'-muh): pus in a cavity

enamel (e-nam'-ul): hard calcium substance that covers the teeth

encephalitis (en-sef-u-liy'-tis): inflammation of the brain

endocarditis (en"-do-kahr-di'-tis): inflammation of the membrane that lines the heart and covers valves

endocardium (en"-do-kahr'-dee-um): membrane lining interior of heart

endocrine gland (en'-doh-krin gland): secretes directly into blood or tissue fluid instead of into a duct

endocrinology (en"-doh-krah-nol'-u-jee): study of physiology and pathology of hormonal system

endometrial cancer (en"-doh-mee'-tree-al kan'-ser): abnormal growth of cells of the lining of the uterus

endometriosis (en"-doh-mee-tree-o'-sis): presence of endometrium, which is normally confined to the uterine cavity, in other areas of the pelvic cavity

endometrium (en"-do-mee'-tree-um): mucous membrane lining uterus

endoplasmic reticulum (en-do-plaz'-mic re-tik'-u-lum): transport system of the cell

endosteum (en-dos'-tee-um): lining of the medullary cavity in the long bone

endothelium (en"-do-theel'-ee-um): epithelial cells lining the blood vessels, heart, and lymph vessels or any closed cavity in the body

endotracheal tube (ET) (en"-do-tra'-ke-al toob): plastic tube that is placed down the throat and into the lungs to help maintain a patent airway for breathing

energy (en'-er-jee): ability to do work

enteral (en-ter'-al): medication administration via the digestive route

enteritis (en-ter-i'-tis): inflammation of the small intestine

enzyme (en'-zime): organic catalyst that initiates and accelerates a chemical reaction

eosinophil (ee"-o-sin'-uh-fil): white blood cell whose granules stain red with eosin or other acid dyes

epidermis (ep"-i-dur'-mis): outermost layer of skin

epididymitis (ep″-i-did′-i-miy-tis): inflammation of epididymis

epididymis (ep″-i-did′-i-mis): portion of the seminal duct lying posterior to the testes; connected by the efferent ductulus of each testis

epidural space (ep″-i-doo′-ral spase): space between the dura mater and the skull that houses cerebral arteries

epigastric (ep-i-gas′-trik): upper region of the abdominal cavity, located just below the sternum

epilepsy (ep-ul-ep′-see): a recurrent paroxysmal disorder of cerebral function

epinephrine (ep″-i-nef′-rin): adrenaline; secretion of adrenal medulla that prepares the body for energetic action

epiphysis (ee-pif′-ah-sis): end of the long bone

episiotomy (e-peez-e-ot′-um-ee): surgical incision into the perineum

epistaxis (ep″-i-stak′-sis): nosebleed

epithelial cells (e-pi-thee′-lee-al selz): cover the body's external and internal surfaces

equilibrium (ee-kwuh-lib′-ree-um): state of balance

ergonomics (er-ga-nom′-iks): application of biology and engineering to the relationship between the worker and the environment; also called biotechnology

erythroblastosis fetalis (e-rith″-ra-blast-o′-sus fe-tal′-es): hemolytic disease of the newborn

erythrocyte (e-rith′-ro-sight): red blood cell

erythropoiesis (e-rith″-ro-poy-ee′-sis): formation or development of red blood cells

esophageal varices (e-sof″-e-je′-al var′-i-sez): distended veins inside the esophagus

esophagus (e-sof′-uh-gus): muscular tube; takes food from the pharynx (mouth) to the stomach

essential amino acids (e-sen′-chul a′-mee′-noh as′-idz): amino acids that are necessary for normal growth and development and are not made in the human body

estrogen (es′-tra-jen): secretion of the ovary; female hormone

ethmoid (eth′-moyd): bone of the cranium located between the eyes

eupnea (yoop′-nee-uh): normal or easy breathing with usual quiet inhalations and exhalations

eustachian tube (yoo-sta′-shen toob): passageway from throat to middle ear; equalizes pressure

excitability (ek-sih′-tah-bil′-eh-tee): ability to respond to stimuli

exocrine gland (ex′-o-krin gland): gland that secretes into a duct

exophthalmos (ek″-sof-thal′-mus): abnormal protrusion of the eyes

expiration (ek″-spir-ay′-shun): act of breathing forth or expelling air from lungs

expiratory reserve volume (ERV) (ek′-sper-ah-toh-re re-serv′ vol′-yoom): amount of air a person can exhale over and above the tidal volume

expressive aphasia (ek-spre′-siv a-fay′-zhuh): inability to speak as a result of the loss of neurological coordination of the muscles involved in speech

extensibility (ek-sten-sih-bil′-ih-tee): ability to be stretched

extension (ek-sten′-shun): act of increasing the angle between two bones

extensor (ek-sten′-sur): muscle that extends or stretches a limb or part

external (ek-ster′-nul): superficial; at or near the surface of the skin

external respiration (ek-ster′-nul res″-pa-ray″-shun): breathing; act of inspiration and expiration

extracellular fluid (ek-stra-sel′-u-lar floo′-id): fluid outside the cell

extrinsic muscles (ek-strin′-sik mus′-ulz): muscles responsible for moving the eye within the orbital socket

fallopian tube (fa-lo′-pee-un toob): uterine tube or oviduct that carries the egg from the ovary to the uterus

fascia (fay′-shuh): thin sheets of fibrous tissue that enclose muscles

fasciotomy (fash″-e-ot′-eh-me): surgical procedure used to reduce swelling in muscle tissue as a result of compartment syndrome

fasciculation (fa-sik″-u-la′-shun): muscle tremor

fat (fat): sometimes called triglyceride; organic compound composed of carbon, hydrogen, and oxygen; made of glycerol and fatty acids

feces (fee′-seez): waste material from the digestive system

femoral artery (fee-mor′-al ar′-ter-ee): artery located in the inguinal or groin area

femoral nerve (fee-mor′-al nerv): part of the lumbar plexus that stimulates the hip and leg

femur (fee′-mur): thighbone

fertilization (fur-til-ah-zay′-shun): process of the union of the egg and sperm

fetal circulation (fet′-ul ser-kyul-a′-shun): brings blood to the fetus

fetal heart tones (fet′-ul hart tonz): the sound of an infant's heartbeat while in the uterus (womb)

fetus (fee′-tus): human young from the third month of the intrauterine period until birth

fiber (fiy′-ber): compound found in plant foods

fibrillation (fib″-ri-lay′-shun): condition in which heart muscle fibers contract at random without coordination

fibrin (fi′-brin): insoluble protein necessary for the clotting of blood

fibrinogen (fi-brin′-o-jen): protein that is converted into fibrin by the action of thrombin

fibrinolytic (fi″-bri-no-lit′-ik): drug that activates enzymes to break up clots

fibroid (fye'-broyd): benign tumor of smooth muscle, especially in the uterus

fibromyalgia (fi-broh-mi-al'-gee-uh): chronic muscle pain

fibula (fib'-yoo-luh): slender bone at outer edge of the lower leg

filtration (fil-tray'-shun): movement of water and particles across a semipermeable membrane by a mechanical force such as blood pressure

fimbriae (fim'-bra-ah): fringelike folds bordering the ovary

fissures (fish'-urz): deep furrows and grooves on the brain's surface

fistula (fis'-choo-luh): abnormal duct from an abscess, cavity, or hollow organ to the body surface or to another hollow organ

flatfeet (flat'-feet): weakening of the leg muscles that support the arch of the foot

flatulence (flach'-uh-lenz): presence of excessive gas in the digestive tract

flexion (fleks'-ee-on): act of bending a limb or decreasing the angle between two bones

flexor (fleks'-or): muscle that bends a joint

follicle stage (fol'-i-kul stayj): first stage of the female menstrual cycle, during which follicle-stimulating hormone (FSH) secreted from the anterior lobe of the pituitary gland is circulated via the bloodstream; FSH reaches an ovary and stimulates several follicles; however, only one matures; as the one follicle grows in size, an egg cell begins to grow inside the follicle

follicle-stimulating hormone (FSH) (fol'-i-kul stim'-yoo-lay-ting hor'-moan): adenohypophyseal hormone that stimulates follicular growth in the ovary

fontanel (fon"-tuh-nel'): gap between the flat bones of an infant's skull; soft spot

foramen (fo-ray'-men): opening in a bone

foreskin (for'-skin): loose fitting skin around the end of the penis

fourth ventricle (forth ven'-tri-kl): cavity in the brain situated below the third ventricle, in front of the cerebellum, and behind the pons and the medulla oblongata

fovea centralis (fo'-ve-ah cen-tral'-is): disc in the eye containing the cones for color vision

fracture (frak'-shure): break in a bone

friable (fri'-a-bel): easily torn tissue

frontal (frunt'-el): pertaining to the forehead

frontal lobe (frunt'-el lowb): area of the brain in the cerebral cortex that controls motor function

full (third-degree) burn (ful [thurd-di'-gree] burn): *see* burn

functional residual capacity (funk'-shun-al re-zid'-u-ahl kah-pa'-sih-te): sum of the expiratory reserve volume plus the residual volume

functional syncytium (funk'-shun-al sin-sish'-e-um): collection of muscles that beat as one unit creating a specific effect

fundus (fun'-dus): part farthest from the opening of an organ

gallstones (gol'-stonz): collection of crystallized cholesterol combined with bile salts and bile pigments

gamete (gah'-met): germ cell; specialized sex cell

gamma globulin (gam'-uh glob'-ye-lin): fractionated part of globulin used to treat infectious diseases

ganglion (gang'-glee-un): mass of nerve cell bodies outside the central nervous system

gangrene (gang-green'): death of body tissue resulting from insufficient blood supply

gastric (gas'-trik): pertaining to the stomach

gastric distention (gas'-trik dis-ten'-shun): excessive air in the stomach

gastric glands (gas'-trik glands): glands lining stomach

gastric tube (gas'-trik toob): a flexible pipe inserted into the stomach to remove gastric contents

gastritis (gas-tri'-tis): inflammation of the stomach

gastrocnemius (gas-trok-nem'-ee-us): calf muscle

gastroenteritis (gas-troh-en"-tur-i'-tis): inflammation of stomach and small intestines

gastroesophageal reflux disease (GERD) (gas-tro-ee-sof'-u-jeel re'-fluks di-zeez'): condition in which stomach contents flow back into the esophagus (e.g., heartburn)

gene (jene): part of the chromosome that transmits a specific hereditary trait

gene mutation (jene mew-tay'-shun): new or altered gene produced to replace a normal preexisting gene

generalized seizure (jen'-ral-izd see'-zure): chaotic disorder of the entire brain's function

genetic disorder (je-net'-ik dis-or'-der): hereditary disorder caused by variation in a genetic pattern

genetics (je-net'-iks): branch of biology that studies the science of heredity and the differences and similarities between parents and offspring

genitals (jen-i-tuls): reproductive organs; also called genitalia

genital herpes (jen'-i-tul hur'-peez): sexually transmitted recurrent disease caused by a virus

genital warts (jen'-i-tul wortz): human papillomavirus; sexually transmitted disease

gestation (jes-tay'-shun): development period of the human young from conception to birth

gigantism (ji-gan'-tizm): hypersecretion of the growth hormone; overgrowth of long bones

gingiva (jin'-jeh-vae): gums

glans penis (glanz pe'-nis): head or tip of the penis

glaucoma (gloh-koh'-muh): increase in interocular eye pressure

glenoid fossa (glee'-noyd fos'-uh): articular surface on scapula for articulation with head of humerus

gliding joint (glid'-ing joynt): nearly flat surfaces of the bone glide across each other, such as is seen in the vertebrae

globin (glo'-bin): protein molecule of hemoglobin

globulin (glob'-yeh-len): plasma protein made in liver; helps in synthesis of antibodies

glomerulonephritis (gla-mer-yul-o-ne-fri'-tis): inflammation of the glomerulus of the kidney

glomerular filtration rate (GFR) (glo-mer'-u-lar fil-tra'-shun rayt): the rate at which the kidneys filter blood as a result of pressures

glomerulus (gla-mer'-yah-lus): part of the nephron; tuft of capillaries situated within Bowman's capsule

glottis (glot'-is): space within the vocal cords of the larynx

glucagon (gloo'-kah-jen): hormone used to increase the level of glucose in the bloodstream

glucocorticoids (G-Cs) (gloo-koh-kor'-ti-koydz): hormones of the adrenal cortex, namely cortisone and cortisol

glucose (gloo'-kos): monosaccharide or simple sugar; the principal blood sugar

gluteal (gloo'-tee-ul): pertaining to the area near the buttocks

glycerin or **glycerol** (glis'-ur-in or glis'-ur-ole): product of fat digestion

glycogen (glye'-kuh-jin): polysaccharide formed and stored largely in the liver

glycosuria (gli"-ko-su'-re-a): large amounts of glucose in the urine

goit (goyt): hypothyroidism

goiter (goy'-ter): enlargement of the thyroid gland

Golgi apparatus (gol'-jee ap-ah-ra'-tus): membranous network that looks like a stack of pancakes; stores and packages secretions to be secreted by the cell

gonads (goh'-nads): sex glands (ovaries or testes)

gonorrhea (gon-eh-ree'-uh): an infectious disease of the genitourinary tract caused by *Neisseria gonorrhoeae*; transmitted mainly by sexual contact

gout (gowt): increase in uric acid crystals in bloodstream, which are deposited in joint cavities, especially the great toe

graafian follicle (graf'-ee-an fol'-e-kel): follicle in the ovary that stores the immature ovum

graft (graft): to transplant tissue into a body part to replace damaged tissue

granulation (gran"-yoo-lay'-shun): tiny red granules that are visible in the base of a healing wound; consists of newly formed capillaries and fibroblasts

granulocyte (gran'-ye-loh-site): granular white blood cell

greater omentum (grat'-er o-men'-tum): double fold of peritoneum that hangs down over the abdominal organs like an apron

greenstick fracture (green'-stik frak'-shure): incomplete fracture of long bone; seen in children; bone is bent but splintered only on convex side

gross anatomy (gros a-nat'-a-me): study of large and easily observable structures of an organism

growth hormone (GH) (growth hor'-moan): or somatotropin; hormone of the pituitary gland responsible for growth and development

growth plate (growth playt): area of bone from which growth of the extremity takes place

gyri (ji'-ree): convolutions in the brain

hair follicle (hayr fol'-i-kul): in the pocketing of the epidermis that holds the hair root

halitosis (hal"-i-to'-sis): bad breath

hammer (malleus) (ham'-er [mal'-e-us]): conductive bone within the ear, essential to hearing

Hangman's fracture (hang'-manz frak'-shure): fracture of the second cervical vertebra

hard of hearing (HOH) (hard of hir'-ing): loss of hearing caused by either acoustic nerve impairment or conductive bone damage

hearing aids (hir'-ing aydz): electro-mechanical device that increases the volume or quality of sound to aid the ear in hearing

heart block (hart blok): interruption of the SA node message to the AV node; lack of coordination between the atria and the ventricles

heartburn (hart'-burn): acid indigestion; results from a backflow of the highly acidic gastric juice into the lower end of the esophagus

heart failure (hart fayl'-yur): condition in which heart ventricles do not contract effectively

hematocrit (hee-mat'-o-krit): amount of red blood cells in a volume of blood

hematoma (hee"-muh-toh'-muh): localized clotted mass of blood formed in an organ, tissue, or space

hematuria (heem-ah-toor'-ee-ah): blood in the urine

heme (heem): iron compound part of the hemoglobin

hemiplegia (hem"-i-plee'-jee-uh): paralysis of one side of the body

Hemoccult (heem'-o-kult): hidden blood

hemodialysis (heem"-oh-di-al'-i-sis): procedure for removing waste products in the circulating blood of patients with kidney failure

hemoglobin (heem'-uh-gloh-bin): oxygen-carrying pigment of the blood

hemolysis (heem-ol'-ah-sis): bursting of red blood cells

hemolytic reaction (heem-ol'-ah-tic re-ak'-shun): destruction of transfused blood by antibodies in the recipient's blood

hemophilia (heem"-oh-fil'-ee-uh): sex-linked, hereditary bleeding disorder occurring only in males but transmitted by females; characterized by a prolonged clotting time and abnormal bleeding

hemorrhage (hem'-ar-ij): bleeding

hemorrhagic stroke (hem'-ar-ij-ik strok): rupture of an artery that results in loss of function in the brain

hemorrhoids (hem'-uh-roydz): enlarged and varicose condition of the veins in the lower part of the anus or rectum and the tissues of the anus

heparin (hep'-uh-rin): substance obtained from the liver that slows blood clotting

hepatic duct (he-pat'-ik dukt): structure from the liver to the common bile duct; carries bile

hepatic-jugular reflex (HJR) (he-pat'-ik-jug'-u-lur ree'-fleks): pressure on the abdomen sends a wave up into the jugular vein as a result of the backup of blood flow into the liver from the heart

hepatic vein (he-pat'-ik vayn): vein that drains blood from liver into inferior vena cava

hepatitis (hep-ah-tit'-is): inflammation of the liver

hepatomegaly (hep"-ah-toh-meg'-ah-lee): enlargement of the liver

hereditary (he-red'-i-tayr-ee): of or pertaining to inheritance; inborn; inherited

Hering-Brewer reflex (heh'-ring brew'-er ree'-fleks): reflex that prevents overstretching of the lungs

hernia (hur'-nee-uh): protrusion of a loop of an organ through an abnormal opening

herpes (hur'-peez): contagious viral infection in which small blisters appear

hiatal hernia (hi-ay'-tal hur'-nee-uh): hernia that occurs when the stomach pushes through the diaphragm

high-density lipoprotein (HDL) (high-den'-si-tee li'-poh-proh-teen) removes excess cholesterol from walls of the artery

hilum (high'-lem): indentation along the medial border of the kidney hinge joint; joint movement in one direction, such as the elbow

hinge joint (hihnj joynt): type of diarthroses joint that moves in one direction or plane, as in knees, elbows, and outer joints of the fingers

histamine (his'-tah-meen): powerful stimulant of acid secretion

histology (his-tol'-uh-jee): microscopic study of living tissues

HIV (h-i-v): human immunodeficiency virus; virus that causes AIDS

Hodgkin's disease (Hoj'-kinz di-zeez'): specific type of cancer of the lymph nodes

homeostasis (ho-me-oh-stay'-ses): state of balance

hormone (hor'-moan): chemical secretion, usually from an endocrine gland

human chorionic gonadotropin (hyu'-man kor"-e-on'-ik go'-na-do-tro'-pin): stimulating hormone produced in the placenta that causes the ovary to produce progestrone

human immunodeficiency virus (hyu'-man im"-u-no-de-fish'-en-se vi'-rus): *see* HIV

humerus (hu'-mer-us): only bone in the upper arm; second largest bone in the body

Huntington's disease (hunt'-ing-tunz di-zeez'): genetic disorder characterized by degeneration of the central nervous system

hyaline (hi'-a-line): type of cartilage that forms the skeleton of the embryo

hydrocephalus (hi-dro-sef'-a-lus): increase in the volume of cerebral spinal fluid within the cerebral ventricles; may occur in fetal development

hydronephrosis (high-droh-nef-roh'-sis): condition in which renal pelvis and calyces become distended as a result of the accumulation of fluid

hydroxide (high-drok'-syd): negatively charged (OH−) ion

hymen (high'-men): membrane at the opening of the vagina

hyoid bone (high'-oyd bone): bone between root of the tongue and larynx, supporting tongue and giving attachment to several muscles

hyperbilirubinemia (hi"-per-bil"-i-roo"-bi-ne'-me-a): excess accumulation of bilirubin

hypercalcemia (hi"-per-kal-se'-me-a): elevated calcium levels

hyperglycemia (hi"-per-gli-see'-me-a): high concentration of glucose in the blood

hyperglycemic (hi"-per-gli-seem'-ic): exhibiting an increase in blood sugar

hyperkalemia (hi"-per-ka-le'-me-a): elevated levels of potassium in the blood

hypermagnesemia (hi"-per-mag"-ne-se'-me-a): elevated levels of magnesium in the blood

hypernatremia (hi"-per-na-tre'-me-a): excessive levels of sodium in the blood

hyperpnea (high-pur'-nee-uh): increase in the depth and rate of breathing accompanied by abnormal exaggeration of respiratory movements

hyperopia (high"-pur-oh'-pee-uh): farsightedness

hypersensitivity (high-per-sen-sah-tiv'-i-tee): abnormal response to a drug or allergen

hypertension (high-pur-ten'-shun): abnormally high blood pressure

hyperthyroidism (high-per-thi'-royd-izm): condition caused by overactivity of the thyroid gland

hypertrophy (high-per'-tra-fee): exercise-induced enlargement of muscle

hyperventilation (high-per-ven-til-ay'-shun): rapid breathing, rapid loss of carbon dioxide; sometimes causes dizziness or fainting

hypocalcemia (hi"-po-kal-se'-me-a): low levels of calcium

hypogastric region (high-poh-gas'-trik re'-jun): lower region of the abdominal area

hypoglycemia (hi"-po-gliy-se'-me-a): low concentration of glucose in the blood

hypokalemia (hi″-po-ka-le′-me-a): condition resulting from very low levels of potassium in the body

hypomagnesemia (hi″-po-mag″-ne-se′-me-a): low magnesium levels in the blood

hyponatremia (hi″-po-na-tre′-me-a): loss of sodium from the blood

hypoperfusion (hi″-po-pur-fu′-shun): decrease in circulation of blood to cells and organs of the body

hypopharynx (hi″-po-far′-inks): area at the back of the throat bordered by the soft palate

hypotension (high″-pho-ten′-shun): reduced or abnormally low blood pressure

hypothalamus (high″-poh-thal′-a-mus): part of the diencephalon, lies below the thalamus

hypothyroidism (high-po-thi′-royd-izm): condition in which the thyroid gland does not secrete sufficient thyroxin

hypovolemia (hi″-po-vo-le′-me-a): loss of fluid volume

hypoxic drive (hi-pok′-sik driv): stimulus to breath comes from low levels of oxygen in the blood

hysterectomy (his″-tur-ek′-tuh-mee): partial or total surgical removal of the uterus

ileocecal valve (il′-ee-o-ce′-kl valv): valve between the small intestine and the cecum

ileum (il′-ee-um): lower part of the small intestine, extending from the jejunum to the large intestine

ilium (il′-ee-um): upper broad portion of the hipbone

immunity (im-yoo′-neh-tee): ability to resist a disease

immunization (im″-yoo-nah-zay′-shun): process of increasing resistance to disease

immunoglobulin (im″-yoo-noh-glob′-ya-lin): protein that acts like an antibody

immunosuppressant (im″-yoo-noh-suh-press′-unt): agent, such as a drug, chemical, or x-ray, used to suppress the immune system of a patient

immunosuppressed (im″-yoo-noh-suh′-pressd): inability of the body to mount an adequate antibody response to infection

impetigo (im-peh-tay′-goh): acute and contagious skin disease

impotence (im′-peh-tens): inability to sustain an erection

incarceration (in-kahr″-ser-a′-shun): entrapment of a loop of small bowel in the muscular abdominal wall

incision (in-sizh′-un): cut made by a knife into the skin; scalpels make a surgical incision

incisor (in-si′-zor): cutting tooth; one of four front teeth of either jaw

incomplete proteins (in″-kum-pleet′ pro′-teens): proteins that lack some or most of the essential amino acids

incontinence (in-kon′-ti-nens): inability to control elimination or excretion

incontinent (in-kon′-tah-nent): unable to control excretory functions of the body

incus (in′-kus): middle ear bone, also called the anvil

indirect force (in′-dye-rekt forse): force that does not directly impact but causes injury to a bone

infarction (in-fahrk′-shun): cell death

infectious mononucleosis (in-fek′-shus mon″-oh-nuk-lee-oh′-sis): contagious disease caused by Epstein-Barr virus, sometimes called the "kissing disease"

inferior (in-feer′-ee-er): below another or lower

inferior concha (in-feer′-ee-er kon′-cha): bones that make up side walls of the nasal cavity

inferior wall (in-feer′-ee-er wall): portion of the left ventricle that lies on top of the diaphragm

infertility (in-fer-til′-ah-tee): incapable of reproduction

inflammation (in″-flah-may′-shun): occurs when tissues are subjected to chemical or physical trauma (cut or heat); invasion by pathogenic microorganisms can cause inflammation; pain, heat, redness, and swelling occur

influenza (in-floo-en′-zah): inflammation of the mucous membrane of the respiratory tract

ingestion (in-jes′-chun): act of taking substances, especially food, into body

inguinal (ing′-gwi-nul): pertaining to the groin

inguinal hernia (ing′-gwi-nul hur′-nee-uh): hernia occurring in the inguinal area of the body

inhalation (in-huh-lay′-shun): taking air into the lungs

innominate bone (in-om′-i-nut bone): hipbone

insertion of muscle (in-sur′-shun of mus′-ul): muscle is attached to the movable part of the bone

inspiration (in″-spih-ray′-shun): drawing in of air; inhalation

inspiratory reserve volume (IRV) (in′-spi-rah-toh-re re-serv′ vol′-yoom): amount of air a person can take in over and above the tidal volume

insulin (in′-sah-lin): hormone produced by the pancreas necessary for glucose metabolism

integumentary system (in-teg′-yoo-men″-tayr-ee sis′-tem): tough, pliable covering; the skin

intercostal muscles (in-tur-kos′-tul mus′-ulz): muscles found between adjacent ribs

interferons (in-ter-feur′-onz): proteins that interfere with virus replication

internal (in-ter′-nal): term specifically used to refer to body cavities and hollow organs

internal respiration (in-ter′-nal res′-paray″-shun): exchange of carbon dioxide and oxygen between the cells and lymph surrounding them

interneuron (in-ter-neur′-on): *see* associative neuron

interstitial cell–stimulating hormone (ICSH) (in″-tur-stish′-ul sell sti′-myu-la-ting hor′-moan): hormone necessary for the production of testosterone in men

interstitial fluid (in″-tur-stish′-ul floo′-id): fluid that bathes the body's cells interstitial tissue (in″-tur-stish′-ul tish′-ew): intercellular connective tissue

interventricular foramen (in″-ter-ven-trik′-u-lar for′-a-men): connects to the two lateral ventricles of the brain

intestinal bowel obstruction (in-tes′-ti-nal bow′-ul obstruk′-shun): inability of food waste to pass through the intestines

intra-aortic balloon pump (IABP) (in″-tra-a-or′-tik baloon′ pump): device that inflates a gas-filled balloon moments after a heartbeat to increase blood flow

intracellular fluid (in-tra-sel′-ya-ler flu′-id): fluid within the cell

intracranial pressure (in″-tra-kra′-ne-al preh′-shur): pressure within the skull

intramuscular (in″-truh-mus′-kew-lur): into the muscle

intraosseous (IO) (in″-tra-os′-e-us): area within the bone

intravenously (in′-truh-vee′-nus-lee): within, or into, the veins

intrinsic muscles (in-trin′-sik mus′-ulz): antagonistic muscles that help the iris control amounts of light entering the pupil

intubation (in″-too-ba′-shun): process of inserting a plastic tube down the throat to assist in breathing

in-vitro fertilization (in-vee′-tro fer″-til-ih-zay′-shun): process of fertilization outside the living organism

involuntary (in-vol′-un-tayr-ee): opposite of voluntary; not within the control of will

involution (in″-vo-lew′-shun): return of an organ to its normal size after enlargement; also the regressive change caused by aging

ion (i′-on): electrically charged particle

ionize (i′-on-iz): conversion of a substance into positively charged hydrogen ions and negatively charged ions of some other element

iris (i′-ris): colored muscular layer surrounding the pupil of the eye

iron deficiency anemia (i′-ern de-fish′-en-se uh-nee′-mee-ah): lack of adequate amounts of iron in the body

irradiation (ir-ay-dee-ay′-shun): exposure to radiation such as infrared, gamma, roentgen, and ultraviolet rays

irritability (ir″-ih-tuh-bil′-ih-tee): ability to react to a stimulus; excitability

ischemia (is-ke′-me-a): oxygen loss resulting in cellular malfunction

ischemic stroke (is-kem′-ik strok): blockage of blood flow to the brain that results in the loss of brain function

ischium (is′-ke-um): lower part of hipbone

islets of Langerhans (i′-letz of lang′-er-hanz): specialized cells in pancreas that produce insulin

isometric (i-soh-meh′-trik): tension in muscle increases but muscle does not shorten

isotonic (i-soh-ton′-ik): muscle contracts and shortens

isotope (i′-soh-tope): atoms of a specific element that have the same number of protons but a different number of neutrons

jaundice (jon′-dis): yellow

joint (joynt): place where two bones meet

jejunum (je-joo′-num): section of small intestine between duodenum and ileum

jugular venous distention (JVD) (jug′-u-lur ve′-nus dis-ten′-shun): backup of blood into the external jugular vein

Kaposi's sarcoma (ka-poh′-siz sahr-koh′-mah): blood vessel malignancy

keratin (ker′-uh-tin): chemical belonging to albuminoid or scleroprotein group found in horny tissue, hair, nails

keto acid (ke′-to as′-id): byproduct of anaerobic metabolism

kidney (kid′-nee): most important excretory organ; makes urine by filtering wastes from the blood

kidney dialysis (kid′-nee di-al′-uh-sis): eliminating excess potassium from the blood through the use of a machine to cleanse the blood

kidney stones (kid′-nee stonz): or renal calculi; stones formed in the kidneys

kilocalorie (kil′-oh-kahl″-or-ee): measurement of heat-producing potential equal to 1000 calories

kilogram (kil′-oh-gram): 1000 grams or approximately 2.2 pounds

kinetic (ki-neh′-tik): pertaining to motion

knee dislocation (nee dis″-lo-ka′-shun): movement of the tibia and fibula off the femur, creating a stepped-off appearance

kneecap dislocation (nee′-kap dis″-lo-ka′-shun): lateral movement of the patella away from the joint

Kussmaul's breathing (koos′-moulz bree′-thing): respiratory pattern that exhibits as regular rapid deep sighing

kyphosis (ki-fose′-is): increasing curvature of the thoracic spine

labia (lay′-bee-uh): lips

labia majora (lay′-bee-uh ma-jor′-a): two folds of adipose (fat) tissue on each side of the vaginal opening (birth canal)

labia minora (lay′-bee-uh mi-nor′-a): two thin folds of skin just outside the vaginal opening (birth canal)

labor (lay′-bor): toning muscular contractions of the uterus in anticipation of childbirth

laceration (las″-er-a′-shun): tear in the skin that involves the entire thickness of the skin

lacrimal (lak′-ri-mul): pertaining to tears

lactated Ringer's solution (LR) (lak-tay′-ted ring′-erz sa-loo′-shun): solution used as a blood substitute;

consists of potassium chloride, sodium chloride, calcium chloride, and lactate

lactation (lak-tay'-shun): secretion of milk from the breasts

lactose (lak'-tose): milk sugar; a disaccharide used in infant formulas

laparoscopy (lap-ah-ros'-ko-pee): minor surgical procedure done to visually examine the abdomen

laryngectomy (lar"-in-jek'-to-me): surgical procedure that creates a permanent opening in the neck

laryngitis (lar-in-ji'-tis): inflammation of the voice box

laryngoscope blade (la-ring'-go-skop blayd): tool used to lift the tongue and jaw out of the line of sight of the vocal cords and trachea; used in intubation

larynx (lar'-inks): voice box; found between trachea and base of tongue; contains the vocal cords

lateral (lat'-ur-ul): toward the side

lateral ventricles (lat'-ur-ul ven'-tri-klz): *see* cerebral ventricles

lateral wall (lat'-ur-ul wall): wall of the left ventricle that lies next to the lateral chest

laxative (laks'-uh-tiv): chemical substance that relieves constipation; a mild purgative

leaflet (leef'-let): flap of the aortic valve

left coronary artery (LCA) (left kor'-o-nair"-ee ar'-ter-ee): artery that supplies blood to the portions of the left ventricle

left ventricle (left ven'-tri-kl): lower chamber of the heart

left ventricular assist device (left ven-trik'-u-lar a-sist' di-vis'): small in-line pump that helps increase the heart's own pumping

lens (lenz): crystal or glass for refraction of light rays

leukemia (lew-ke'-me-ah): cancerous condition characterized by an increase of white blood cells

leukocyte (lew'-ko-sight): white blood cell

leukocytosis (lew"-ko-sigh-tow'-sis): increase in the white blood cell count, above 10,000 cells per cubic millimeter (mm^3)

leukopenia (lew"-ko-pee'-nee-uh): decrease in the normal number of white blood cells (leukocytes)

leukorrhea (lew"-ko-ree'-uh): whitish, mucopurulent discharge from vagina

life functions (lif funk'-shunz): series of highly organized and related activities that help living organisms live, grow, and maintain themselves

ligament (lig'-uh-ment): band of fibrous tissue connecting bones or supporting organs

ligamentum arteriosus (lig"-a-men'-tum ahr-ter"-e-o'-sis): closure of the ductus arteriosus and conversion into the ligament that attaches the aorta to the heart

lingua (ling'-wa): pertaining to the tongue

lipase (lip'-ase): enzyme that changes fats into fatty acids and glycerol

lipid (lip'-id): fatty compound

liver spots (liv'-ur spotz): dark, yellowish-brown markings on the hands; generally seen in older people

lobule (lob'-yool): small lobe or a small section of a lobe

locomotion (lo"-kuh-moh'-shun): act of moving from place to place

loop of Henle (lup of hehn'-le): tubule descending into the medulla that contains a straight descending limb, a loop, and a straight ascending limb

lordosis (lor-do'-sis): forward curvature of lumbar region of spine

low-density lipoprotein (LDL) (lo din'-si-tee lip'-oh-pro"-teens): composed mostly of cholesterol; carry fat to cells

lubb dupp (lub dup): sound made by the heart valves when they close

lumbago (lum-bay'-go): backache occurring in lower lumbar or lumbosacral area of the spinal column

lumbar (lum'-bahr): pertaining to the loins; region between the posterior thorax and sacrum

lumbar puncture (lum'-bahr punk'-tur): removal of cerebrospinal fluid for diagnostic purposes

lumbar vertebrae (lum'-bahr vur'-te-bray): five vertebrae associated with lower part of back

lumen (lew'-min): internal diameter of an artery

lumpectomy (lum-pek'-to-me): removal of a small portion of the breast to remove cancerous tissue

luteinizing hormone (LH) (lew'-ten-i'-zing hor'-moan): hormone of the pituitary gland that stimulates the corpus luteum to produce progesterone in females

lymph (limf): watery fluid in the lymphatic vessels

lymphadenitis (lim-fa"-den-i'-tis): inflammation of the lymph nodes

lymphadenopathy (lim-fa"-den-op'-ah-the): lymph node enlargement

lymphatic (lim-fat'-ik): vessel carrying lymph

lymphatic system (lim-fat'-ik sis'-tum): system of vessels and nodes supplemental to blood circulatory system carrying lymph

lymphedema (lim"-fe-de'-ma): swelling in the arm resulting from a backup of fluid after the removal of lymph nodes

lymph nodes (limf nodz): tiny oval-shaped structures in a stationary collection found all over the body

lymphocyte (lim'-foh-sight): type of white blood cell

lymphoma (lim-foh'-mah): cancer-causing tumors in the brain

lymph vessels (limf ve'-sulz): tubes that transport lymph from tissues to the circulatory system

lysis (li"-sis): break up

lysosome (lye"-so-sohm): cytoplasmic organelle containing digestive enzymes

macrophage (mak'-rah-faj): large phagocytic cell that can wall off and isolate an infected area macular degeneration (mak'-yu-ler de-jen"-er-ay'-shun): condition in which thinning of retinal layer of eye or leakage develops under retina, disturbing sharp central vision

magnesium (Mg+) (mag-ne'-ze-um): electrolyte found in bones and extracellular fluid; aids in cellular metabolism, activation of enzymes, and contraction of skeletal muscle

magnum foramen (mag'-num): opening in the skull through which the spinal nerves leave the brain and enter the spinal column

malabsorption syndrome (mal"-ab-sorp'-shun sin'-drome): impaired absorption of nutrients from the gastrointestinal tract

malaise (mah'-layz): fatigue

malignant (mah-lig'-nent): rapidly spreading; cancerous

malleus (mal'-ee-us): largest of three middle ear bones; also called the hammer

maltose (mawl'-tose): disaccharide formed by the hydrolysis of starch

mammary (mam'-ur-ree): pertaining to the breast

mammogram (mam'-e-gram): x-ray of the breast

mandible (man'-dih-bul): lower jawbone

manubrium (mah-new'-bree-um): (1) handlelike process; (2) upper part of the sternum (breastbone)

mastectomy (mas-tek'-ta-mee): removal of a breast

mastication (mas"-ti-kay'-shun): process of chewing

matrix (ma'-triks): part of the fingernail bed where the nail is formed

matter (mat'-ur): anything that has weight and occupies space

maturation (match"-oo-ray'-shun): process of coming to full development

maxilla (mak-sil'-a): bone of the upper jaw

McBurney's point (mik-bur'-neez poynt): area at the middle of a triangle formed by the symphysis pubis, iliac crest, and umbilicus

meatus (mee-ay'-tus): passageway or opening

medial (mee'-dee-ul): toward the midline of body

mediastinum (mee"-dee-as'-tih-num): intrapleural space separating the sternum in front and the vertebral column behind

medulla (mah-dul'-uh): inner portion of an organ

medulla oblongata (mah-dul'-uh ob'-lon-gah'-tuh): part of the brainstem; contains the nuclei for vital functions; location of respiratory center

medullary canal (med'-ul-er-ee ka-nal'): center of the shaft of long bone

meiosis (mi-yo'-sis): cell division of gamete or cells; there is a reduction in the number of chromosomes

melanin (mel'-a-nin): pigment that gives color to hair, skin, and eyes

melanocytes (mel'-a-no-sytz): cells that give color to the skin

melatonin (mel-eh-toh'-nin): hormone produced by the pineal gland

membrane (mem'-brayn): thin layer of tissue that covers a surface or divides an organ

membrane excitability (mem'-brayn ek-si"-tah-bil'-ih-tee): process of creating electric impulses through the nerves

memory (mem'-eh-ree): process by which we store information we have learned

menarche (me-nahr'-kee): time when menstruation begins

Meniere's disease (man-arz' di-zeez'): condition affecting the semicircular canals of the inner ear

meninges (men-en'-jez): any of three linings enclosing the brain and spinal cord

meningitis (men"-in-ji'-tis): inflammation or infection of the membranes surrounding the brain

menopause (men'-o-pawz): physiological termination of menstruation, generally between 50 and 55 years of age

menstrual cycle (men'-stroo-ul si'-kul): recurring series of changes that take place in the ovaries, uterus, and accessory sexual structures during menstruation

menstruation (men"-stroo-ay'-shun): monthly shedding of endometrial lining if ovum is not fertilized

mesentery (mez'-en-ter-ee): peritoneum attached to posterior wall of the abdominal cavity

metabolism (me-tab'-oh-liz-em): sum total of processes of digestion, absorption, and the resulting release of energy

metacarpal (met"-uh-kahr'-pal): bones of wrist

metastases (me-tas'-tuh-ses): transfer of malignant cells from an original site to a distant one through the circulatory system or lymph vessels

metatarsal (met"-uh-tahr'-sal): sole of foot; forms the arch

metered-dose inhaler (MDI) (me'-terd-dos in-hai'-ler): handheld device for the administration of medication; often includes a spacer for dispersing the medication over a volume of air before inhalation

microbe (migh'-krobe): microscopic organisms, especially bacterium

microscopic anatomy (migh-kro-skop'-ic a-nat'-a-me): using a microscope to study gross anatomy

microsurgery (mi'-kro-sur"-jur-e): surgery aided by the use of a microscope

micturition (mich"-tew-rish'-un): voiding, urinating

midaxillary line (MAL) (mid-ak"-si-lar'-e lyn): line of reference that runs from the middle of the armpit parallel to the midline

midclavicular line (MCL) (mid-kla"-vi-cu'-lar lyn): line of reference, beginning at the midpoint of the collarbone, that runs parallel to the midline

midline (mid'-lyn): line of reference that runs down the center of the body, dividing it into two equal parts

midsagittal plane (mid-saj'-eh-tel plane): imaginary line dividing the body into equal right and left halves

milliequivalent (mEq) (mil"-eh-e-kwiv'-a-lent): measure used to determine the amount of electrolytes in a certain volume of fluid (e.g., mEq per liter)

mineral (min'-ur-ul): inorganic, solid chemical compound found in nature

mineralocorticoids (M-Cs) (min'-ur-ul-o-cort'-ih-coydz): hormones of the adrenal cortex, namely aldosterone

miotic (miy-ot'-ik): causing contraction of pupil

miscarriage (mis'-kar-ej): premature loss of pregnancy; lay term for abortion

mitochondria (miy-toh-kon'-dree-a): organelle that supplies energy to the cell

mitosis (migh-toe'-sis): cell division is divided into two distinct processes: (1) mitosis—the exact duplication of the nucleus to form two identical nuclei; (2) cytoplasmic division—after nuclear division, the cytoplasm is divided into two approximately equal parts

mitral valve prolapse (miy'-tral valv proh'-laps): improper closure of the valve between the left atrium and the left ventricle

mittelschmerz (mit'-el-shmertz): sharp pain felt in the lower abdomen at the time of ovulation

mixed nerve (mikst nerv): nerve composed of both afferent (sensory) fibers and efferent (motor) fibers

modified Trendelenburg position (mod'-i-fyd tren'-de-len-burg pa-zi'-shun): positioning a patient supine with the legs elevated

molar (moh'-lar): teeth designed for crushing and tearing

molecule (mol'-uh-kyool): smallest unit of a compound that still has the properties of the compound

monocyte (mon'-oh-sight): large mononuclear leukocyte with deeply indented nucleus, slate gray cytoplasm and fine bluish granulations

monorchidism (mon-or'-kid-izm): presence of only one testis

monosaccharide (mon"-oh-sack'-uh-ride): simple sugar; glucose

mons pubis (monz pu'-bis): large pad of fat covered with coarse hair on the mature female

morphology (mor-fol'-ah-jee): study of the shape of an organism

motor aphasia (moh'-ter a-fay'-zhuh): inability to speak as a result of the loss of muscle control

motor nerve (moh'-ter nerv): or efferent neuron; carries messages from brain and spinal cord to muscles and glands

motor unit (moh'-ter u'-nit): motor nerve plus all the muscle fibers it stimulates

mucilaginous (mew"-si-ladj'-ih-nus): gumlike consistency

mucin (mew'-sin): mixture of glycoproteins forming basis of mucus

mucosa (mew-koh'-suh): mucous membrane

mucous membrane (mew'-kus mem'-bran): layers of tissue that lubricate and protect linings of the respiratory, digestive, reproductive, and urinary systems

mucous plug (mew'-kus plug): blockage created from dried secretions in the airway

multicellular (mul-ti-sel'-u-lar): many celled

multiple sclerosis (mul'-tih-pul skle-roh'-sis): chronic inflammatory disease in which the immune cells attack the myelin sheath of a nerve

murmur (mur'-mer): gurgling or hissing sound from heart valves failing to close properly

muscarinic receptor (mus"-ka-rin'-ik ree-sep'-tur): cholinergic receptor that causes slowing of the heart rate, dilation of arteries, increased gastrointestinal activity, increased mucous production, and constriction of pupils

muscle fatigue (mus'-ul fah-teeg'): caused by an accumulation of lactic acid in the muscle

muscle spasm (mus'-ul spa'-zum): sustained muscle contraction

muscle tissue (mus'-ul tis'-ew): contains cell material that has the ability to contract and move the body

muscle tone (mus'-ul tone): muscles always in a state of partial contraction

muscular dystrophy (mus'-kew-ler dis'-tre-fee): muscle disease in which the muscle cells deteriorate

mutagenic agent (mew"-tuh-jen'-ik ay'-junt): any substance causing a genetic mutation

mutate (mew-tate'): to change or alter a characteristic that will make it different from that of the parental type

mutation (mew-tay'-shun): appearance of a new and different organic trait caused by the inheritance of a mutated gene or chromosome

myalgia (migh-al'-juh): muscular pain

myasthenia gravis (migh-es-the'-nee-a gra'vis): disease in which there is abnormal weakness and eventual paralysis of muscles

myelin (migh'-e-lin): lipoid substance found in the sheath around nerve fibers

myelin sheath (neurilemma) (migh'-e-lin sheeth [noor"-i-lem'-a]): fat covering over axon of nerve cell that aids in speed of conduction of impulse

myeloblast (migh'-eh-loh-blast): cells that synthesize granulocytes in bone marrow

myocardial infarction (migh"-o-kahr'-de-al in-fark'-shun): blockage of a coronary artery, resulting in the lack of blood supply to the heart muscle; heart attack

myocarditis (migh"-o-kahr-dye'-tis): inflammation of muscular tissue of heart

myocardium (migh"-o-kahr'-de-um): muscle of the heart

myometrium (migh"-o-mee'-tree-um): uterine muscular structure

myopia (migh-o'-pee-uh): nearsightedness

myositis (migh'-oh-sigh'-tis): inflammation of muscle tissue, generally voluntary muscle

myotonia (migh"-oh-toh'-nee-uh): condition in which there is an abnormally slow muscle relaxation after voluntary muscle contraction

myringotomy (mir-en-got'-oh-mee): opening into the tympanic membrane

myxedema (mik-se-de'-ma): hypofunction of the thyroid gland; swelling around nose and lips

nasal (nay'-zul): nose

nasal cavity (nay'-zul ka'-vih-tee): one of the pair of cavities between anterior nares and nasopharynx

nasal polyp (nay'-zul pol'-ip): growth that occurs in sinus cavity

nasal septum (nay'-zul sep'-tum): partition between the two nasal cavities

natural acquired immunity (na'-chur-al a-kwi'-erd i-mu'-ni-tee): immunity that is the result of having the disease and recovering

natural immunity (na'-chur-al i-mu'-ni-tee): immunity with which a person is born

navicular bone (na-vik'-u-lar bone): small carpal bone next to the thumb

neck of tooth (nek of tooth): that part of a tooth at the gum line

needle decompression (nee'-del de"-kom-presh'-un): method used to decrease pressure built up in the chest

negative feedback (neg'-uh-tiv feed'-bak): return of part of the output to the source or beginning; this leads to an adjustment in the system; may occur in hormonal or nervous control systems

neoplasm (nee'-o-plaz-em): tumor; can be benign or malignant

nephron (nef'-ron): functional unit of the kidney; contains glomerulus, Bowman's capsule, proximal distal tubule, loop of Henle, and distal tubule

nervous tissue (nur'-vus tis'-yoo): contains cells that react to stimuli and conduct an impulse

neuralgia (noo-ral'-ja): severe stabbing pain along the pathway of a nerve

neuritis (noo-rih'-tis): inflammation of a nerve

neurogenic bladder (noor-o-jen'-ik blad'-ur): condition caused by damaged nerves that control the bladder

neuroglia (noo-rog'-lee-ah): network of cells that insulate, support, and protect the nerves of the central nervous system

neurohypophysis (new"-roh-high-pof'-ih-sis): posterior lobe of the pituitary gland; stores two hormones produced by the hypothalamus: antidiuretic hormone and oxytocin

neurology (noo-rol'-ah-jee): study of the physiology and pathology of the nervous system

neuromuscular blocking agent (noor'-oh-mus'-kya-lur blok'-ing ay'-junt): chemical that interferes with neurotransmitters by blocking the acetylcholine receptor, thus paralyzing the patient

neuromuscular junction (noor-oh-mus'-kya-lur junk'-shun): point between the motor nerve axon and the muscle cell membrane

neuron (new'-ron): nerve cell, including its processes

neurotransmitter (noor-o-trans'-mit-er): chemical messenger in the nervous system

neutralization (noo-tral-ah-zay'-shun): an acid and a base combine to form a salt and water

neutrophil (noo'-trah-fil): multilobed white blood cell that phagocytizes bacteria; sometimes called "polys"

nicotinic receptor (nik"-o-tin'-ik ree-sep'-tur): cholinergic receptor that causes muscle contraction

noncompliance (non"-kom-ply'-anz): failure to take medications as prescribed

nongravid (non"-grav'-id): not pregnant

nonpathogenic (non"-path-o-jen'-ik): incapable of producing disease

norepinephrine (nor"-eh-pin-eh'-frihn): chemical messenger in the sympathetic nerves

normal saline (nor'-mal say'-leen): solution used to replace blood lost; also known as 0.9 NaCl in sterile water

nuclear membrane (noo'-klee-er mem'-brayn): double-layered membrane that surrounds the nucleus

nucleic acid (noo-klay'-ik as'-id): organic compound containing carbon, hydrogen, oxygen, nitrogen, and phosphorous (e.g., DNA, RNA)

nucleolus (new-klee-uh'-lus): small spherical structure within cell nucleus

nucleoplasm (new'-klee-o-plazm): protoplasm of the nucleus; also called nuclear sap or karyolymph

nucleus (new'-klee-us): core or center of a cell containing large quantities of DNA

nutrient (new'-tree-unt): affording nutrition

nystagmus (ni-stag'-mis): rapid involuntary movement of the eyeball

obesity (oh-bee'-sih-tee): increase of body weight caused by fat accumulation of 10% to 20% above normal range for the specific age, height, and sex

occipital (ok-sip'-i-tal): area at rear of skull

occipital lobe (ok-sip'-i-tal lowb): area of the brain that controls eyesight

occiput (ok'-sih-put): pertaining to the back of the head

occlusive stroke (o-kloo'-siv strok): stoppage of blood flow to an area of the brain because of a blockage

olecranon process (oh-lek'-ruh-non pro'-ses): large projection at upper extremity of ulna

olfactory (ol-fak'-tur-ee): pertaining to the sense of smell

olfactory nerve (ol-fak'-tur-ee nerv): nerve that conducts the sense of smell from the smell receptors to the brain for interpretation

oogenesis (o"-oh-jen'-e-sis): process of origin, growth, and formation of ovum in ovary during preparation for fertilization

ophthalmic (op-thal'-mik): referring to the eyes

opportunistic infection (op'-er-toon-is"-tik in-fek'-shun): an infection that may occur because a person's immune system dysfunctions

optic disc (op'-tik disk): disc containing nerve fibers from the retina; blind spot

oral cavity (or'-el ka'-vih-tee): encloses the teeth and tongue

orbital cavity (or'-bi-tel ka'-vih-tee): contains the eye and its external structures

orchitis (or-ki'-tis): inflammation of testis

organ (or'-gan): group of tissues that together perform a specific function within the body

organ of Corti (or'-gan of kor'-tee): hearing organ

organ system (or'-gan sis'-tem): group of tissues and organs, organized according to structure, that function together

organic catalyst (or-gan'-ik kat'-ahl-ist): affects the rate or speed of a chemical reaction without itself being changed

organic compound (or-gan'-ik kom'-pownd): compound that contains the element carbon

organelle (or-guh-nel'): microscopic specialized structure within the cell having a special function or capacity

origin (or'-eh-jin): part of the skeletal muscle that is attached to the fixed part of the bone

oropharynx (or"-o-fayr'-inks): oral pharynx, found below the level of the lower border of the soft palate and above the larynx

orthopnea (or"-thup'-nee-uh): difficult or labored breathing

osmoreceptor (oz"-moh-ree-sep'-tur): structure found in the hypothalamus; sensitive to changes in the osmotic blood pressure and controls the release of antidiuretic hormone (ADH)

osmosis (oz-moh'-sis): passage of fluid through a membrane

osmotic pressure (oz-mot'-ik preh'-shur): pressure developed when two solutions of different concentrations of the solute are separated by a membrane permeable only to the solvent

ossa carpi (os'-sa kahr'-pye): eight bones of the wrist

osseous (os'-ee-us): bony; composed of or resembling bone

ossicle (os'-ih-kul): small bone; usually refers to the three small bones of the middle ear

ossification (os"-eh-fi-kay'-shun): process of bone formation

osteitis (os"-tee-eye'-tis): inflammation of bone tissue

osteoarthritis (os"-tee-oh-ahr-thry'-tis): degenerative joint disease

osteoblast (os'-tee-oh-blast): cells involved in formation of bony tissue

osteoclast (os'-tee-oh-klast): cells involved in resorption of bony tissue

osteocyte (os'-tee-oh-site): bone cell

osteomyelitis (os-tee-o-mie-lit'-is): inflammation of the bone

osteoporosis (os"-tee-oh-pour-oh'-sis): loss of calcium in bone, causing brittleness; occurs mainly in females after menopause

osteosarcoma (os-tee-oh-sar-koh'-mah): bone cancer

otitis media (oh-ti'-tis me'-de-ah): infection of the middle ear

otorrhea (o"-to-re'-a): fluid leaking from the ears

otosclerosis (ah"-toh-skle-roh'-sis): chronic, progressive ear disorder in which the bone in the region of the oval window first becomes spongy and then hardened, causing the stirrup, or stapes, to become fixed or immobile

ova (o'-va): female reproductive cells

ovarian cancer (o-var'-ee-an kan'-ser): abnormal cell growth in the ovary

ovary (o'-veh-ree): female reproductive organ produces ova, estrogen, and progesterone

ovulation stage (ah"-vyoo-lay'-shun stayj): second stage of the menstrual cycle, when a ripe egg cell is released from an ovarian follicle cell

oxygenate (ok"-si-ji'-nate): to saturate a substance with oxygen, either by chemical combination or by mixture

oxyhemoglobin (ok"-see-hee'-muh-gloh"-bin): hemoglobin combined with oxygen

oxytocin (ok"-si-to'-sin): hormone released during childbirth, causing strong contractions of the uterus

palate (pal'-ut): roof of the mouth

palatine (pal-ah-teen'): facial bones that form the hard palate of the mouth

palpitation (pal"-pah-tay'-shun): an awareness of one's own heartbeat, usually felt in tachycardias

pancreas (pan'-kree-as): organ of digestion lies behind the stomach; produces digestive juices, insulin, and glucagon

pancreatitis (pan"-kre-ah-ti'-tis): inflammation of the pancreas

Pap smear (pap smir): cytological, diagnostic cancer technique that studies exfoliated cells, especially those from vagina

papilla (pa-pil'-uh): small, nipple-shaped elevations

paralysis (pah-ral'-ih-sis): loss of motion or sensation

paraplegia (par"-eh-plee'-jee-a): complete paralysis of the lower body, including both legs

parasympathetic nervous system (par'-ah-sim'-pah-thet'-ik nerv'-us sis'-tem): division of the autonomic nervous system; inhibits or opposes the effects of the sympathetic nervous system

parathormone (par″-uh-thor′-moan): hormone that controls the concentration of calcium in blood

parathyroid gland (par″-uh-thiy′-royd gland): four small endocrine glands embedded in the thyroid gland; secretes parathormone

parenteral (per′-in-ter″-ul): medication administration via routes that bypass the digestive system

paresis (pa-re′-sis): muscular weakness

paresthesia (par″-es-theez′-shuh): loss of sensation

parietal (pa-ri′-a-tal): roof of the skull

parietal lobe (pa-ri′-a-tal lowb): area of the brain that controls sensory function

parietal membrane (pa-ri′-a-tal mem′-brayn): lining of a body cavity

Parkinson's disease (par′-kin-senz di-zeez′): marked tremors may be due to decrease of neurotransmitter dopamine

parotid gland (pah-rot′-id gland): largest of the salivary glands

partial (second-degree) burn (pahr′-shel burn): *see* burn

partial seizure (pahr′-shel see′-zure): chaotic nervous activity in a portion of the brain

passive acquired immunity (pas′-iv a-kwi′-erd i-mu′-ni-tee): borrowed immunity; has a temporary effect (e.g., gamma globulin)

patella (pah-tel′-uh): kneecap

pathogenic (path″-uh-jen′-ik): disease causing

pathogens (path′-o-jenz): microorganisms

pearl (purl): abbreviation for a test of pupillary reaction

pecking order (pek′-ing or′-der): process of selective perfusion

pectoral (pek′-tuh-rul): pertaining to the chest

pectoralis major (pek-to-ral′-is ma′-jor): muscle of the upper extremity that flexes the upper arm and helps to abduct the upper arm

pedal edema (ped′-al e-de′-ma): swelling in the feet and ankles

pelvic cavity (pel′-vik ka′-vih-tee): body cavity containing the urinary bladder, reproductive organs, rectum, part of the large intestine, and appendix

pelvic inflammatory disease (PID) (pel′-vik in-flam′-a-tor″-ee di-zeez′): infections that occur in the reproductive organs and spread to the fallopian tubes and peritoneal cavity

pelvis (pel′-vis): any basin-shaped structure or cavity

pelviscopy (pel-vis′-ko-pe): visual inspection of the internal pelvis using a flexible tube

penile shaft (pe′-nyl shaft): fold in the penis

penis (pe′-nis): external male organ through which both urine and semen leave the body

penumbra (pe-num′-bra): overlap of cell injury, ischemia, and death, appearing in a bull's-eye pattern

peptic ulcer (pep′-tik ul′-ser): sore on the mucous membrane lining in the stomach or small intestine

perfusion (per-fu′-zhun): blood flow to all cells of the body

pericarditis (per″-ih-kahr-di′-tis): inflammation of the outer membrane covering of the heart

pericardium (per″-ih-kahr′-dee-um): or pericardial membrane; closed membranous sac surrounding heart cavity that protects the heart

perineum (per′-ah-nee-um): area between the vagina and the rectum

periodontal membrane (per-ee-o-dan′-tel mem′-brayn): membrane that anchors a tooth in place

perioral paresthesia (per″-ee-or′-al par″-es-the′-zha): numbness around the mouth

periosteum (per-ee-os′-tee-um): fibrous tissue covering the bone

peripheral (pe-rif′-er-al): outside surface, or the area away from the center

peripheral edema (pe-rif′-er-al e-de′-ma): swelling in the extremities

peripheral nervous system (pe-rif′-er-al): made up of 12 pairs of cranial nerves and 31 pairs of spinal nerves

peripheral vascular disease (pe-rif′-er-al vas′-kul-ar di-zeez′): blockage of arteries, usually in the legs

peristalsis (per″-ih-stal′-sis): progressive wave of contraction in tubular structures provided with longitudinal and transverse muscular fibers, as in esophagus, stomach, and small and large intestines

peritoneum (per-ih-toh′-nee-um): or peritoneal membrane; serous membrane lining of the abdominal cavity that protects the abdominal organs

peritonitis (per″-ih-ton-i′-tis): inflammation of the lining of the abdominal cavity

pernicious anemia (per-nish′-us uh-nee′-mee-a): condition caused by a decrease of B_{12} or lack of intrinsic factor in the stomach

peroxisomes (per-ee-oks′-i-somz): membranous sacs containing oxidase enzymes that help digest fats and detoxify harmful substances

pertussis (per-tus′-is): *see* whooping cough

phagocyte (fag′-oh-sight): cell having the property of engulfing and digesting foreign particles or cells harmful to body

phagocytosis (fag″-oh-si-toh′-sis): ingestion of foreign or other particles by certain cells

phalanges (fah-lan′-jez): bones of fingers and toes

pharyngitis (fair′-in-ji′-tis): inflammation of the throat

pharynx (fair′-inks): throat

phenylketonuria (PKU) (fen″-il-kee-toh-new′-ree-uh): metabolic disorder in which the body cannot make an enzyme needed for normal metabolism or breakdown of the amino acid phenylalanine; excess phenylalanine disrupts the normal development of neurons in the brain

pheochromocytoma (fe″-o-kro″-mo-si-to′-ma): tumor of the adrenal gland

phlebitis (fle-bye'-tis): inflammation of a vein, with or without infection and thrombus formation

phospholipids (fos'-foh-lip'-ids): fats that contain carbon, hydrogen, oxygen, and phosphorous

phototherapy (fo"-to-ther'-uh-pee): use of light to alleviate neonatal physiologic jaundice

phrenic nerve (fren'-ik nerv): stimulates the diaphragm

pH scale (p-h scayl): measures hydrogen ion concentration of solution or air mixture; potential of hydrogen

physiologic jaundice (fiz"-ee-o-lah'-jik- jon'-dis): disorder in infants in which the liver cannot excrete bilirubin into the bile

physiology (fiz"-ee-ol'-uh-jee): science that studies functions of living organisms and their parts

physiotherapy (fiz"-ee-oh-ther'-uh-pee): treatment of disease and injury by physical means, using light, heat, cold, water, electricity, massage, and exercise

pia mater (pee'-uh may'-tur): innermost vascular covering of brain and spinal cord

pigment (pig'-ment): (1) dye or coloring matter; (2) organic coloring matter of body

pineal gland (pin'-ee-al gland): located in the third ventricle of the brain; produces melatonin

pinna (pin'-ah): outer ear

pinocytic vessel (pin"-oh-si'-tik ves'-el): formed by having the cell membrane fold inward to form a pocket

pinocytosis (pin"-oh-sye-toh'-sis): process of engulfing large molecules in solution and taking them into the cell

pituitary gland (pi-too'-e-tayr'-ee gland): small gland located in the sphenoid bone in the cranium; its hormones affect all other glandular activity; it is called the master gland

pivot joint (piv'-et joynt): joint in which an extension of one bone rotates in a second arch-shaped bone

placenta (pla-sen'-ta): a spongy, blood-filled organ that supplies nourishment to the developing fetus in the uterus

placenta previa (pla-sen'-ta preh'-vi-ah): implantation of the placenta low in the uterus, over the opening of the uterus blocking the vaginal birth canal

planes (playnz): imaginary, anatomical dividing lines useful in separating body structures

plasma (plaz'-muh): liquid part of blood containing corpuscles

pleura (ploor'-uh): or pleural membrane; serous membrane protecting the lungs and lining the internal surface of thoracic cavity

pleural fluid (ploor'-al flu'-id): *see* serous fluid

pleurisy (ploor'-ih-see): inflammation of pleura

plexus (plek'-sus): network of spinal nerves

premenstrual syndrome (PMS) (pre-men'-stroo-ul sin'-drome): symptoms that are exhibited just prior to the menstrual cycle

pneumonia (noo-mon'-ya): infection of the lung

pneumothorax (noo-mo-tho'-raks): abnormal accumulation of air in the pleural cavity

point of maximum intensity (PMI) (poynt of mak'-see-mum in-ten'-si-tee): area in which the heartbeat can best be felt or heard

point tenderness (poynt ten'-der-ness): acute pain at one spot

poliomyelitis (po"-le-o-mye-lye'-tis): disease of nerve pathways of spinal cord; rarely seen because of polio vaccines

polycythemia (pol"-eh-si-thee'-mee-ah): too many red blood cells

polydipsia (pol'-eh-dip'-see-ah): excessive thirst

polymorphonuclear leukocyte (pol"-e-morf-o-nu'-kle-ar lu'-ko-sit): granulated white blood cell that phagocytizes bacteria with lysosomal enzymes

polyphagia (pol'-e-fay'-jah): excessive hunger

polypnea (pol"-ip-nee'-uh): very rapid respiration or panting resulting from increased muscular activity or emotional trauma

polysaccharide (pol"-ee-sak'-uh-ride): complex sugar

polyuria (pol'-e-yoor'-ee-ah): excessive urination

pons (ponz): part of the brainstem

popliteal (pop-lit'-ee-ul): area behind the knee

popliteal artery (pop-lit'-ee-ul ar'-ter-ee): artery behind the knee

pores (porz): (1) very small openings on a surface; (2) opening ducts of a sweat gland

portal circulation (por'-tul sir-ku-lay'-shun): brings blood from the organs of digestion through the portal vein to the liver

portal hypertension (por'-tul hi'-pur-ten"-shun): condition resulting from blood backing up into the portal vein

portal vein (por'-tul vayn): collects blood and delivers it to the liver

posterior (pos-teer'-ee-ur): located behind or at the back; opposite to anterior

posterior chamber (pos-teer'-ee-ur chaym'-bur): the portion of the eye behind the iris

posterior pituitary lobe (pos-teer'-ee-ur pih-tu'-ih-tar-ee lowb): part of the pituitary gland that stores hormones produced by the hypothalamus

posterior wall (pos-teer'-ee-ur wall): base of the heart where the valves are located

postictal (post-ik'-tal): period after seizure activity stops

potassium (K+) (po-tas'-ee-um): electrolyte found inside the cell that controls cellular functions such as osmosis and acid-base balance

potential energy (po-ten'-shal en'-er-gee): energy in the body waiting to be released

preeclampsia (pre"-e-klamp'-see-a): condition occurring between the twentieth week of pregnancy and the first week after delivery, exhibited by excessive edema, weight gain, protein in urine, and hypotension

pregnancy (preg'-nan-see): fetus is carried in the uterus until birth; to be gravid (i.e., heavy with child)

pre-ictal (pre-ik'-tal): the first phase of a seizure, in which the person may experience an aura and loss of consciousness

presbycusis (prez"-be-kyu'-sis): condition that causes deafness as a result of the aging process

presbyopia (prez"-bee-oh'-pee-uh): farsightedness of advanced age caused by loss of elasticity in the lens

priapism (pri'-a-piz"-um): painful sustained erection

primary repair (pri'-mar-ee re-payr'): type of epithelial tissue repair that takes place on clean wounds

prime mover (prime muv'-er): muscle that provides movement in a single direction

progesterone (pro-jes'-tur-ohn): steroid hormone secreted by the ovary from the corpus luteum to help maintain pregnancy

progressive atherosclerosis (pro-gres'-iv ath"-er-o-sklah-ro'-sis): buildup of fatty layers called plaque within the arteries

prolactin hormone (PR) (pro-lak'-tin hor'moan): hormone that develops breast tissue and stimulates the production of milk after childbirth

prolapsed uterus (pro-lapst' yoo'-tur-us): condition in which normal supportive structures around the uterus weaken and allow the uterus to fall from its normal position

pronation (pro-nay'-shun): (1) condition of being prone; (2) turning of palm of hand downward

prostaglandin (pros-tah-glan'-din): hormones secreted by various tissues; their function depends on which tissue excretes them

prostatectomy (pros"-tuh-tek'-tuh-mee): surgical removal of all or part of the prostate

prostate gland (pros'-tate gland): gland located just under the urinary bladder; secretes a thin, milky alkaline fluid that enhances sperm motility

prostate cancer (pros'-tate kan'-ser): abnormal cell growth within the prostate

prostatic urethra (pros'-tat-ik yoo-ree'-thruh): area at the beginning of the urethra, surrounded by the prostate gland

prostatitis (pros"-ta-ti'-tis): inflammation or infection of the prostate

protease (pro'-teez): pancreatic juices that break down protein to amino acids

protein synthesis (pro'-teen sin'-the-sis): process in which cells containing DNA produce proteins

prothrombin (pro-throm'-bin): chemical substance formed in the liver that helps the blood clotting process

protoplasm (pro'-tuh-plazm): living colloid material of the cell; contains proteins, lipids, inorganic salts, and carbohydrates

proximal (prok'-sih-mul): located nearest the center of the body; point of attachment of a structure

pruritus (proo-rye'-tes): itching

psoriasis (so-rye'-ah-sis): chronic inflammatory skin disease with silvery patches

psychic (sigh'-kik): (1) pertaining to psyche, which is the mind or self as a functional unit, helping a person adjust to the changes, demands, or needs of the environment; (2) sensitive to nonphysical forces; (3) mental

ptyalin (tayl'-in): saliva that converts starches into sugar

puberty (pew'-bur-tee): age when reproductive organs become functional

pubis (pew'-bis): pubic bone; portion of hipbone forming front of pelvis

public access defibrillation (PAD) (pub-lik' ack'-ses de-fib"-ri-lay'-shun): lay persons who implement automated external defibrillation in public places

pulmonary artery (pool-'ma-ner-ee ar'-ter-ee): structure takes blood from the right ventricle to the lungs

pulmonary circulation (pool-'ma-ner-ee ser-kyul-a'-shun): blood pathway through the lungs only

pulmonary edema (pool-'ma-ner-ee e-de'-ma): backup of blood into the lungs from the left-side of the heart

pulmonary embolism (pool-'ma-ner-ee em'-bol-izm): blockage in pulmonary artery or one of its branches

pulmonary semilunar valve (pool-'ma-ner-e sem-i-lu'-nar valv): lets blood travel from the right ventricle into the pulmonary artery, then into the lungs

pulmonary veins (pool-'ma-ner-ee vayns): structures that takes blood from the lungs to the right atrium

pulp cavity (pulp ka'-vih-tee): inside of the tooth; contains blood vessels and nerves

pulse (puls): measures the number of times the heart beats per minute; the rhythmic flow of blood

pulselessness (puls'-less-ness): loss of circulation

pulse points (puls poyntz): areas of the body in which the pulse can be felt by compressing the artery against a bone

pulse pressure (puls presh'-ur): difference between the systolic and diastolic blood pressure

puncture (pungk'-chur): wound breaking the entire thickness of the skin; caused by a pointed or sharp object

pupil (pew'-pil): opening in the iris of the eye for passage of light

Purkinje fibers (per-kin'-jee fye'-burs): conduction fibers that conduct impulses through the ventricles of the heart

pus (pus): product of inflammation; cream-colored liquid that is a combination of dead tissue, dead and living bacteria, dead white blood cells, and blood plasma

pyelonephritis (pye-loh-nef-right'-is): inflammation of the kidneys and the pelvis of the ureter

pyloric sphincter (pye-lo'-rik sfink'-tur): valve that regulates the entrance of food

pyloric stenosis (pye-lo'-rik ste-no'-sis): narrowing of the pyloric sphincter; occurs most often in infants

pylorospasm (pye-lor'-o-spazm): abnormal condition when the pyloric sphincter fails to relax; food remaining in stomach does not get completely digested and eventually is vomited

pylorus (pye-lo'-rus): circular opening of stomach into duodenum

pyrexia (pye-rek'-see-uh): fever

pyrogen (pye'-ra-jen): any fever-producing agent

pyuria (pi-yoor'-ee-a): pus in the urine

quadriplegia (kwod"-ra-ple'-ja): loss of movement in all four extremities

quickening (kwik'-en-ing): the first awareness of movement of the fetus within the uterus

raccoon's eyes (ra-koonz' iyz): bilateral periorbital ecchymosis; two black eyes

radial artery (ra'-dee-al ar'-ter-ee): pulse point at the wrist, on the same side as the thumb

radial nerve (ra'-dee-al nerv): part of the brachial plexus that stimulates the wrist and hand

radioactive (ra'dee-oh-ak'-tiv): capable of emitting energy in the form of radiation

radius (ra'-dee-us): bone on the thumb side of the forearm

recommended dietary allowance (RDA) (rek'-o-mend"-ed die'-ih-tare'-ee ah-lau'-ans): contains the daily allowances for protein, fat-soluble vitamins, water-soluble vitamins, and minerals as recommended by the Food and Nutrition Board

rebound tenderness (re'-bound ten'-der-ness): pain upon recoil of the abdomen during palpation

receptive aphasia (ree-sep'-tiv a-fay'-zhuh): inability to understand the spoken word

receptor (ree-sep'-tur): sensory nerve that receives a stimulus and transmits it to the CNS

recombinant DNA (re-kom'-bi-nant d-n-a): sophisticated technology used to isolate a desired gene

rectum (rek'-tum): end of the colon; opens to the anus

red muscle (red mus'-ul): muscle that appears red in the fresh state because of the presence of muscle hemoglobin

referred pain (re'-furd payne): pain that is felt in an area other than the injured area

reflex (ree'-fleks): involuntary action; automatic response

reflex arc (ree'-fleks ahrk): pathway traveled by an impulse during reflex action, going from receptor to effector

reflexive emptying (ri-flek'-siv emp'-tee-ing): automatic emptying of the bowels or bladder

reflux (ree'-fluks): return flow

regurgitation (re-gur"-ji-ta'-shun): vomiting

rehabilitation (ree-ha-bil-eh-tay'-shun): the process of restoring function through therapeutic exercise

renal (ree'-nul): pertaining to the kidney

renal columns (ree'-nul col'-umz): interpyramidal cortical supports, interspersed with renal pyramids

renal compensation (ree'-nul kom"-pen-sa'-shun): excretion of hydrogen in the form of acid or retention of bicarbonate by the kidneys to maintain acid-base balance

renal fascia (ree'-nul fash'-ah): tough, fibrous tissue surrounding each kidney and the adipose capsule

renal pelvis (ree'-nul pel'-vis): funnel-shaped structure at the beginning of the ureter

renal pyramids (ree'-nul peer'-ah-midz): radially striated cones interspersed with renal columns

rennin (ren'-in): milk-coagulating enzyme found in gastric juice of infants; not present in the adult human stomach

relative hypovolemia (re'-la-tiv hi"-po-vo-le'-me-a): condition in which blood volume is misplaced within the blood vessels because of excessive expansion (dilation) or failure in the integrity of the walls of the vessels

residual volume (re-zi'-du-al vol'-yoom): amount of air that cannot be voluntarily expelled in the lungs

respiratory arrest (res'-peh-ruh-tor-ee uh-rest'): condition in which a person stops breathing

respiratory compensation (res'-peh-ruh-tor-ee kom"-pen-sa'-shun): increased ventilation to return blood to a normal pH through elimination of carbon dioxide

respiratory distress syndrome (res'-peh-ruh-tor-ee dis-tres' sin'-drome): condition that generally affects premature babies; characterized by the formation of a hyaline-like false membrane within the alveoli, which causes the alveoli to collapse

retina (ret'-in-ah): innermost layer of the eye contains the rods and cones

retract (re'-trakt): to withdraw

retroperitoneal (ret"-ro-per"-i-toh-nee'-ul): located behind the peritoneum

retroperitoneal cavity (ret"-ro-per"-i-toh-nee'-ul ka'-vih-tee): space behind the abdominal cavity

rheumatic heart disease (roo-mah'-tic hart di-zeez'): infectious disease of the heart; treated with antibiotic therapy

rheumatoid arthritis (roo'-mah-toyd arth-ri'-tis): chronic inflammatory disease affects connective tissue and joints

Rh factor (r-h fak'-tor): antigen found in red blood cells

rhinitis (rih-ni'-tis): inflammation of the lining of the nose

rhinorrhea (rye"-noh-ree'-uh): discharge of thin, watery fluid from the nose

RhoGAM (ro'-gam): specific preparation of immune globulin

ribonucleic acid (rye'-boh-noo-kley'-ik as'-id): RNA; type of nucleic acid

ribosome (rye'-bo-sohm): submicroscopic particle attached to endoplasmic reticulum; site of protein synthesis in cytoplasm of cell

rickets (rik'-its): disorder in which bones soften as a result of lack of vitamin D

right coronary artery (RCA) (ryt kor'-o-nair"-ee ar'-ter-ee): artery that supplies blood to the ventricle

right lymphatic duct (ryt lim-fat'-ik dukt): short channel where the lymph nodes empty into the inferior vena cava

right ventricle (ryt ven'-tri-kl): lower chamber of the heart; pumps to pulmonary circulation

Ringer's solution (ring'-erz sa-loo'-shun): solution containing potassium chloride, sodium chloride, and calcium chloride; acts as a blood substitute

ringworm (ring'-worm): contagious fungal infection with raised circular patches

rods (rodz): cells in the retina; sensitive to dim light

root (root): (1) part of hair that is implanted in the skin; (2) embedded in the alveolar processes of the jaw

rotation (roh-tay'-shun): allows a bone to move around a central axis

rotator cuff disease (roh-tay'-tor kuf di-zeez'): inflammation of a group of tendons that fuse together and surround the shoulder joint

rugae (roo'-jee): wrinkles or folds

rule of nines (rool of nynz): measures the percent of the body burned

S_3 (S-three): the extra sound the heart makes as a result of asynchronous contraction of the left and right ventricles; also called a ventricular gallop

sacral edema (sa'-kral e-de'-ma): swelling in the small of the back

sacroiliac joint (say"-kro-il'-ee-ak joynt): joint between sacrum and ilium

sacrum (sa'-krum): wedge-shaped bone below the lumbar vertebra at the end of the spinal column

sagittal plane (sadj'-ih-tul plane): longitudinal plane dividing the body into two parts

salivary gland (sal'-ah-ver-ee gland): gland located in the mouth that secretes saliva; there are three pairs

salpingitis (sal-pin-ji'-tis): inflammation of the fallopian tubes

salt (salt): compound formed when a negative ion of acid combines with a positive ion of a base

sarcolemma (sar-koh'-lem-mah): muscle cell membrane

sarcoplasm (sahr'-ko-plazm): hyaline or finely granular interfibrillar material of muscle tissue

sartorius (sahr-to'-ree-us): thigh muscle

scab (skab): capillary fluid that dries and seals a wound

scapula (skap'-yoo-luh): large, flat, triangular bone forming back of shoulder

scar (skar) *see* cicatrix

sciatica (siy-at'-ik-ah): neuritis of the sciatic nerve

sciatic nerve (siy-at'-ik nerv): largest nerve in the body originates in the sacral plexus; runs through the pelvis and down the leg

sclera (skleer'-uh): tough, white covering, part of external coat of eye

scoliosis (skoh"-lee-oh'-sis): lateral curvature of the spine

scrotum (skro'-tum): pouch that contains the testicles

sebaceous gland (se-bay'-shus gland): gland that secretes sebum, a fatty material

sebum (see'-bum): secretion of sebaceous glands that lubricate the skin

secondary repair (seh'-kon-dayr-ee re-payr'): epithelial tissue repair that includes the granulation process to heal large open wounds

secretin (suh-kree'-tin): hormone secreted by the epithelial cells that line the duodenum; stimulated by the acidic gastric juice and the partially digested proteins from the stomach

section (sek'-shun): cut made through the body in the direction of a certain plane

sedimentation rate (sed"-e-men-tay'-shun rayt): time it takes red blood cells to settle to the bottom in an upright tube

segmented movement (seg'-men-ted moov'-ment): single segments of the intestine alternate between contraction and relaxation

seizure (see'-shur): disruption of brain function

selectively permeable membrane (se-lek'-tiv-lee per'-mee-ah-bul mem'-brayn): barrier that allows only particular substances to pass from one side of a membrane to the other

sella turcica (sel'-uh tur'-si-kuh): saddle-shaped depression in sphenoid bone

semen (see'-mun): male reproductive fluid containing sperm

semicircular canals (sem'-ih-sir'-kuh-lar kan-alz'): structures in the inner ear involved with equilibrium

semilunar (sem"-ih-lew'-nur): half-moon–shaped valve of aorta and pulmonary artery

seminal vesicles (sem'-i-nul ves'-i-kuls): two highly convoluted membranous tubes that produce substances found to help nourish and protect sperm on its journey up the female reproductive system

seminiferous tubules (sem-ih-nih'-fer-us tu'-bulz): tiny, twisted tubule found in the testicular lobe

senescence (se-nes'-unce): old age; senility

sensory neuron (sen'-soh-ree neur'-on): *see* afferent nerve

sentinel nodes (sen'-ten-el nodz): the first lymph nodes that entrap disseminating cancer cells

septal wall (sep'-tal wall): wall shared between the right and left sides of the heart

septicemia (sep"-tih-see'-mee-a): presence of pathogenic organisms in the blood

septum (sep'-tum): partition; dividing wall between two spaces or cavities, such as the septum between left and right side of heart or nose

serous fluid (seer'-us floo'-id): (1) normal lymph fluid; (2) thin, watery body fluid

serous membrane (seer'-us mem'-brayn): double-walled membrane that produces serous fluid

serum (seer'-um): clear, pale yellow fluid that separates from a clot of blood; plasma that contains no fibrinogen

shaft (shaft): (1) part of the hair that extends from the skin surface; (2) diaphysis of the long bone

shingles (shing'-elz): herpes zoster, a virus infection of the nerve endings

shin splints (shin splintz): injury to muscle tendon in front of the shins

shock (shok): disorder characterized by low blood pressure and loss of circulating blood volume

shock syndrome (shok sin'-drome): process of depriving certain organs of oxygen-rich blood (hypoperfusion) to save other organs (core organs)

shunting (shun'-teen): redirection of blood flow away from or toward an organ

sickle cell anemia (sick'-ul sel uh-nee'-mee-uh): blood disorder; shape of the red blood cell is a sickle shape, which makes the red blood cells clump together

SIDS (sidz): see sudden infant death syndrome

sigmoid (sig'-moyd): shaped like the letter S; distal, S-shaped part of colon

silicosis (sil'-ah-koh'-sis): lung condition caused by breathing dust containing silicon dioxide; lungs become fibrotic

simple partial seizure (sim'-pul par'-shel see'-zure): involvement of only one small portion of the brain

sinoatrial (SA) node (sigh"-no-ay'-tree-ul node): dense network of fibers of conduction at the junction of the superior vena cava and the right atrium that serves as the dominant pacemaker in the heart

sinus (sigh'-nus): recessed cavity or hollow space

sinus of Valsalva (sigh'-nus of Val-salv"-ah): hollow behind the aortic valve

sinusitis (sigh-new-si'-tis): infection of the mucous membrane that lines the sinus cavities

six cardinal gazes (siks kar'-den-al gay'-zez): primary directions of eye movement

skeletal muscle (skel'-e-tal mus'-ul): muscle attached to a bone or bones of the skeleton and concerned in body movements; also known as voluntary or striated muscle

skeletal system (skel'-e-tul sis'-tem): system composed of the bony framework in the body

slipped (herniated) disk (slipt [hur'-nee-a-ted] disk): cartilage disk between the vertebrae that ruptures or protrudes out of place

small-volume nebulizer (SVN) (smaal vol'-yoom neb'-u-liz-er): handheld device used to administer medication for inhalation

smooth muscle (smooth mus'-ul): nonstriated involuntary muscle

sodium (Na+) (so'-de-um): electrolyte found outside the cell that controls nervous impulse and contraction of muscle

0.9% sodium chloride (0.9 NaCl) (so'-de-um klor'-id): solution used to replace blood lost; also known as normal saline

3% sodium chloride (so'-de-um klor'-id): super-saline solution used to pull fluid from the cells into the bloodstream

sodium-potassium pump (so'-de-um-po-tas'-ee-um pump): ability of cells to push sodium into the cell and potassium out of the cell after the cell has been stimulated

solute (sol'-yoot): dissolved substance in a solution

somatic cell (soh-mat'-ik sel): all the body cells except for sex cells (egg and sperm)

somatic pain (soh-mat'-ik payne): pain with an exact location on the body

somatotropin (soh'-ma-te-troh'-pin): growth hormone

spastic quadriplegia (spas'-tik kwod'-re-plee'-ja): spastic paralysis of all four limbs

sperm (spurm): reproductive cell of the male

spermatic cord (spur-mat'-ik kord): cord that extends from the testis to the deep inguinal ring; contains the ductus deferens, the blood vessels and nerves of the testis and epididymis, and the surrounding connective tissue

spermatogenesis (spur'-mat'-ah-jen'ah-sis): process of the formation of sperm

spermatozoa (spur-mat"-ah-zo'-ah): male gametes produced by one of the testes

sphenoid (sfen'-oid): key bone of the skull

sphincter (sfink'-tur): circular muscle, such as the anus

spilling sugar (spil'-ing shu'-gur): passage of sugar in urine

spina bifida (spye'-nuh bye'-fi-duh): congenital defect in closure of the spinal canal, with hernial protrusion of the meninges of the spinal cord

spinal canal (spye'-nel ka-nal'): passage inside the spinal column that houses the spinal nerves

spinal cavity (spye'-nel ka'-vih-tee): area of body containing the spinal cord

spinal cord (spye'-nel kord): part of the central nervous system within the spinal column; begins at foramen magnum of the occipital bone and continues to the second lumbar vertebra spinal nerves (spye'-nul nervz): thirty-one pairs, originating in the spinal cord

spinal shock (spye'-nel shok): disorder characterized by low blood pressure and loss of circulating blood volume as a result of injury to the spinal cord; also called neurogenic shock

spirometer (spi-rom'-eh-ter): apparatus that measures inhaled and exhaled air

spleen (spleen): lymph organ situated below and behind the stomach

splenomegaly (splen-oh-meg'-ah-lee): enlarged spleen

spondylitis (spon"-di-lye'-tis): inflammation of the vertebrae

spongy bone (spon'-jee bone): when hard bone breaks down, it leaves spongy bone

spontaneous abortion (spon-ta'-nee-us ah-bor'-shun): the body's ridding itself of a non-viable pregnancy; a miscarriage

sprain (sprayn): wrenching of a joint, producing a stretching or laceration of ligaments

standard precautions (stand'-ard pre-caw'-shuns): guidelines used during patient care and cleaning to prevent spread of disease

stapes (stay'-peez): stirrup-shaped bone in the middle ear

Starling's law (stahr'-lingz law): principle that the maximum distention of the ventricles results in the greatest force of contraction

status epilepticus (sta'-tus ep"-i-lep'-ti-kus): one prolonged seizure or a series of seizures without an intervening period of consciousness

steapsin (stee-ap'-sin): pancreatic lipase

sterile (ster'-el): incapable of reproducing, or free from bacteria or other microorganisms

sternocleidomastoid (stur"-no-klyd-o-mas'-toyd): large muscle extends down side of neck

sternum (stur'-num): flat, narrow bone in median line in front of chest; composed of three parts: manubrium, body, and xiphoid process

steroid (ster'-oyd): lipids or fats containing cholesterol

stethoscope (steth'-uh-skope): instrument used for detection and study of sounds arising within the body

stimulus (stim'-ye-lus): any change in environment

stirrup (stir'-rup): or stapes; a bone that transmits sound waves from the eardrum to the inner ear

stomach (stum'-ik): major organ of digestion; a pouch-like structure located in the upper left quadrant of the abdominal cavity, between the esophagus and the duodenum

stomatitis (sto-me-tiy'-tis): inflammation of the mucous membrane of the mouth

strabismus (strah-bis'-mus): condition in which the muscles of the eyeball do not coordinate their actions ("cross eyes")

strain (strayn): tear in a muscle or stress

stratum corneum (strah'-tum kor'-ne-yum): slightly acidic cellular layer of the epidermis that defends the body against invading bacteria

stratum germinativum (strah'-tum ger-min-a'-tiv-um): layer of the epidermis that replaces cells and pushes them upward toward the epidermis

strength (strenth): capacity to do work

stroke (strok): loss of function in a portion of the brain; *see* cerebrovascular accident

stroke volume (strok vol'-yoom): entire volume of blood ejected from the ventricles in a single heartbeat

sty (stye): infection of gland along the eyelid

subarachnoid space (sub"-a-rak'-noid spase): space between the arachnoid mater and the brain that houses a network of capillaries

subdural space (sub-doo'-ral spase): space between the dura mater and the arachnoid mater that houses cerebral veins

subluxation (sub"-luk-say'-shun): incomplete dislocation

sudden infant death syndrome (su'-den in'-fant deth sin'-drome): crib death; sudden, unexplainable death of an infant during sleep

sudoriferous (sue"-dur-if'-ur-us): producing perspiration

sulci (sul'-ce): fissure or grooves separating cerebral convolutions

superficial (su-per-fih'-shal): describes a structure or organ on or near the surface of the body

superficial (first-degree) burn (su-per-fih'-shal [furst duh-gree] burn): *see* burn

superior (su-peer'-ee-ur): in anatomy, higher; denoting the upper of two parts, toward vertex

supination (suh-pih-nay'-shun): turning of the palm of the hand upward; condition of being supine (lying on back)

supine hypotensive syndrome (suh'-pyn high"-po-ten'-siv sin'-drome): condition occurring in pregnancy as a result of pressure on the vena cava; exhibited by a drop in blood pressure and dizziness

suppository (su-poz'-i-tor-ee): medication in a waxlike form that is administered rectally

surfactant (sur-fak'-tunt): lipid material that covers the inner surfaces of the lungs' alveoli

suspensory ligaments (sus-pen'-soh-re lig'-ah-mentz): muscles that hold the lens in place behind the pupil

suture (sue'-chur): (1) in osteology, a line of connection or closure between bones, as in a cranial suture; (2) in surgery, a fine threadlike catgut or silk used to repair or close a wound

symbol board (sim'-bowl bord): a communication device that depicts meanings in symbols and pictures

sympathetic nervous system (sim-pah-theh'-tik ner'-vus sis'-tem): division of autonomic nervous system

synapse (sin'-aps): space between adjacent neurons through which an impulse is transmitted

synaptic cleft (si-nap'-tik kleft): space between the axon of one neuron and the dendrite of another

synarthroses (sin-ar-thro'-ses): immovable joints connected by fibrous connective tissue

syndrome of inappropriate antidiuretic hormone (SIADH) (sin'-drome of in'-ah-pro"-pre-et an"-ti-di"-u-ret'-ik hor'-moan): disorder that results when the posterior lobe of the pituitary excretes excessive amounts of ADH, which results in excessive water retention

synergist (sin'-er-jist): muscles that help steady a joint

synovial cavity (si-noh'-vee-al ka'-vih-tee): area between the two articular cartilages

synovial fluid (si-noh'-vee-al flu'-id): viscid fluid present in joint cavities

synovial membrane (si-noh'-vee-al mem'-brayn): double layer of connective tissue; lines joint cavities and produces synovial fluid

synthesis (sin'-the-sis): in chemistry, processes and operations necessary to build up a compound; in general, a reaction or series of reactions in which a complex compound is obtained from elements or simple compounds

syphilis (sif'-eh-lis): infectious disease transmitted by sexual contact

systemic anatomy (sis-te'-mik a-nat'-a-me): study of the structure and function of body organs

systemic circulation (sis-te'-mik sur-kyu-lay'-shun): route of circulation that carries blood around the body

systole (sis'-tuh-lee): contraction of ventricles, forcing blood into the aorta and pulmonary artery

systolic blood pressure (sis-tol'-ik blud preh'-shur): pressure measured at the greatest moment of concentration

tachycardia (tak"-i-kahr'-dee-uh): abnormally rapid heartbeat

tachypnea (tack-ip'-nee-uh): abnormally rapid rate of breathing

talus (tay'-lus): ankle bone that articulates with the bones of the leg

tarsal (tahr'-sal): ankle bone

tarsus (tahr'-sus): instep

taste buds (tayst budz): cells on the papillae of the tongue that can distinguish salt, bitter, sweet, and sour qualities of dissolved substances

Tay-Sachs disease (tay-saks' di-zeez'): genetic mutation caused by lack of a particular enzyme (hexosaminidase) needed for the breakdown of lipid molecules in the brain

temporal (tem'-per-el): side of the head

temporal artery (tem'-per-el ar'-ter-ee): located slightly above the outer edge of the eye

temporal lobe (tem'-per-el lowb): area of the brain that controls hearing

tendon (ten'-dun): cord of fibrous connective tissue that attaches a muscle to a bone or other structure

tennis elbow (ten'-is el'-boh): inflammation of the tendon that connects the arm muscles to the elbow

tension pneumothorax (ten'-shun noo-mo-tho'-raks): condition in which trapped air builds up pressure in the chest and causes compression of the heart

teratogen (ter'-a-to-jen): any infection or toxin that causes abnormal development of the embryo resulting in a birth defect

testes (tes'-tis): male reproductive organ produces sperm and testosterone

testosterone (tes-tos'-te-rohn): male sex hormone responsible for male secondary sex characteristics

tetanus (tet'-uh-nus): infectious disease, usually fatal, characterized by spasm of voluntary muscles and convulsions caused by toxin from tetanus bacillus (*Clostridium tetani*)

tetany (tet'-uh-ne): intermittent spasms resulting from hypofunctioning of the parathyroid glands

thalamus (thal'-a-mus): part of the diencephalon; relays sensory stimuli to the cerebral cortex

therapeutic level (ther"-a-pu'-tik le'-vul): dosage of medication given to maintain an adequate blood level of medication

third ventricle (third ven'-tri-kl) *see* cerebral ventricles

thoracic cavity (thor-rah-sik ka'-vih-tee): upper portion of the ventral cavity containing the esophagus, bronchi, lungs, trachea, thymus gland, and heart

thoracic duct (thor-rah'-sik dukt): left lymphatic duct; largest lymph vessel in the body

thoracic vertebrae (thor-rah-sik ver'-teh-bra): one section of the vertebral column in the chest; includes 12 vertebrae

thoracentesis (thor"-ruh-sen-tee'-sis): aspiration of chest cavity for removal of fluid, usually for empyema

thorax (tho'-raks): chest; portion of the trunk above the diaphragm and below the neck

threshold (thresh'-hold): term used to describe the limit of reabsorption

thrombin (throm'-bin): enzyme found in blood; produced from an inactive precursor, prothrombin, inducing clotting by converting fibrinogen to fibrin

thrombocyte (throm'-bah-site): platelet; part of megakaryocyte cells necessary for blood clotting

thrombocytopenia (throm"-bah-siy-toh-pen'-ee-ah): decrease in the number of platelets

thrombolytic (throm'-bo-li"-tic): drug used to break up blood clots

thromboplastin (throm'-boh-plas-tin): substance secreted by platelets when tissue is injured; necessary for blood clotting

thrombosis (throm-boh'-sis): formation of a clot in a blood vessel

thrombotic stroke (throm-bot'-ik strok): stroke caused by a blood clot

thrombus (throm'-bus): blood clot

thymus (thi'-mus): endocrine gland located under the sternum; produces T-lymphocytes

thyroid gland (thi'-royd gland): endocrine gland located on anterior portion of the neck; produces thyroxine, triiodothyronine, and calcitonin

thyroid-stimulating hormone (TSH) (thi'-royd-sti'-myu-lay-teen hor'-moan): hormone of the pituitary gland that stimulates growth and secretion of the adrenal cortex

thyroxine (T₄) (thi-rok'-seen): hormone secreted by the thyroid gland or prepared synthetically

TIA (t-i-a): *see* transient ischemic attacks

tibia (tib'-ee-uh): larger, inner bone of the leg, below the knee

tic (tik): uncontrollable rhythmic contraction of a muscle

tidal volume (ti'-dal vol'-yoom): amount of air that moves in and out of the lungs with each breath

tinnitus (tin-i'-tus): ringing sensation in one or both ears

tissue (tish'-yoo): cells grouped according to size, shape, and function; epithelial, connective, muscle, and nerve

T-lymphocytes (te-limf'-o-site): type of white blood cell found in the thymus gland

tonic phase (ton'-ik fase): contraction of the muscles of the body

tonometer (ton-om'-eh-ter): instrument that measures intraocular eye pressure

tonsillitis (ton-sihl-i'-tis): condition characterized by enlarged tonsils, difficulty in swallowing, severe sore throat, elevated temperature, and chills

tonsils (ton'-silz): mass of lymph tissue in the back of the throat that produces lymphocytes

topographic anatomy (top"-o-graf'-ik a-nat'-a-me): study of the relationship of one body part to another

torticollis (tor-ti-kol'-is): contracted state of the neck muscles producing an unnatural position of the head; also called wryneck

total lung capacity (to'-tal lung kah-pa'-sih-te): includes tidal volume, inspiratory reserve, expiratory reserve, and residual air

toxic shock syndrome (tok'-sik shok sin'-drome): rare but often fatal disease caused by infection with certain strains of bacteria

trace elements (trayse el'-eh-mentz): zinc, copper, iodine, cobalt, manganese, selenium, chromium, molybdenum, and fluorine; present in the body in small amounts

trachea (tray'-kee-ah): thin-walled tube between the larynx and the bronchi; conducts air to the lungs

tracheostomy (tray"-kee-os'-to-mee): surgical procedure that creates an opening in the trachea

traction device (trak'-shun di-vis'): tool used to keep a fracture of a long bone in proper alignment to promote healing

trait (trayt): any characteristic, feature, quality, or property of an organism

transection (tran-sek'-shun): cut

transient ischemic attack (tran'-see-ent is-kem'-ik a-tak'): temporary interruption of the blood flow in the brain; a ministroke

transmit (tranz'-mit): to pass on to another person, place, or thing

transverse (tranz-vurs'): crosswise; at right angles to longitudinal axis of body

transverse colon (tranz-vurs' ko'-luhn): portion of the colon that is located across the abdominal cavity below the spleen

triceps (tri'-seps): three-headed muscle on the back of the upper arm

tricuspid valve (tri-kus'-pid valv): three-part valve located between the right atrium and right ventricle

trigeminal neuralgia (tri-jem'-i-nel noo-ral'-ja): painful condition affecting the fifth cranial nerve; also known as tic douloureux

triiodothyronine (T₃): hormone in the bloodstream that serves to regulate the system

trimester (tri-mes'-ter): the division of pregnancy into three parts, each about three months long

trisomy 21 (tri'-so-mee 21): Down syndrome; common chromosomal abnormalities involving an extra chromosome, designated as chromosome 21

true ribs (tru ribz): first seven pairs of ribs, which are attached to the sternum by costal cartilage

trypsin (trip'-sin): one of four protein-digesting enzymes found in pancreatic juice

trypsinogen (trip-sin'-uh-jen): inactive form of trypsin; in the small intestine, trypsinogen is converted to trypsin by the influence of enterokinase, an intestinal enzyme that is secreted by glands lining the small intestine

tuberculosis (too-bur"-kya-loh'-sis): infectious disease caused by tubercle bacillus; mainly affects lung

tumor (too'-mer): abnormal and uncontrolled growth of cell

tunica (too'-ni-kah): layer of tissue found in the blood vessels and specified as tunica adventitia (externa), the outer lining; tunica media, the middle lining; and tunica interna, the inner lining

tunica albuginea (too'-ni-kuh al-bew-jin'-ee-uh): fibrous tissue covering the testes

turbinate (tur'-bin-ut): nasal conchae bones that divide the nasal cavity into three passageways

tympanic membrane (tim-pan'-ik mem'-brayn): membrane separating the external ear from the middle ear

type and crossmatch (typ and cros'-mach): test that determines the blood type and Rh factor of blood between a donor and recipient

ulcer (ul'-sur): inflammation that occurs on the mucosal skin surface

ulna (ul'-nuh): bone on inner forearm

umbilicus (um-bill'-li-kis): navel

unicellular (yoo"-nih-sel'-yoo-lur): composed of one cell

unilateral (yoo"-nih-lat'-ur-ul): pertaining to or affecting one side

universal donor (yoo"-nih-ver'-sal do'-nur): type O blood; has no A or B antigens; can be donated to all blood types

universal recipient (yoo"-nih-vur'-sul re-sip'-ee-unt): individual belonging to the AB blood group

uremia (yoo-ree'-mee-ah): presence of urea and excess waste products in the blood

ureter (yoor'-ah-ter): long, narrow tube that conveys urine from the kidney to the urinary bladder

urethra (yoo-re'-thra): tube that takes urine from the bladder to the outside of the body

urinalysis (yoor-i-nal'-ah-sis): chemical analysis of urine

urinary bladder (yoor'-i-ner-ee blad'-er): muscular, membrane-lined sac situated in the anterior part of the pelvic cavity that holds urine

urinary meatus (yoor'-i-ner-ee mee'-tus): external opening to the urethra

urticaria (ur"-ti-kar'-ee-a): skin condition characterized by itching wheals or welts and usually caused by an allergic reaction; also known as hives

uvula (yoo'-vew-luh): projection hanging from soft palate in the back of the throat, blocking the nasal passages during swallowing

vacuole (vak'-yoo-ole): (1) clear space in a cell; (2) cavity bound by a single membrane; usually a storage area for fat, glycogen, secretions, liquid, or debris

vagina (va-ji'-nuh): part of the female reproductive system; sheathlike structure; tube extending from the uterus to the vulva

vaginitis (vaj"-eh-ni'-tis): inflammation of the vagina

vagus nerve (va'-gus nerv): nerve that controls heart rate

vallecula (va-lek'-u-la): space above the epiglottis and proximal to the hyoid bone

valve (valv): structure that permits flow of a fluid in only one direction

varicose veins (var'-i-kose vayns): veins that have become abnormally dilated and tortuous as a result of interference with venous drainage or weakness of their walls

vasopressin (vay"-zo-pres'-in): hormone secreted by the posterior pituitary gland; has an antidiuretic effect; also called antidiuretic hormone (ADH)

vasopressor (vay"-zo-pres'-or): blood vessel constrictor

vasotonia (va"-zo-to'-ne-a): process by which the vasomotor muscle fibers work to ensure continuous uninterrupted blood flow

vein (vayn): vessel that carries blood toward the heart

vena cava (ve'-na ka'-va): large blood vessel that returns blood to the right atrium; there are two: superior and inferior

ventral (ven'-trul): front or anterior; opposite of posterior or dorsal

ventricle (ven'-tri-kl): small cavity or chamber, as in the heart or the brain

ventricular bundle (ven-tri-ku-lar bun'-dl): collection of muscle fibers making up the ventricles

ventricular fibrillation (ven-tri'-ku-lar fib"-ri-lay'-shun): chaotic electrical activity within the ventricles

ventricular gallop (ven-tri'-ku-lar gal'-op): sound the heart makes because of an asynchronous beating of the heart; S_3

venule (ven'-yoo-ul): small vein

vermiform appendix (vur'-mi-form a-pen'-diks): small, blind gut projecting from cecum

vertigo (vur'-ti-go): sensation of dizziness

vestibule (ves'-ti-bul): small space in front of a passage

villi (vil'-eye): hairlike projections, as in intestinal mucous membrane

viscera (vis'-er-ah): internal organs

visceral membrane (vis'-er-al mem'-brayn): membrane covering each organ in a body cavity

visceral pain (vis'-er-al payne): pain that is within the body, usually associated with an organ

vital lung capacity (vi'-tal lung kah-pa'-sih-te): total amount of air involved with tidal volume, inspiratory reserve volume, and expiratory reserve volume

vitamin (vye'-tuh-min): any of a group of organic compounds found in very small amounts in natural food; needed for the normal growth and maintenance of an organism

vitreous humor (vit'-ree-us hew'-mur): transparent, gelatin-like substance filling the greater part of the eyeball

VLDL (v-l-d-l): a lipoprotein

voluntary (vol'-un-ter"-ee): under control of the will

vomer (vo'-mer): flat, thin bone that forms part of the nasal septum

wart (wart): benign tumor of the epithelial tissue

water intoxication (wa'-tur in-tok"-si-ka'-shun): excess amounts of water in the body

weapons of mass destruction (we'-ponz of mas de-struk'-shun): weapons that are designed to harm or endanger large groups of people

Wernicke's area (ver'-ni-keez air'-ee-a): area in the temporal lobe of the brain

Wernicke's encephalopathy (ver'-ni-keez en-sef"-a-lop'-a-thee): dysfunction of the brain and central nervous system

wheezing (we'-zing): sound produced by a rush of air through a narrowed passageway

whiplash injury (wip'-lash in'-jer-ee): trauma to cervical vertebrae

white muscle (white mus'-ul): skeletal muscle that appears paler in the fresh state than red muscle

whooping cough (hoop'-ing kof): infectious disease characterized by repeated coughing attacks that end in a "whooping" sound; also called pertussis

whorl (hwerl): muscular bundles of the heart that form a double-loop spiral-like configuration

wisdom tooth (wiz'-dum tooth): third molar tooth in adult mouth

wound (woond): breech of the skin's protective covering as a result of trauma or violence

zona pellucida (so'-nuh pe-lew'-si-duh): thick, solid, elastic envelope of ovum

zygomatic (zye"-go-mah'-tik): two facial bones that form the prominence of the cheek

zygote (zye'-gote): organism produced by union of two gametes

Index